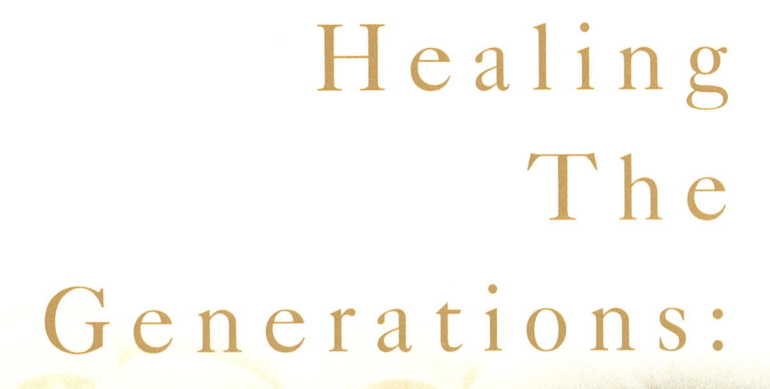

# Healing The Generations: A History Of Physical Therapy And The American Physical Therapy Association

*By Wendy Murphy*

PHOTOGRAPHY CREDITS

| | |
|---|---|
| p. 11 | from Nicholas Andry *L'Orthopédie*. First Edition 1741 |
| pp. 33, 39, 125 | courtesy of the Smithsonian Institution, NMAH/Medical Sciences |
| p. 38 | courtesy of The Cotting School |
| p. 52 | courtesy of Northeastern University |
| pp. 116, 117 | courtesy of Bella Abramowitz Fisher |
| p. 151 | courtesy of Vilma Evans |
| p. 156 | courtesy of Indiana University School of Allied Health Sciences Physical Therapy Program |
| p. 161 | left, courtesy of *Time Inc.* |
| p. 227 | courtesy of Professional Sportscare |

pp. 6, 40, 54, 59, 60, 64, 69, 103 courtesy of Mary Farrell

pp. 7-10, 14, 22, 23, 27, 28, 32, 35, 36, 37 courtesy of the National Library of Medicine

All other photographs and historical items courtesy of the American Physical Therapy Association Archives

Photography of American Physical Therapy Association artifacts by Timothy J. Connolly

© 1995 American Physical Therapy Association. All rights reserved.

Printed and bound in the United States of America. No part of this publication may be reproduced or transmitted in any form or by any means, electronic or mechanical, including photocopying, recording, or any information storage and retrieval system now known or to be invented, without permission in writing from the American Physical Therapy Association, 1111 North Fairfax Street, Alexandria, VA 22314-1488, except by a reviewer who wishes to quote brief passages in connection with a review written for inclusion in a magazine, newspaper, or broadcast.

Produced and published by Greenwich Publishing Group, Inc.
*Lyme, Connecticut*

Design by Bill Brown Design
*Madison, Connecticut*

Separation & film assembly by Silver Eagle Graphics, Inc.

Library of Congress Catalog Card Number: 95-76492

ISBN: 0-944641-13-X

First Printing: June 1995

10 9 8 7 6 5 4 3 2 1

# Table of Contents

*Foreword* — 5

**Chapter One**
*Through A Glass Darkly: The Past As Prologue* — 6

**Chapter Two**
*Mary McMillan And Wartime "Reconstruction": 1914-1919* — 40

**Chapter Threee**
*With Vision, Faith, And Courage: 1920-1939* — 70

**Chapter Four**
*The World War Two Years: 1939-1946* — 104

**Chapter Five**
*"Progress Is A Relay Race": 1946-1959* — 136

**Chapter Six**
*The Golden Years: 1959-1979* — 178

**Chapter Seven**
*The Diamond Jubilee Years: 1980-1996* — 216

*Timeline* — 248

*Past Presidents, Executive Directors, And Journal Editors* — 250

*Honors And Awards* — 250

*Index* — 253

*Acknowledgments* — 256

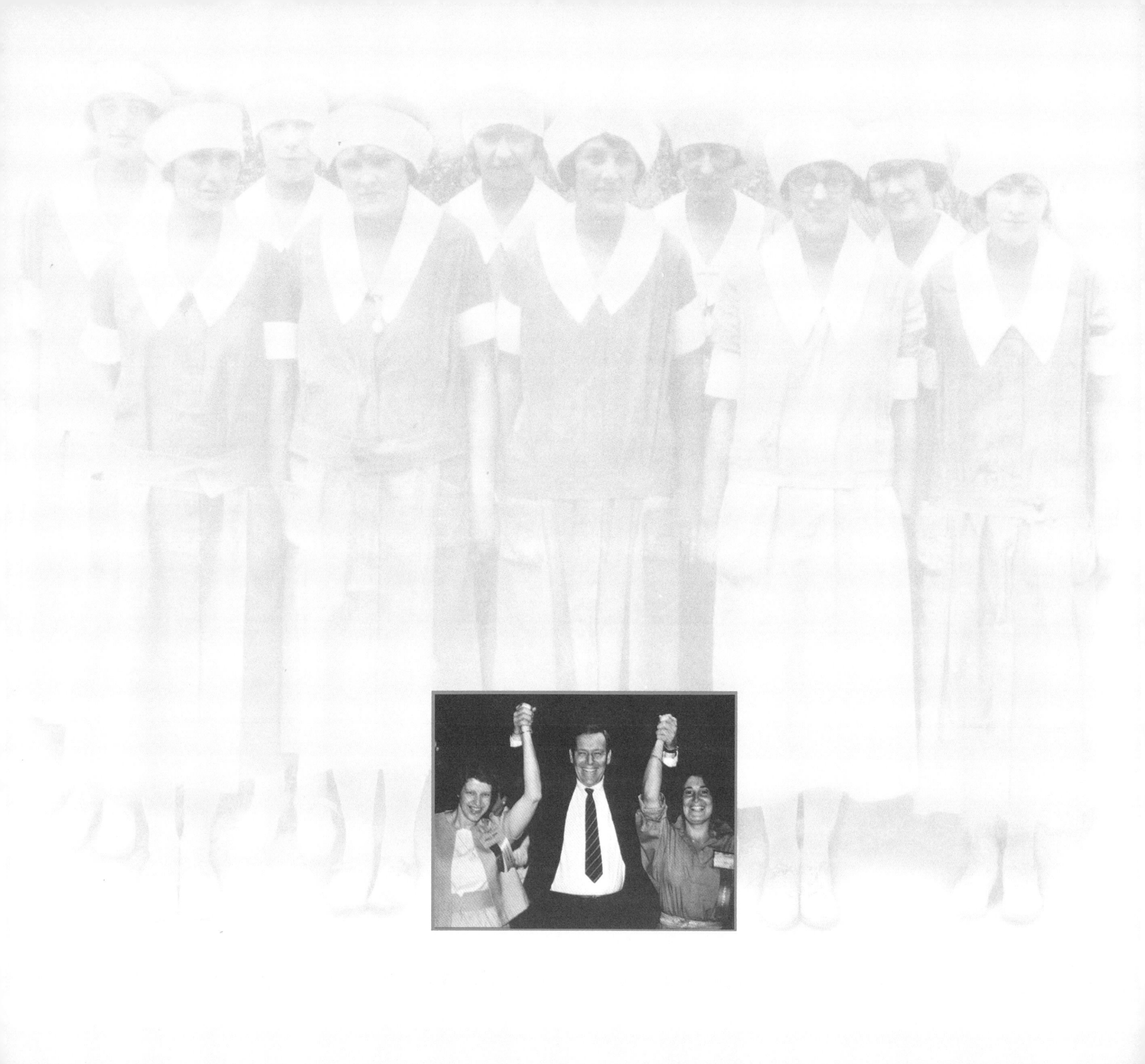

# *Foreword*

It has often been said that history must be, first of all, a good story. If this is true, then the story of physical therapy is history at its best.

*Healing the Generations: A History of Physical Therapy and the American Physical Therapy Association* was commissioned by the APTA Board of Directors in celebration of the Association's 75th Anniversary in 1996, and it is truly a compelling account of the profession's history. The book tells the story of physical therapy's beginnings, complete with heroines and heroes, scientific mysteries and discoveries, political plot twists, and captivating human dramas. Throughout that story, the reader is reminded of the role of physical therapy professionals in "healing" in the truest sense of the term — that is, "helping to overcome."

The Association is grateful to the following individuals for their dedication to the creation of this work:

Wendy Murphy, the author, who interviewed more than 200 APTA members and others and combed through mountains of archival materials in search of the information on which to base her engaging story.

Members of APTA's Committee on History from 1991 to 1995, as well as the Board liaisons to the Committee, who collectively provided valuable counsel and individually served as manuscript reviewers.

The following members, who committed their time and energy to reviewing the manuscript and who provided important information and perspectives: Vilma Evans, PT, EdD, FACCE, FAAPT; Charles Magistro, PT, FAPTA; Eugene Michels, PT, FAPTA; Dorothy Pinkston, PT, PhD, FAPTA; Jay Schleichkorn, PT, PhD; Rosemary Scully, PT, EdD, FAPTA; and Jane M. Walter, PT, EdD, FAPTA.

The following APTA members, who reviewed the initial outline and/or provided much-needed advice or information — often on very short notice — as the manuscript neared completion: Samuel M. Brown, PT; Robert Harden, PT, MS; Harold R. "Rick" Hawkins, PT; Geneva Johnson, PT, PhD, FAPTA; Florence P. Kendall, PT, FAPTA; Virginia Metcalf, PT, MA; Arthur J. Nelson, PT, PhD, FAPTA; Roger M. Nelson, PT, PhD; Inez Peacock, PT; Eric D. "Rick" Reuss, PT; Jules M. Rothstein, PT, PhD, FAPTA; and Jane K. Sweeney, PT, PhD, PCS.

Greenwich Publishing Group, in the persons of R. Mowry Mann, Christine Huberty, Bronwyn Evans, and Tim Connolly, and designer Bill Brown, who maintained their professionalism and their sense of humor throughout this project.

And the following members of the APTA staff: Francis J. Mallon, Esq.; Nancy Perkin Beaumont, CAE; Andrea Blake; Heather Hohlowski; and Sandra McDonald.

*Marilyn Moffat, PT, PhD, FAPTA*
*President*
*American Physical Therapy Association*

CHAPTER 1

# Through A Glass Darkly

*Boston-born and British-educated, Mary "Mollie" McMillan was at the forefront of the physical therapy movement launched in the first decades of the twentieth century. The first president and generally considered the founder of the American Physical Therapy Association, McMillan, shown here in 1918, left a legacy to tens of thousands of physical therapists who are members of APTA today.*

In the spring of 1905, a young American pathfinder named Mary McMillan completed her studies in physical education at Liverpool University and traveled to London to enroll in a series of post-graduate courses. She trained under several of the most distinguished clinical and theoretical instructors of the day, taking courses in electrotherapy, therapeutic exercise, massage, anatomy, and an assortment of pre-medical courses. As she and her fellow students made the rounds of the city's hospitals and clinics, she also had a chance to observe progressive-minded women like herself in challenging, worthwhile careers, their responsibilities well defined, their standing within the medical community as "trained masseuses" and "medical rubbers" protected by a ten-year-old professional society.

These were exciting, even inspiring, times to be young and full of idealism, and they proved the making of Mary McMillan. In a larger sense, they were also the making of physical therapy in America, for as later chapters will relate, McMillan returned to the United States in 1916 to begin a new odyssey. Singled out for her unique combination of knowledge, hands-on experience, and personal charisma, she was asked by the U.S. Army Surgeon General to lend a hand in the World War I emergency. The army needed hundreds of young women to assist in "reconstructing" the wounded and disabled, and no American knew more about the new science of physical therapeutics than McMillan. Would she teach others?

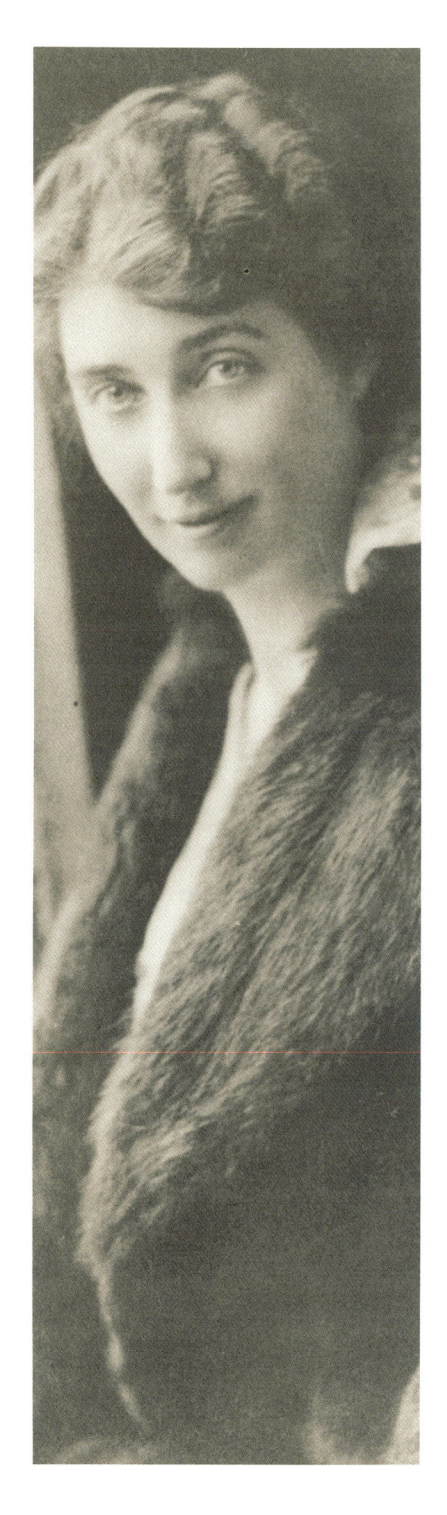

McMillan threw herself into the work with tremendous energy, personally preparing more than 200 young women for duty and later taking over the administration of the innovative army program. When the war ended and the work seemed destined for dismantling, McMillan became the prime mover in organizing her "girls" into a permanent professional organization capable of keeping physical therapeutics alive and growing. Since 1921, when it was founded, the American Physical Therapy Association has grown into one of the largest and most influential health care organizations in the United States, and the profession it represents has grown into one of the primary components of rehabilitation and preventive health care.

McMillan's life can thus be appreciated not only on its own considerable merits, but also as a critical link between physical therapy's Old World beginnings and its transplantation into the New World. She played a substantial role in the development of physical therapy from the trial-and-error empiricism it had followed for centuries toward the modern discipline it is today. To understand how all these pieces fit together and to see our modern knowledge in the context of what has come before, we can do no better than to start at the beginning. As physical therapy has developed upon the particular traditions of Western medicine, this history must properly commence in ancient Greece, though certainly the basic modalities of heat, cold, water, light, exercise, and massage — the basic armamentarium of physical therapy — were being used to lessen man's physical ills as long ago as prehistoric times.

### In The Beginning . . .

Therapeutic exercise and massage with aromatic oils were probably the first therapeutic modalities to be applied consciously. The Greeks saw physical and spiritual health as ideally indivisible. Health and sickness were functions of the balance among the four elements — fire, water, air, and earth; their complementary qualities — hot, moist, cold, and dry; and the body's four humors or fluids — blood, phlegm, and black and yellow bile. When imbalances occurred, usually attributed to supernatural interference, disease or debility arose. The Greek physician was expected to assist nature by helping his patient to restore a healthy balance through generally physical means, which could include bleeding and purging as well as the gentler therapeutics.

Medical treatment had a distinctly religious cast, and physicians were often connected with temples. In that setting, *exercise*, a word derived from the Greek and translating loosely as "freed movement," followed by relaxed bathing, could be performed in

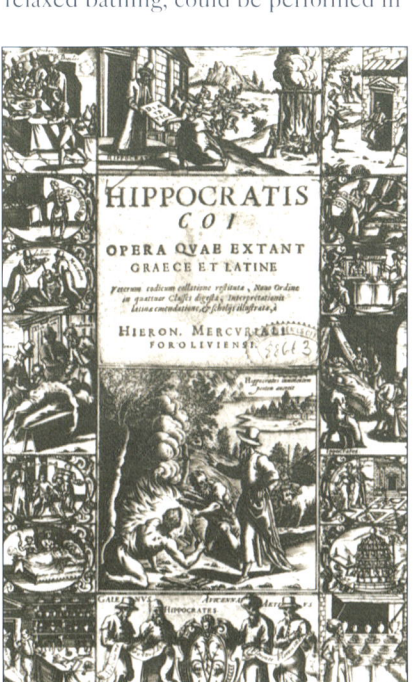

*The teachings of Hippocrates, the ancient Greek physician who is often called the father of Western medicine, have resonated through the ages. Shown here is the title page of a collection of his works written in Latin and published in Venice in 1588.*

*Massage, bathing, walking, hydrotherapy, and an ample diet of wine were among the favored treatments for the majority of ailments in earlier times. In this sixteenth-century woodcut from an Italian medical text, a healer massages his patient's aching back.*

a state of undress *(gymnos)* in an enclosure called a gymnasium. Hippocrates, the fifth-century B.C. physician who gave to ancient Greek medicine its scientific spirit of inquiry and its ethical ideals, was the first to prescribe therapeutic exercise specifically as a "restorative." Writing in *On Articulations*, Hippocrates accurately defined the common causes of muscle wasting: "Generally speaking, all parts of the body which have a function, if used in moderation and exercised in labors to which each is accustomed, become thereby healthy and well developed and age slowly; but if unused and left idle, they become liable to disease, defective in growth, and age quickly. This is especially the case with joints and ligaments, if one does not use them. In those who are neglected and never use the leg to walk but keep it up in the air, the bones are more atrophied than in those who do use it; and the tissues are much more atrophied than in those who use the leg."

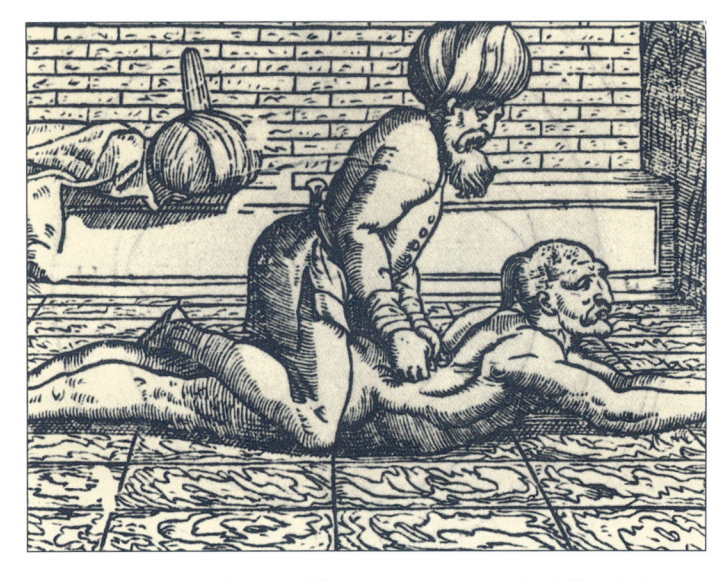

A believer in massage for the treatment of many conditions, Hippocrates is thought to have used friction in the treatment of sprains and dislocations and used kneading as a therapy for constipation. He also gave considerable attention to correcting problems in the skeletal system, including manipulations to stretch the scoliotic spine and to treat clubfoot. Asclepiades, an eminent Greek physician of the second century B.C., was less captivated than was Hippocrates by the theory of humoral balance; he believed primarily in systematic intervention in disease states and relied above all else on massage, exercise, and bathing as curatives.

Hippocrates's skills in observation, and to a lesser extent the Greeks' fondness for exercise and massage, were passed on to the Romans, who further systematized the humoral doctrine of medicine and health. Galen, physician to the imperial gladiators in the second century A.D., became an authority on traumatic surgery and musculoskeletal injuries and understood better than anyone else in his time the roles that anatomy and physiology played in movement. His voluminous writings became the definitive work on medicine for twelve centuries. Caelius Aurelianus, who lived circa 400 A.D. and was the last of the great classical healers, recognized the value of hydrogymnastics, suspension, and kinesitherapy and used weights and pulleys, particularly in rehabilitating immobilized joints. He also advocated postoperative exercises following wound surgery. In all, his writings contained a catalog of more than 60 exercise routines treating every part of the body. As for recognizing the therapeutic value of massage, the most famous Roman of all, Julius Caesar, is said to have been treated for his neuralgia with daily pinching and rubbing. Pliny, the great Roman naturalist, reported that massage relieved his own chronic asthma.

### THE RENAISSANCE OF PHYSICAL THERAPEUTICS

For nearly 10 centuries after the fall of the Roman Empire, medical inquiry stagnated in the Christianized West. Humoral theory provided a total view of the human being, even down to his temperament, which was diagnosed as choleric, splenetic, bilious, or sanguinary. Physical exercise and massage as therapeutic measures were officially abandoned by the medical profession, though it is presumed that many of the most effective treatments were kept alive by folk healers — the part-time midwives, sprain-rubbers, and bonesetters who tended ordinary folks. (Bonesetters had a virtual monopoly on the repair of fractures and dislocations. One of the most famous English bonesetters was the formidable Mrs. Sarah Mapp, better known to her early-eighteenth-century clients as Crazy Sally. Mrs. Mapp is reputed to have reset a dislocated shoulder with the force of her own two hands and to have lengthened a man's leg by six inches after hip and knee had been misaligned for some 20 years!)

Not until the end of the Renaissance did scientists and physicians begin to challenge humoral doctrine with any vigor, and not until the nineteenth century did it cease to be an influential force in the pursuit of better medicine. The names and contributions of those involved in advancing the science of corrective exercise and massage are legion, but a few examples suffice to show how knowledge evolved.

In 1543 Andreas Vesalius of Padua published his landmark text on human anatomy, *De Humanis Corporis Fabrica*, thereby inaugurating the modern science of anatomy. Two years later, the Parisian Ambroise Paré, royal surgeon to Charles IX, wrote the first modern classic on wound treatment and subsequently became a trailblazer in amputative surgery and a host of other procedures. A great exponent of the forgotten art of massage, he was so persuasive in his writings on

*A sixteenth-century stained glass panel, once used to illuminate a Swiss practitioner's office, depicts the many faces of hydrotherapy.*

*The Swiss-born medical iconoclast Paracelsus wrote eloquently about the value of the therapeutic bath. In this illustration from his* Opus chyrurgicus, *1565, a man and woman are shown in treatment. Seated in a sauna, their feet soak in tubs of water. The application of small cups to the patient's arms and legs, or "cupping," was a treatment used to produce healing hyperemia.*

the subject that he is credited with having made French the international language of massage terminology, as it remains today. In 1569 Hieronymus Mercurialis of Padua wrote the first important modern book on exercise, *De Arte Gymnastic*. This was followed by dozens of other seventeenth-century works in the same vein published in many other parts of Europe. By the eighteenth century, medical knowledge had advanced far enough to spawn the specialty of orthopedics, a word coined in 1741 by French surgeon Nicolas Andry, whose *L'Orthopédie* became the first basic textbook on the art of correcting childhood deformities through splinting, massage, and prostheses.

Occupational therapy was given its first exposition in 1781, when another Frenchman, Joseph-Clément Tissot, wrote extensively on the specific correlation between certain occupational arts-and-crafts activities and the rehabilitation of groups of muscles. Tissot, who served as surgeon-in-chief in Napoleon's Italian campaign, also made innovative suggestions regarding mobilization of postsurgical patients. He was a vigorous opponent of bed rest and had advanced notions for respiratory exercises, for the treatment of arthritis with mild massage, and for the rehabilitation of patients recovering from stroke. Tissot posited correctly, well in advance of the neurological research to support his theory, that "The important point in the treatment of stroke consists in reawakening the weakened control of the brain by bringing into play all those body elements that sustain wakefulness. Motion can help in this urgent indication." He went on to argue, "The apoplectic must not be kept in bed. . . . The horizontal position will serve as a continuous incentive to remain inactive. . . . We are obliged to keep him occupied, even to the point of annoying him. . . . Experience has shown that continued exercises taken for a certain period each day have been more useful to these patients than all the meaningless remedies which they have taken while stretched out on an easy chair or bed."

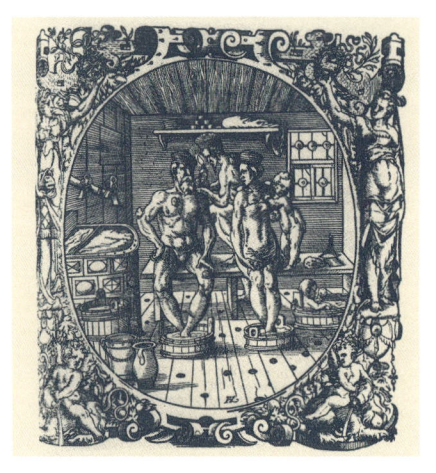

The first elaborate exercise equipment also dates from the end of the eighteenth century. Notable are a vibrating chair, a rocking horse, and a machine that was probably of the assistive treadle-and-pulley design. The last was said to be so clever that its inventor, anatomist John Pugh, would not depict it in his otherwise lavishly illustrated *Treatise on the Utility . . . of Muscular Action for Restoring the Power of Limbs*, for fear of having his idea stolen by competitors.

A generation later, John Shaw of London became the first to apply a regimen of gymnastics and massage to treat scoliosis. Shaw devised the protocol, which was diametrically opposed to the traditional policies of immobilization and bed rest, after studying scores of museum specimens and becoming convinced that spinal deformities were not always caused by rickets or muscle spasms, as widely assumed. His hypothesis was that weak spinal

10  *Healing The Generations*

muscles were the causative factor, which explained why some patients who sought relief from "rubbers" often fared better than those in the care of physicians. Shaw's prescription for correcting spinal deformity consisted of manipulating the spine and vertebrae into an increasingly normal position, along with exercise that strengthened the associated muscles to the point at which they could retain the spine in such alignment on their own, without artificial bracing.

Shaw's French contemporary, orthopedic surgeon Jacques Delpech, also took up the subject of scoliosis. To maximize his experimental base, he opened a school for girls with scoliosis in Montpelier where he carried out all manner of remedial work, much of it involving exercise apparatuses and graded exercises. Looking first to the approaches recommended by others, he declared as misguided the prescription of unequal weights as a means of balancing curvature and argued, "Such a procedure will aggravate one or both of the curves as a direct result of the weights carried." He preferred suspension: "The advantages of suspension of the body by the hands from very elastic objects have seemed so great to us that we have incorporated it into most of our sports and have pursued this thought completely." Delpech also experimented with suspension in water and built a swimming pool for the purpose.

The nineteenth-century Englishman William John Little pioneered the treatment of several other childhood deformities and published five books on his findings. Little brought to his work a personal viewpoint, for he had a foot that was congenitally deformed (then called clubfoot). Through the surgical intervention of Georg F. L. Stromeyer, a prominent German surgeon who had developed the procedure of subcutaneous tenotomy, the 26-year-old Little had finally been cured of his lameness. He resolved to show his gratitude by carrying on Stromeyer's art in his homeland. In 1838 Little founded England's first hospital devoted to the specialty of orthopedics (the future Royal National Orthopaedic Hospital) and subsequently undertook the study of the disordered action of muscles. Little is credited with identifying the common connection between abnormal parturition and deformities in children. His observations also laid the foundation for much of what later became known about the causes and treatment of cerebral palsy, a condition promptly termed, for lack of a better designation, "Little's Disease."

Like Shaw and Delpech, Little also found time to consider scoliosis, the treatment of which, he said, was all too often left to charlatans. In his 1868 text *On Spinal Weakness and Spinal Curvature*, Little described the horrors inflicted on adolescent girls "who exhibit the slightest trace of deformity" and said he had personally had occasion to release several patients who had worn "uninterruptedly, during one, two, or three years, spinal machines or supports consisting of clumsy, rude scaffolding or ornamented iron bars, weighing five to nine pounds, variously mystified by straps, screws, and cogwheels." In place of the bracing, Little offered methods of restoration involving exercise, mechanical instruments, and massage that he claimed were superior in comfort and result.

*The methodology of correcting skeletal deformities through the application of mechanical devices, or osteosynthesis, was first presented in detail by Nicolas Andry, an eighteenth-century French medical professor. Here, from the title page of Andry's classic 1741 textbook L'Orthopédie, is a graphic representation of that premise, later adopted as the symbol of orthopedic surgery.*

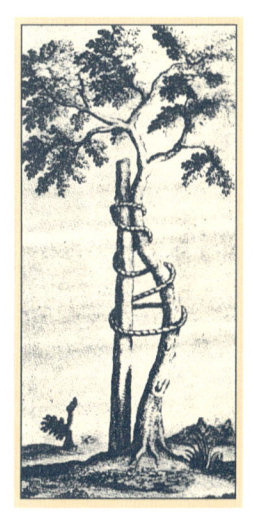

### The Art Of "Swedish Movements"

Still greater advances in medical exercises and "movement cures" came in the early nineteenth century when several men more or less simultaneously developed systematic gymnastics, a forerunner of muscle reeducation as we know it today. Of these, the most influential by far was Pehr Henrik Ling of Sweden. In his student days, Ling had studied in Copenhagen, where he took his exercise in a private school for gymnastics instructors managed by Franz Nachtegall that followed the then-popular principles of German military calisthenics. Ling found the idea of exercises salutary, but he thought many of the prescribed movements were unnecessarily complicated. He favored freer movement that was "more easily adaptable to the bodily peculiarities of individuals" and could be carried out with less cumbersome equipment than the heavy bars, ropes, masts, and vaulting horses favored by the Germans.

Returning to Lund, where he became an instructor in fencing and Norse culture at the university, Ling developed a system of "free exercise" routines. Though he drew upon fencing maneuvers, he emphasized movements anatomically "in harmony with the human body." Some were "pedagogical," by which he meant they were designed to maintain health; others were "medical" and intended to relieve specific ailments and support recovery. Each kind of exercise was prescribed according to strict rules of dosage and degrees of movement and was applied to the particular gymnast or patient only after his unique needs had been analyzed, an approach which represented a significant therapeutic advance over German gymnastics. Ling also studied the nature of movement. He first broke down each movement into its smallest components and then reassembled them as reproducible acts. He concluded that all voluntary motion is produced by an agonist group of muscles moderated by an antagonist group and that the basic mechanisms of contraction consisted of concentric and eccentric actions.

In 1813 Ling obtained a royal license to open the Central Gymnastic Institute (CGI) in Stockholm. Here, under government sponsorship, he developed and taught the approach that became known as the "Ling System" or the "Swedish Movement Treatment," which included gymnastics and "Swedish massage." (Ling knew the value of massage firsthand, having reportedly cured himself of rheumatism in his arm by self-administered percussive massage.) At first, only male students were trained at the CGI, but 16 years after Ling's death, with his son Henrik Ling as director, the Institute accepted women students.

One student of the Ling system was a Swedish physician named Gustav Zander. In 1857 Zander became a part-time teacher of gymnastics at a Swedish boarding school, where he became interested in the problem of remediating scoliosis. Concerned that medical gymnastics as taught by Ling required the almost constant attention of a personal trainer, a costly luxury for Zander's students and certainly a drain on his own energies, the physician looked for a more economical alternative. He eventually combined levers, wheels, and weights in a series of ingenious mechanical exercise machines that could be managed by patients with little or no assistance. Calling his system "mechanotherapy," Zander opened his Medico-Mechanical Institute in 1864, offering 27 different instruments for active exercise (the patient moves the machine), passive exercise (the machine moves the patient), and massage. Many of his machines were equipped with a performance monitor to register the force exerted, and most were adjustable to offer variable rates and degrees of movement. Professor Zander went on to devise nearly 50 additional devices, some employing steam and electricity for motive power. The machines were so well received that protégés recreated Zander Institutes in virtually every other country in Europe, and these remained popular up to World War I. Zander's apparati were also much used in American spas and sanitaria, which were multiplying in emulation of Europe's health and exercise craze.

Meanwhile, graduates of Ling's Central Gymnastics Institute were much sought after. In the latter half of the nineteenth century, many found their way to England, where concern about the physical condition of military conscripts, who came from an increasingly urban environment, made many upper-class Englishmen seek some form of exercise training. With the passage of the 1870 Education Act, a far larger and more diverse body of English children, including girls and young women, suddenly became eligible and in need of remedial gymnastics. As there were scarcely any gymnastics teachers ready and able to carry out the work, particularly as it applied to women, Ling graduates were entrusted with training England's first generation of women gymnastics teachers. Some of these women would go on to found Britain's professional physiotherapy organization.

Ling's teachings also had a significant and long-lasting impact on American medicine and American physical education. Shortly before the Civil War, George Taylor, a student of Ling, opened the Remedial Hygienic Institute in New York for the treatment of a broad range of disabilities. Professor Dio Lewis popularized the "Swedish Movement Cure" through his Normal Institute for Physical Education founded in Boston in 1861, the first school devoted to training teachers of physical education in America. This was followed in 1878 by Dudley Allen Sargent's Hygienic Institute and School of Physical Culture, forerunner of the pioneer Sargent School and of modern physical education/physical therapy training. As in England, America's physical education schools became the principal training grounds for the professional masseurs and corrective exercise "nurses" who were the essential support technicians of orthopedists and neurologists prior to World War I.

As exercise became an accepted adjunct to preserving health and treating some musculoskeletal diseases, it was only a matter of time before medical researchers began to investigate its application in other conditions. Although they were less celebrated than Ling as precursors of modern physical therapy, Rubens Hirschberg of Paris and H. S. Frenkel of Switzerland were pioneers in the medical application of exercise. Writing in 1903, Hirschberg analyzed stroke according to its recovery stages and recommend-

*Mechanical exercise machines, initially devised by Swedish physician Gustav Zander circa 1864, enjoyed broad popularity for more than half a century. They were part of the equipment provided in this World War I U.S. Army Evacuation Hospital in Coblenz, Germany.*

ed targeted exercise as a treatment. Immediately following the "attack," he said, patients needed absolute rest. During the second phase, which he said began somewhat less than a week later, passive motion should be instituted to avoid ankylosis. "The third period is the time for muscle reeducation," Hirschberg observed. "The most important symptom is contracture, which sets in rather rapidly." He said that where paralysis was not complete, the commencement of active motion, in which the patient is persuaded to move some part of his body and the therapist offers mild resistance, has the potential to "excite function" in adjoining muscles when repeated systematically. He also recommended methods of exercise that would promote the gradual resumption of walking.

Frenkel had a specific interest in the use of exercise to rehabilitate cases of locomotor ataxia, a more common condition in the era of untreated syphilis. In the 1890s Frenkel wrote several influential papers setting forth his method of retraining ataxic patients in the complicated patterns of walking "through the differentiation of tactile impressions of minute strength." Patients in small groups were literally taken through their paces, the successive placement of each foot marked on the floor, until they had achieved satisfactory patterns of locomotion. Progressive as his ideas were, they were not widely adopted for several decades.

Emphasis on physical conditioning led naturally to the development of calibrated devices for measuring strength and flexibility. The first medical dynamometers, which measure voluntary muscle strength, probably were introduced by the French sometime in the first half of the nineteenth century and were widely imitated thereafter. The Salter one-handed device and its 1885 improvement by Graeme Hammond were among several sold in the United States.

### Spinal Manipulations

To some practitioners within orthodox medical practice, exercise treatments held considerable medical promise in treating various musculoskeletal problems. Yet many Americans were attracted to techniques of "spinal manipulation," chiefly osteopathy and chiropractic, both homegrown, nineteenth-century developments.

Osteopathy as a medical system was introduced by Andrew Taylor Still, a self-taught itinerant Missouri physician. After practicing conventional medicine for several years, he began to seek alternative methods that he believed would be more in tune with the body's own internal healing mechanisms. Advertising himself first as a "magnetic healer" and later as a "lightning bonesetter," he gradually formulated a system of treatment based on correcting biomechanical dysfunction. Professor Still declared that disease was due to the imbalance of internal fluids, the result of an obstruction in some artery or vein, and that this could be traced to "a bone out of place," most probably in the spinal column. Treatment therefore involved discovery of strain or dislocation points followed by manipulation to correct them. Though his personal appearance and manner were decidedly eccentric, his reputation for relieving physical complaints was sufficient to attract many patients. Not only did he treat the usual assortment of backaches and muscle atrophy, but he applied his unique form of palpation and manipulation to headache, heart disease, lumbago, sciatica, rheumatism, local paralysis, and a host of other chronic conditions with reportedly favorable results. He called his method of cure *osteo*, for bone, and *pathos*, for suffering or disease.

In 1892, Still opened the American School of Osteopathy in Kirksville, Missouri, and in 1897 his students, Doctors of Osteopathy, or D.O.s, established the American Osteopathic Association to oversee the profession. Before the turn of the century, Kirksville had become a veritable mecca of healing, with as many as 500 patients undergoing treatment at any one time. Not surprisingly, orthodox medicine became sufficiently concerned to demand that Missouri authorities set some standards for practice and the granting of D.O. certificates. In an effort to give osteopathy a firmer scientific foundation, some of Still's followers searched medical literature and found what they asserted were precedents, chiefly in the use of medical massage advocated by George Taylor, Weir Mitchell, and Douglas Graham, all respected American physicians.

In time, they enlarged the training of D.O.s until it included much of what was taught in orthodox medical schools, including the use of surgery, drugs, x-ray treatments, and other standard practices, although its fundamentally holistic approach remained intact. Today, some 35,000 osteopaths are licensed to practice medicine in the United States, and they participate in all federal health programs.

*Chiropractic*, a term derived from the Greek words for "done by hand," also was born in the Midwest in the late nineteenth century. Its founder, a self-taught "magnetic" healer from Davenport, Iowa, named Daniel David Palmer, discovered his system of spinal manipulation while treating a local janitor who had lost his hearing coincident with a back injury. Palmer found that the janitor had a lump on his back and, believing it to be a displaced vertebra, applied firm pressure until the lump slipped back into place. The man's hearing reportedly returned. Later, Palmer also used spinal manipulation to relieve symptoms of heart disease and apparently achieved success.

Palmer came to believe that a flow of energy from the brain was the essential life-giving force in the human body and that interference with this flow, chiefly through displaced vertebrae that impinge upon nerves, was the chief cause of disease. Stories of his remarkable cures naturally attracted patients, as well as students wishing to learn his techniques, and in 1898 he founded the Palmer School of Chiropractic in Davenport. Today, there are 15 accredited colleges of chiropractic and 50,000 practitioners at work. Unlike osteopaths, they have not expanded their arsenal of treatments much beyond Palmer's original spinal manipulations; they are, however, licensed in all states and recognized for reimbursement in all federal programs.

Still another contributor to the discussion of spinal manipulations was the German physician Rudolph Klapp, who came along somewhat later and never gained a particular following, though some of his ideas have since been incorporated into other programs. In 1904 Klapp introduced "creeping exercises" as a treatment for children with scoliosis during their formative years. Klapp's regimen, which involved extended periods of walking on all fours in the manner of quadrupeds, was based on his contention that prone posture mobilizes the spine and develops trunk muscles in a manner superior to the normal human stance.

### Turning "Rubbers" Into Medical Masseurs

Meanwhile, massage, which had been incorporated into Pehr Ling's System as just one of many therapeutic activities, was gaining support as a worthy treatment in its own right. French surgeon Just Marie Marcellin Lucas-Championnière was the first to elucidate the value of massage as a follow-up to orthopedic surgery and bonesetting. Lucas-Championnière's report in *Massage and Mobilization in the Treatment of Fractures*, published in 1889, was based on his observation that a broken arm bone in one of his patients had healed both faster and stronger than expected despite failure to have it immobilized following injury. From this surprising finding, Lucas-Championnière deduced that movement had played a positive role, and he gradually abandoned splinting in favor of massage as a controlled form of motion in many of his orthopedic cases. He confidently stated that "early motion . . . maintains flexibility and increases the circulation and nutrition of the part." He went on to prescribe mild massage to the surrounding soft tissue, stating that pain typically disappeared more rapidly, swelling was reduced, and the recovery of function was accelerated. The older method, he added firmly, inevitably produced stiff joints and deformity.

Orthopedist William Bennett brought the revolutionary treatment to England, introducing medical massage at London's St. George's Hospital. Bennett, in turn, influenced Robert Jones, who became his country's most influential orthopedist in the last decade of the nineteenth century as president of the British Orthopaedic Association. Jones mentored British colleague James B. Mennell, who would become one of the most effective spokesmen for scientific massage in the first quarter of the twentieth century. (Mennell's text, *Physical Treatment by Movement, Manipulation and Massage*, published in 1917, is still read by American students as an authoritative source in its fifth edition.) Also influential in spreading Lucas-Championnière's ideas were orthopedists Albert J. Hoffa and Douglas Graham. Hoffa, who introduced a well-known surgical procedure for correcting congenital hip dislocations, wrote what has been described as the most basic of all texts on massage, *Technik der Massage*, in 1900. Graham was the author of the 1902 *Treatise on Massage, Its History, Mode of Application and Effects*, which first aroused the interest of American orthopedists in this form of aftercare.

Massage was also central to the so-called Weir Mitchell Rest Cure, an American innovation that was widely adopted in England and on the Continent in the late nineteenth century. Mitchell's treatment employed medical rubbers to treat nervous complaints, reportedly epidemic among middle- and upper-class women in the 1870s and 1880s. Frequently attributed to the "rush of modern life," the condition more likely resulted from women's increasing frustrations with their repressed lives. Mitchell, a clinical neurologist at the Philadelphia Orthopedic Hospital and Infirmary for Nervous Diseases, described his approach to neurasthenia in the rather clumsily titled *Fat and Blood and How to Make Them*, published in 1877. Mitchell put his depressed and listless patients to bed for six to 12 weeks, literally stuffed them with huge quantities of nourishing food, and prescribed prolonged doses of "massage and electricity" as a means of getting them back on their feet.

A modified version of the Rest Cure, which included graduated exercise, was introduced into England by W. S. Playfair, professor of obstetric medicine at the London Hospital. Playfair achieved several well-publicized cures of so-called "sofa mothers," invalid women suffering from extended postpartum depression. So fashionable did the Rest Cure become among the gentry that many women, including some with no discernible medical complaints, engaged personal masseuses daily in their homes as a form of preventive medicine. Gentlemen did much the same, also ostensibly for medical reasons, though usually taking treatment at one of the comfortable and clubby West End massage "parlors."

With demand for masseurs and masseuses growing yearly in Britain and no regulation of the practice, people from many venues readily found employment. One group kept busy were the old-fashioned rubbers, the massage equivalent of the self-proclaimed bonesetters. Bennett described the rubbers as mostly women, "very respectable people, rather portly in figure as a rule, strictly honest according to their lights, their main purpose seemed to be the rubbing away of knots in muscles, which were not apparent, and the dispersing of curious conditions of the veins, which were also of doubtful existence. In addition, they were much concerned in the removal of humors from all parts of the body, which lay more in the imagination of the rubber than in the person of the patient. But they . . . supplied a want and did some good. They found their clientele chiefly in the neighborhood and by word of mouth."

Modern orthopedists and physicians like Playfair generally required "a better class" of rubber. Skills in practical nursing and a basic knowledge of anatomy, along with a strong

## The Beginnings Of Physical Therapy Education In America

Physical therapy in America owes a tremendous debt to the early schools of physical education, which turned out a generation or more of well-trained "medical gymnasts" well before the profession came into formal existence. Although their curricula have little in common with modern physical therapy education they offered rigorous schooling in basic anatomy, physiology, and kinesiology, and equally importantly, they gave their women students the sense that they could and should take up careers.

The first in the pantheon of institutions was the Sargent School, founded in Boston in 1881 by physician Dudley Allen Sargent. Sargent was director of Harvard's Hemenway Gymnasium, a post he had held for two years when he began the school. Sargent brought to his life's work an eclectic background that included experience as a seaman, circus gymnast, and founder of the Hygienic Institute in New York. He had a deep-seated conviction that what he termed "preventive medicine" could best be practiced through an emphasis on individualized physical training. Sargent's "System," which was offered to every Harvard student, was based on a thorough examination and measurement of heart and lung capacity, muscular strength, personal history, and occupation as they might impinge on susceptibility to any particular disease. Based on his findings, Sargent prescribed specific exercises to strengthen deficient muscle groups.

Sargent's novel program at Harvard brought him national recognition at a time when a spate of newly founded women's colleges and schools were seeking women teachers to train their students. Starting on a very small scale, the Sargent School sought to fill that need, providing a one-year postgraduate course in anatomy, physiology, and various activity skills to young women preparing to teach. The program was expanded five years later to two years with the addition of anthropometry, body mechanics, nutrition, physical diagnosis, and the study of mind-body interactions. When it became apparent that Sargent graduates were ideally suited to assist orthopedists in postsurgical rehabilitation, Sargent actively sought affiliations with the medical community. Beginning in 1886, his students were able to do clinical observations at Boston Children's Hospital. Shortly after the turn of the century, the link grew stronger when BCH's Elliott Brackett and Robert Lovett joined the Sargent faculty.

Eight years after the establishment of the Sargent School, the Massachusetts Institute of Technology in Cambridge became the site of a huge conference on physical training attended by doctors, theologians, educators, and social reformers. One participant, Amy Homans, promptly opened the Boston Normal School of Gymnastics (BNSG) on the other bank of the Charles River. Homans claimed to offer "the best instruction in Swedish gymnastics to be found this side of Sweden." Though her immediate objective, like Sargent's, was to train physical education teachers, she had a larger agenda that specifically included preparing students for professional careers in a world that was still suspicious of, if not hostile to, working women.

Thanks to the generous financial support of Boston philanthropist Mary Hemenway, Homans was able to hire instructors of the most unimpeachable academic credentials — Harvard University, Harvard Medical School, and MIT — to teach a rigorous two-year curriculum that was heavily weighted toward science. In addition to the expected anatomy, physiology, and practical gymnastics courses, BNSG "girls" studied kinesiology, chemistry, histology, growth, reproduction, metabolism, sensation, and reflex actions. To eliminate "any traits or habits which would militate against success," Homans personally monitored the comportment of her students. No one was allowed to graduate who did not look, speak, and act the part of a self-assured, competent, "womanly" professional.

In 1909, the BNSG merged with nearby Wellesley College, becoming the Department of Hygiene and Physical Education and offering a four-year liberal arts education with an optional fifth year of physical education specialization. In 1914, six BNSG graduates, believing there was a continuing need for a two-year professional course, established a third institution, the Boston School of Physical Education. Marjorie Bouvé was named director and Marguerite Sanderson taught corrective physical education. After several transmogrifications, this school would emerge as Bouvé-Boston, associated with Simmons College (1930-1942), Tufts University (1942-1966), and subsequently Northeastern University. Sargent College, also experiencing winds of change in the educational field, left Wellesley to seek incorporation with a larger degree-granting institution and in 1929 became part of Boston University. Other early schools included the New Haven Normal School of Gymnastics in Connecticut, the origins of which trace to 1886; the Battle Creek Normal School of Physical Education, Battle Creek, Michigan, which began in 1909 as an outgrowth of J. H. Kellogg's sanitarium; and Columbia University's program, which originated in 1889 as part of the New York College for the Training of Teachers.

physical constitution, a refined nature, cheerful demeanor, good conversational skills, and punctuality, were all deemed necessary attributes of this group. To meet the demands, some physicians underwrote short-term workshops at which would-be apprentices could understudy with experienced masseuses. Others attended the new Swedish-inspired schools of physical education. As the revival of medical massage coincided with the rise of "new women," most of the trainees were well-bred (by late-Victorian standards), idealistic, and possessed of a spirit of personal independence and self-worth unknown to their mothers' generation. The young women saw in medical massage not only a useful occupation outside the home but also a challenging new frontier in which they might make a genuine contribution to British society. Many, like Rosalind Paget and Rosabella Fynes-Clinton, had taken Florence Nightingale as their role model and had first become hospital-trained nurses. Others, like Lucy Robinson, were medically trained midwives. Always interested in expanding their knowledge, the new masseuses kept in touch with one another and with news of their "profession" through *Nursing Notes*, a British publication started by Paget in 1887.

In *Nursing Notes* Paget contributed a regular column devoted to scientific "massing" as it was often termed, full of advice on everything from how to dress appropriately when administering massage to suitable behavior (no strong spirits consumed on the job) and new applications for particular massage strokes. In one article, Paget included a description of the "perfect hand," in which she quoted from Dr. Stretch Dowse, chief of physical treatment at West End Hospital for Nervous Diseases and owner of one of the medical massage training schools. According to Dowse, the best tools for delivering massage were squarish, powerful hands possessed of "suppleness, pliability, flexibility, firmness of grip, compliancy to yield readily, impressibility, smoothness, fineness, warmth, even delicacy and freedom from moisture." Elsewhere Paget wrote of the wonderful improvements lately achieved with massage, citing among many an instance in which "lateral curvature [was] perfectly cured, and little feet that had been born completely turned in and useless until three years old [had been made] as active as any others after two years treatment." Paget urged her sister medical masseuses to pursue the study of anatomy, to beware of overtiring clients, and to avoid being both nurse and masseuse to the same patient — especially those undergoing the Weir Mitchell treatment, as anyone enduring therapeutic imprisonment was sure to benefit from seeing two fresh faces rather than one.

Paget's readers were high-minded individuals with a vocation to serve the prescribing physician and their patients conscientiously, and so were the majority of the old-time rubbers. However, the chronic shortages of trained specialists had created a vacuum into which many others were drawn. Some of this last group were ill-suited to the work by temperament or physical constitution; others were downright disreputable. By the 1890s, they were attracting enough negative attention to risk the reputation of the best rubbers and massage-givers. As described in fascinating detail in Jean Barclay's *In Good Hands*, the centennial history of the Chartered Society of Physiotherapy published in 1995, concerns were first raised in the prestigious *British Medical Journal*, in which it was reported that many massage establishments were in reality "houses of ill-fame." Their employees, carrying names like "Nurse Dolly" and "Nurse Kitty," were nothing less than prostitutes masquerading under "a cloak of massage." The *BMJ* went on to say that it was abandoning its plan to offer physicians a periodic directory of qualified masseuses because the field had become so crowded with charlatans that they no longer felt confident to judge. An alarmed medical community called on the British Home Secretary and on Scotland Yard to investigate, and this was followed within the month by debate in the House of Commons about how to close down the "aristocratic bagnios" in London's West End.

Even more concerned about the "massage scandals" were Paget and her friends, who feared that if the unregulated sector were allowed to continue, doctors would be reluctant to prescribe massage in the future. Ten of the respectable ladies, forming a "council," decided to counterattack. In late 1894, the council held several meetings at the Midwives' Institute and Trained Nurses' Club in London, and the following January, they announced the formation of a separate Society of Trained Masseuses (STM). The society's stated purpose was the setting of uniform standards of proficiency, technique, and conduct for women in their profession and the establishment of a certification process by which truly qualified women could separate themselves from the crowd. (There were few male rubbers at the time and fewer still involved in medical massage; STM's founders presumed that the men neither wanted nor needed their help.)

The society sent a circular to hospitals, nursing homes, and members of the medical profession detailing the group's four cardinal rules of conduct: members would not undertake massage except under medical direction; members would not provide any sort of massage to male patients that might compromise propriety, by which was meant "general" or body massage; members would not advertise their services except in professional journals; and members would not under any circumstances provide drugs to patients. In February 1895 and again in April, the STM held its first certifying examinations, asking a dozen questions such as: "Give the position, origin and insertion, and use of four leading muscles" and "What do you understand by the 'Weir Mitchell' treatment?" Thirteen candidates received certification; three others were pronounced unqualified. With these first momentous steps, the profession of physiotherapy in Britain was formally launched, and the model was set for the eventual establishment of like organizations of skilled physiotherapists in Australia (1906), Canada (1920), America (1921), and other nations.

Weir Mitchell's "cure," it was noted above, went beyond massage to include the application of "electricity." As a matter of practice, progressive physicians increasingly prescribed two or more therapeutic modalities as

*Benjamin Franklin, as much scientist as statesman, experimented at length with the medical uses of electricity. He is said to have cured a 14-year-old Philadelphia girl of chronic convulsive fits through repeated application of electric shock therapy in 1752.*

adjuncts to basic therapeutic exercise and massage. In the late nineteenth century, these modalities included electricity, light therapy, heat therapy, and hydrotherapy, as they do today. Advancing independently as scientifically based treatments, each has a fascinating history all its own and deserves our brief attention.

## "Medical Electrics"

The earliest use of electricity in medicine was reported by Hippocrates. He recommended that the torpedo fish, which was equipped to stun its prey with an electrical charge of up to 80 volts, be served up as part of a therapeutic breakfast for asthmatics. The same fish also got high marks from the Roman physician Scribonius Largus, who prescribed using the fish as a poultice to treat headache and gout, an idea that seems to anticipate transcutaneous nerve stimulation for pain relief. But it was not until the middle of the eighteenth century — when a Dutch physicist invented the Leyden Jar, the first convenient means of generating and storing an electrical charge — that medical scientists finally had a practical means of exploring the therapeutic applications of electricity with any seriousness. The first device, a static electricity machine, produced a one-directional current of very high voltage (about 100,000 volts) and of minimal amperage (no more than 1 milliampere).

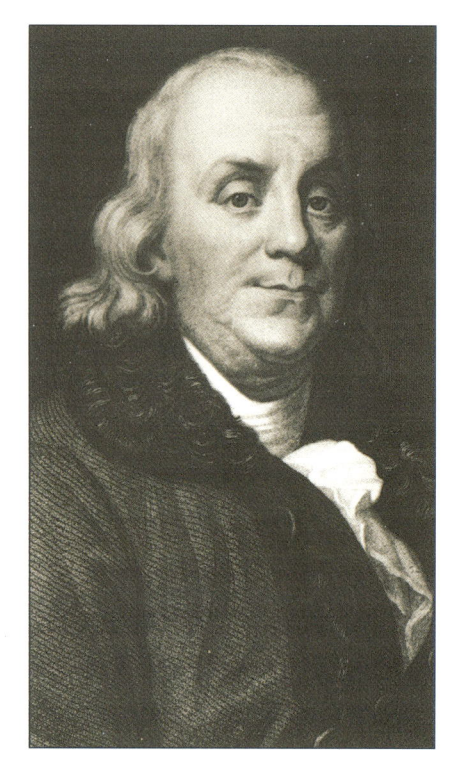

One of the first physicians to experiment was Christian Kratzenstein, a German physician, who in 1744 found that static electricity applied to his hand increased his pulse rate and made him sleep more soundly.

Another was the Swiss physician Jean Jallabert, who reported success in treating a locksmith who had lost the use of his hand in a shop accident. In 1746 Jallabert experimented with a combination of warm water bath, massage, and electrical stimulation to his patient's atrophied muscles and reportedly restored sufficient tone to get the hand working again. Benjamin Franklin, another to be intrigued by the potentials of electricity, ordered an electrical "influence machine" from England in 1757, applied its static charges to several individuals suffering muscle paralysis, and concluded that it produced only some "lifting of the spirits." But there was much enthusiasm elsewhere, particularly in France and England where palsy, sciatica, kidney stones, hysteria, convulsions, and angina pectoris were among the many conditions treated in some of the more scientifically venturesome hospitals and doctors' offices. The medical literature reflected this interest, too, carrying anecdotal reports of remarkable cures, as in the instance of "lockjaw abruptly terminated" and "obstinate St. Vitus' dance cured" by single doses of static electricity. One particularly influential practitioner, Franz Anton Mesmer of Austria, took a slightly different fix on electrical treatments in that he treated magnetic imbalances in his patients, using electricity as just one of many curatives. The term "mesmerize" to describe quack hypnosis memorializes this highly popular, if suspect, practitioner.

Not surprisingly, disillusionment set in eventually when electrotherapy did not prove to be the heralded panacea, and by 1800 the number of physicians still using it had fallen off sharply. However, work going on in Italy on the nature of electricity eventually provided enough new information to reinvigorate medical interest and to make the requisite electrical machinery more reliable. The first to contribute to this revival was Luigi Galvani, an obstetrician in Pavia, who undertook a study of the action of animal muscle and nerve and concluded that electricity is intrinsic to muscle-nerve preparation. He followed up in 1786 by describing a mechanism by which electricity might be used therapeutically. Next came Alessandro Volta, a professor of physics in Bologna, who produced the first electrical battery and the first continuous flow of electricity, widely known thereafter as galvanic or direct current (DC).

These major discoveries were followed by Englishman Michael Faraday's simple contrivance for inducing alternating electric current (AC) by means of an induction coil. Faraday built the first crude electric generator in 1831. Some three decades later, his Laws of Electromagnetic Induction were summarized and made coherent by Scotsman James Maxwell, who was able to show that electromagnetic waves and light waves are all parts of a single system. As a result of such research, the practice of medical electricity was no longer based solely on subjective observations but on a solid body of scientific facts.

Volta had noticed during his experiments that when he applied direct current to a muscle by means of a needle, the muscle contracted. Emil DuBois-Reymond of Germany took the understanding of motor activity another major step forward around 1848 when he was able to differentiate currents of injury from normal electrical potentials recorded during muscle contraction. French neurologist Guillaume Duchenne saw in this same phenomenon an opportunity to use galvanic current to treat painful muscle and nerve disorders. Duchenne quickly determined that the practice of puncturing the skin to enhance contact between electrodes and underlying tissues was unnecessarily painful. Instead, he inserted a wet sponge between the intact skin and the elec-

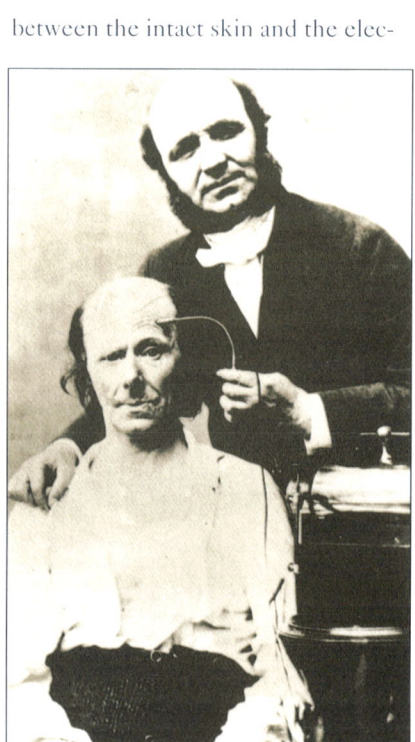

*French neurologist Guillaume Duchenne, frequently termed the father of modern electrotherapy, made extensive studies of the physiology underlying electrotherapy, identifying motor points and muscle actions. Here, he probes the reaction of the frontalis to faradic current circa 1860.*

*Through A Glass Darkly* 23

trode, a procedure he dubbed "faradization" in tribute to his intellectual progenitor, and found it worked fully as well. Also troubling the observant physician were his patients' muscular responses. They often seemed at such variance with what he had been taught at medical school that he began to suspect much of anatomical theory was either incomplete or wholly inaccurate. He decided to devote the rest of his life to correcting these deficiencies.

Duchenne first set out to classify the electrophysiology of the entire muscular system, identifying the motor points and muscle actions of isolated muscles in relation to each bodily movement, from the mechanisms of facial expression and paralyses to the workings of the healthy and flat foot. He then went on to assess the effect of faradization on paralyzed muscle and concluded that it was not the cure-all it was claimed to be but rather a tool to be applied only when voluntary control was on the point of returning. To track the repair process more accurately, he developed a sequential description of nerve recovery, starting with hyperesthesia of the affected part and following through a slight rise in temperature and improved nutrition to the return of voluntary control.

Still another Frenchman, Louis LaPicque, capitalized on the general observation that paralyzed muscle responded to galvanic current and that the duration of the current flow played a critical role in the degree of muscle contraction elicited. A few short years later, this observation would provide the basis for establishing strength-duration curves for healthy and diseased muscle, and this, in turn, would become the basis for assessing the excitability and integrity of motor units. Meanwhile, German investigators Robert Remak and Hugo von Ziemssen refined Duchenne's mapping efforts, making it possible eventually to distinguish between direct stimulation of muscles (placement of the electrode directly on the muscle itself) and indirect stimulation (placing the electrode on the area of skin nearest the motor nerve).

Once the battery and induction coil were readily available, medical electricity became a subject of intense interest, first in Europe and somewhat later in the United States, where it had to shake off its strong associations with quackery. Leading the parade in the United States were George M. Beard and Alphonso David Rockwell (the latter, incidentally, the inventor of the "electric chair" used in capital punishment). Beard and Rockwell had begun their investigation in 1865 "in a deliberate and systematic way, for the purpose of determining as far as possible the real therapeutic value of electricity." The results were far more promising than expected, and this prompted them to collaborate on *Medical and Surgical Electricity*, a comprehensive textbook that was published in 1871 and quickly went through 10 editions.

One reader who was persuaded of electricity's merits was Weir Mitchell, the Rest Cure proponent, whose further experiments with induced current proved to him "that it is in some way an active agent, capable of positively influencing the nutritive changes of the body." By 1895, five teaching hospitals in London and two in Scotland had "electrical departments" in which such procedures as electrolysis, ionic medication, and electrocautery were carried out along with muscle testing and obesity reduction, this last in a vibrating "Bergonié chair." Electrotherapy also had a following among some obstetricians and gynecologists as a treatment for uterine disease and tumors.

The teaching of electrical therapeutics and the manufacture and sale of electrotherapeutic devices gained momentum in the United States, and it was not long before the idea of organizing an exclusive society of interested American practitioners arose. In 1891 the American Electro-Therapeutic Association came into being, the forerunner of the modern specialty of physical medicine and rehabilitation. A second national society, drawn exclusively from the field of homeopathy, was organized in 1892. In spite of their differences, the two groups agreed on one issue: lay practitioners ministering under the authority of mail-order diplomas and using all manner of illegitimate electrical devices and procedures posed a threat to serious electrotherapeutists. Separately, the organizations campaigned for better, specialized training based on scientific research and better, more reliable equipment. Their efforts were only partially effective, however. Men calling themselves physicians and therapists touted electrical belts, girdles, hair brushes, liniments, rings, and other "stimulators" as curatives for everything from heart disease and "slow blood" to sexual impotence and hair loss.

A similar mix of the scientific and the fraudulent developed in England. The standard offerings among serious physicians included both "galvanism" and "faradism." In the former treatment, the physician or his trained technician provided "hand-surging with faradic stroking," which was when the current passed through the technician before it entered the patient's body in treatments that might be applied locally or bodywide with a damp sponge, depending upon the condition to be treated. In the "faradic" cure, alternating current was delivered directly to a patient seated or standing with feet upon a large electrode, while the attendant wielding a second electrode wand delivered sometimes jolting "earth shocks" to various parts of the body. One particularly difficult treatment, for constipation, involved rectal faradization. It says much about the fortitude of patients and the persuasiveness of their therapists that such treatments were tolerated by either party for long.

Electricity as a diagnostic tool developed somewhat more slowly. DuBois-Reymond's study of biologic electricity in the 1840s had led him to devise a highly sensitive galvanometer capable of detecting changes in action potential when an impulse passed down a nerve trunk; with that, the concept of electromyography was born. Liverpool physician Richard Caton built upon these ideas to seek and discover electrical activity emanating from the brain, and in the process, he developed the first electroencephalogram in 1875. As the result of many small discoveries about the electrical forces produced by heart muscle activity, Dutch physicist Willem Einthoven produced the extremely sensitive string galvanometer in 1903. Unlike Caton's prototype of the EEG, which never went beyond animal experimentation, Einthoven's electrocardiogram, or

EKG, was rapidly adopted as a fundamental tool for diagnosing heart disease. The electroencephalograph was not taken up as a medical diagnostic tool until the 1930s, by which time Caton's name was forgotten.

### SHEDDING HEAT AND LIGHT

Hot stones, hot irons, hot mud packs, and hot water bottles were some of the most common forms of thermotherapy used historically in connection with healing injured tissue. All are applied to the skin and achieve their effects by means of conduction. The heat is transmitted only shallowly, however, because of the skin's poor conduction capabilities, and it has little or no therapeutic effect on deep-seated injuries.

Sunlight, or heliotherapy, rich in ultraviolet and infrared rays, is another kind of thermotherapy with ancient antecedents. Conferring heat principally through radiation, heliotherapy penetrates somewhat deeper than conduction heat. It was first exploited as a specific treatment by the ancient Greeks, who found it therapeutic for several chronic diseases, including rickets and muscular wasting. The Greek historian Herodotus was perhaps the first to record the folk wisdom that exposure to sunshine is a contributing factor in strengthening bone tissue. He realized this when he observed a battlefield strewn with the bleached bones of fallen warriors, the Persian invaders on one side, the Egyptian defenders on the other. He wrote subsequently, "The skulls of the Persians were so fragile that a mere pebble thrown at them would penetrate. But those of the Egyptians were so strong that you could hardly break them with a stone. The cause of this, so the people said, . . . is that from childhood the Egyptians shave their heads, and the bone is thickened by exposure to the sun. . . . And the reason why the Persians have weak skulls is that they cover their heads all their lives with felt hoods."

Over the next millennium and a half, the sun was alternately lauded and ignored for its health-giving properties. The sun's stock soared to new heights, however, in the nineteenth century. By that time, substantial parts of the population were living in environments in which polluted air, windowless buildings, and endless work days kept the working classes permanently underexposed to sunlight. At the same time, scientists were beginning to appreciate the actinic or photochemical properties of sunlight, particularly as they applied to deficiency diseases such as rickets and tuberculosis, which were increasing at a frightening rate. For those who could afford it, medical treatment by systematic exposure to sunlight at a Swiss Alpine clinic was considered the best possible treatment for tuberculosis, with Auguste Rollier's "Ecole au Soleil" near Leysin, which opened in 1903, being one of the later and more celebrated of many such places.

It took only a short leap of imagination and the availability of electrical power to investigate the therapeutic possibilities of using artificial sunlight to cure various ills more conveniently. The leading American pioneer in artificial heliotherapy, as in many other physical modalities, was John Harvey Kellogg, a surgeon who became medical superintendent of the Seventh-Day Adventists' Western Health Reform Institute, renamed the Battle Creek Medical and Surgical Sanitarium, in Michigan in 1876.

At Kellogg's sanitarium, the emphasis was on intelligent diet (Kellogg's flaked cereal preparations were featured) and natural medicines, including sun baths. Although Battle Creek's living conditions were pleasant enough, its northerly location made it uncommonly short on natural sun in the winter months, which in Kellogg's mind was just as likely to deprive one of health as living in the shadow of an industrial smokestack. Kellogg came up with an artificial light bath cabinet in 1891, soon after Thomas Edison made the carbon filament light bulb practical. One of Kellogg's cabinets was displayed in the Chicago Exposition of 1893 and described in a paper read before the fourth annual meeting of the American Electro-Therapeutic Association in 1894. Observers were much taken with the idea, and a foreign manufacturer copied and began manufacturing the Kellogg light cabinet in whole-body and portable units specific to arms, legs, and torsos. When the cabinets began appearing in some American health spas, Kellogg decided it was time to get into the business himself. His Sanitarium Equipment Company offered full-body cabinets in four models equipped with between 24 and 40 incandescent, 60-watt bulbs and mirrors. Kellogg prescribed heliotherapy for lumbago, sciatica, rheumatism, jaundice, neuraesthenia, Bright's disease, and consumption, as well as many other conditions.

Coincident with Kellogg's helio inventions, a Danish physician named Niels Finsen and a German physicist named Wilhelm Roentgen made two other discoveries in the area of electromagnetic waves. Finsen went looking for a light treatment that did not

*While a patient receives therapeutic heat by means of a powerful solar arc lamp, the therapist massages tight muscles. The therapeutic benefits of sunlight have been professed throughout history, but the discovery that artificial light provides similar results, called artificial heliotherapy, in the late nineteenth century was a scientific breakthrough.*

*John Harvey Kellogg popularized the use of hydrotherapy, light therapy, massage and therapeutic exercise in turn-of-the-century America. Kellogg is shown here in the ceremonial garb of his position: superintendent of Battle Creek Sanitarium and its associated college for health practitioners.*

involve the high levels of heat found in incandescent exposure. He first obtained "cold" ultraviolet light — the wavelengths just beyond the shortest visible light rays — by filtering natural light through blue-colored water. Finding this ultimately impractical, he turned to the carbon arc lamp, a source of concentrated ultraviolet light. After a year of promising results in treating lupus vulgaris, a tuberculous condition of the skin, Finsen established the Finsen Medical Light Institute in Copenhagen to conduct research into phototherapy. A second Finsen Institute was opened by two American physicians in Chicago in 1903, but as carbon arc lamps had many drawbacks, they were soon superseded by newer mercury arc lamps, which became commercially available in 1910.

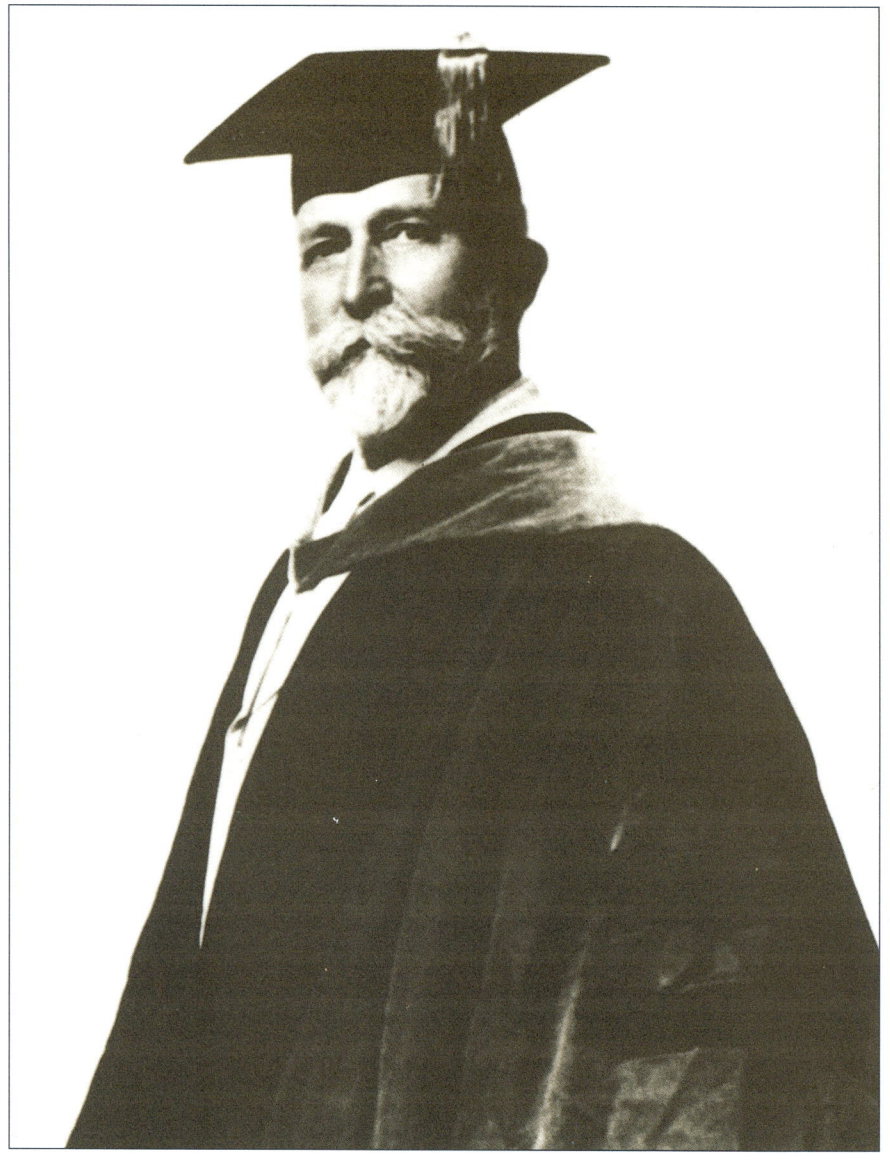

Roentgen's work in electromagnetism led, quite by accident, to the discovery in 1895 of a still shorter band of invisible waves. Known today as x-rays but dubbed "Roentgen waves" in their time, the rays were absorbed differently as they passed through bone, muscle, and organs of varying densities. This made it possible to peer inside the workings of the body without making a surgical opening, a tremendous advantage in diagnostics. Just two years after this discovery, a rudimentary machine went to war aboard a U.S. Army hospital ship, where it became the surgeons' key tool in locating bullets and shell fragments in the wounded of the Spanish-American War. Thanks to the development of special photographic paper and contrast media, "roentgenology" quickly found many other applications. Particularly appreciative were the orthopedists, who found x-rays invaluable in examining and repairing fractures. Fluoroscopy, which came along in 1897 and combined Roentgen's observation with technology developed by Thomas Edison, took orthopedic diagnostics one step further in that it permitted the doctor to see the body's internal parts in action, much like an x-ray motion picture.

Another important tool in heat/light therapy, introduced around the turn of the century, was diathermy. The first experiments with diathermy occurred in the 1890s after Nikola Tesla, a Croatian-American, suggested in an American scientific journal that currents of high frequency were capable of increasing body temperature without other obvious physiological effects. This led Jacques-Arsène D'Arsonval, a French physicist, to explore the potential effect of high-frequency, oscillating electrical currents on the metabolic processes of the body. D'Arsonval recognized that while lower frequencies of electricity induced muscle contractions, higher frequencies in the range of several hundred thousand cycles per second had other, deep-seated physiological effects. He thought they might be used to treat diabetes, gout, or obesity.

Evidently similar work was pursued in the United States by Professor Elihu Thomson, a consulting engineer at the General Electric Company in the 1890s. Thomson delivered a paper on deep-heating to the fourth annual meeting of the American Electro-Therapeutic Association in 1894, but according to electro-therapeutist G. Betton Massey, who was present, the paper prompted no curiosity, much less discussion, because "the facts and their medical applications were not understood by the hearers." Massey went on to write that it was only several years later, after the society had visited Professor Thomson's laboratory in Lynn, Massachusetts, that the medical significance of what he was doing became apparent to the group. Perhaps it was this research that inspired the first claimed clinical application of diathermy in the United States, a collaboration between Frederick de Kraft and New York physician William Benham Snow in 1906. (Snow was the most prominent electro-therapeutist of his day. He died 24 years later, allegedly one of the multitude of progressive physicians who became "x-ray martyrs," learning too late of the dangers of excessive exposure.)

In any case, metabolic applications ultimately proved to be ineffective. The incidental deep warming action of the "D'Arsonval current," however, led Karl Franz Nagelschmidt, a Berlin physician, to further experiments, and in 1907 he proved conclusively that such currents had a salutary effect on diseases of the joints and circulatory system. He named the procedure *Durchwarmung*, which translates literally as "through heat," and from this developed the term *diathermy*. Within a short time, the modality was taken up enthusiastically by physicians on both sides of the Atlantic.

In diathermy, the patient becomes part of the circuit between two condenser electrodes placed on either side of the area targeted for treatment.

When diathermy is skillfully applied, the intervening tissue presents resistance to the current, and this, in turn, causes deep heating up to temperatures in the tolerable range of 104°F. Due to insufficient knowledge of the phenomenon in the early years, however, commercial equipment and techniques put patients and technicians at some risk. Shocks, superficial burns and sparks at electrode sites, and energy transmitted into tissues not intended for treatment were frequent occurrences. Equipment capacity was also highly variable, with large, noisy machines providing "long-wave" oscillation rates of 400,000 to 3,000,000 cycles per second. Nonetheless, the fundamental concept of Nagelschmidt's diathermy was clearly a good one, and improvements were soon making treatment a more predictable event for all concerned.

### "Wetting And Sweating"

Water, used externally, is another modality within physical therapy that is older than civilization. Historically it was supplied principally through fresh water bathing and immersion—in springs, lakes, and rivers and later in formalized settings called *thermae* or baths. In some instances, the water had unusual natural properties — bubbles, color, odor, extreme heat or cold, mineral content — said to contribute to its curative powers. Invariably the waters were treated with a certain reverence in the belief that their ultimate source was supernatural.

Explicit records of hydrotherapy's use abound from the time of the Greeks, when warriors often took the water cure to overcome fatigue, heal injuries, or combat melancholy, perhaps under the supervision of a temple priest or healer. The Romans, following suit, so invested water with these powers that they built extraordinary public and private baths throughout the empire, offering facilities for exercise, steam, hot and cold plunges (contrast baths), and massage. Among the most celebrated were the Baths of Caracalla, which covered 33 acres of the Roman capital; and Aqua Sulis (modern-day Bath, England), which featured several mineral springs, one reportedly delivering a half-million gallons of water per day at a temperature of 120°F. Following the fall of Rome and the rise of Christianity, however, all such places were branded as centers of licentiousness and abandoned by respectable people.

Fresh and saltwater baths, spas, and other forms of hydrotherapy did not fully revive as a therapeutic option in the West until the nineteenth century, when "taking the waters" became a favorite health regimen of the wealthy, who went in search of cures all over Europe. By that time there were already several medical works on the subject, perhaps the most influential being *Medical Reports on the Effects of Water, Cold and Warm*, published in 1797 by Liverpool physician James Currie. America also had its early proponents, led by Philadelphian John Bell, whose *Journal of Health* contained frequent references to the beneficial effects of cold water to reduce swelling, to treat headache, to reduce pain and irritation, and to mitigate inflammation.

Physicians nominally ran the most fashionable spas, but enterprising laymen were not averse to promising miraculous cures wherever water bubbled forth. Such a figure was Austria's Vincent Priessnitz, a farmer's son who is commonly recognized as the founder of modern hydrotherapy. Priessnitz had been introduced to cold-water therapy as a folk cure for his family's dairy cows. Believing that the therapy had a positive effect, he later applied the same treatment to himself, wrapping his torso in wet toweling after suffering a serious accident that fractured his ribs. When the young man made a remarkably swift and full recovery, others came to his Graefenberg farm seeking cures for a multitude of physical complaints. Reportedly, many went away well satisfied, and by the late 1820s, Priessnitz was running a formal water-cure establishment offering a regimen of wet sponging, sheet packs, friction, sweating, vigorous massage, and various specialized baths and showers for chronic conditions.

The theory behind Priessnitz's approach was an updated version of the old humoral theories of disease causation: internal "bad stuff," as he called it, was the source of every ill; the cold-water cure simply aided nature by stirring up the bad stuff, inducing a "crisis," and sending the undesirable matter through the skin's pores to be washed away. Considering that modern antibiotics had not been developed, internal and external methods of flushing out disease were in fact the best method of treatment for many disease conditions. At any one time, as many as 500 patients were under Priessnitz's care, including many who were themselves doctors with physical ills.

As the fame of Priessnitz's systemic water stimuli spread, imitators appeared. The first hydropathic institute in America opened in New York City in 1843, and by 1848 there were 21 such institutions and a *Water Cure Journal* to inform them. The numbers give only scant indications of hydropathy's popularity, however, because it was a system that could be practiced at home, with or without the supervision of one of the more than 300 independent hydropathic physicians said to be practicing at mid-century. (Patent applications for all manner of home hydroapparatuses flooded the U.S. Patent Office; fixed and portable steam-bed baths were a perennial favorite.)

Hydropathy remained a popular alternative to conventional medicine in America for many decades, but it gradually became enfolded within a larger natural health movement that included diet reform, exercise, temperance, clothing reform, and a renunciation of heroic medicine and its excesses. One American medical hydropath stands out: Simon Baruch, a general practitioner trained in conventional medicine at the Medical College of Virginia. Baruch, a former Confederate Army field surgeon, began experimenting with hydrotherapy in the 1870s after reading about the uses of cold and graduated-temperature baths as an antipyretic for typhoid and as an anti-inflammatory for rheumatism and pneumonia. He was encouraged by what he found, but it was only after 1884, when he was made staff chairman at New York's Montefiore Home for Chronic Invalids, that he had an opportunity to become a true propagandist for water and other physical therapeutics.

At Montefiore, an institution dealing exclusively with patients deemed "incurable," Baruch introduced systematic hydrotherapy, reportedly rehabilitating scores of patients. Among

*Simon Baruch was a nineteenth-century proselytizer for hydrotherapy in the United States. His foremost contribution to the medical use of water treatments was his 1895 "douche table," which was equipped with an array of control valves, thermometers, pressure gauges, and short hoses, useful in delivering water under a variety of pressures and temperatures.*

the devices used was the "douche table," consisting of a stand equipped with multiple control valves, thermometers, pressure gauges, and short hoses by which an attendant directed water in a variety of pressures and temperatures to the patient being treated. Baruch went on to author several texts on hydrotherapeutics, the most widely read being *Principles and Practice of Hydrotherapy*, 1898, which went into three English-language and several foreign editions.

More importantly, perhaps, Baruch used his medical pulpit — he was professor of hydrotherapy in the College of Physicians and Surgeons, Columbia University, and a popular lecturer on the medical society circuit — to argue for more systematic study and reporting of the results of non-medicinal therapeutic treatments. "No remedial agent is entitled to confidence," Baruch told his colleagues repeatedly, "unless its action has a rational basis, unless it may be administered in measured dosage, and unless its clinical results are convincing." He pronounced physiological therapeutics, including rest, exercise, diet, and water, as "remedies which have demonstrated their value in all epochs of medical history," adding that "their use and abuse should be studied with at least as much care and bedside observation as the medicinal agents which are issuing in rapid succession from our good friends the pharmacists. . . . Prove all and choose the best . . . with the aid of physiological and pathological experiment, so that posterity may not flounder in the mire of uncertainty as our predecessors have done." Baruch's words and goals still resonate within the physical therapy community.

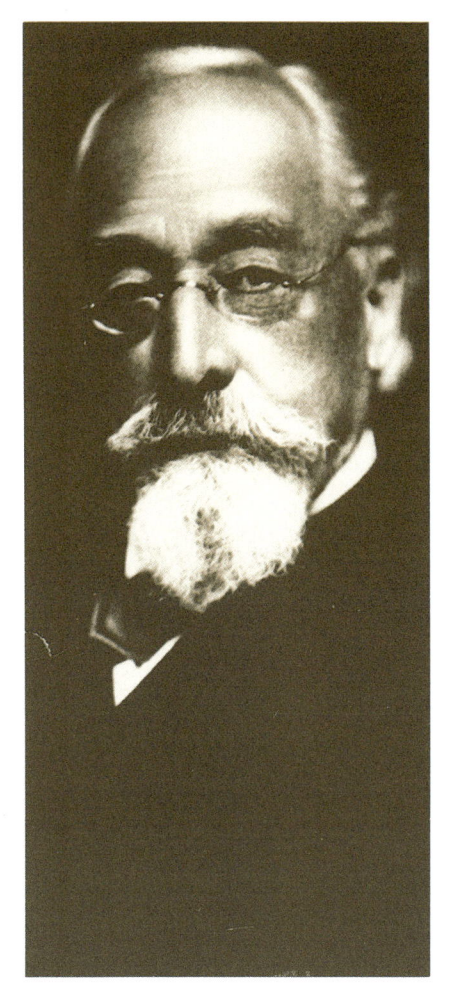

Another critical step in the evolution of hydrotherapy was made with the discovery of underwater exercise, or "hydrogymnastics." The initiators were physicians Ernst von Leyden and Alfred Goldscheider, who published a paper on "bath kineto-therapeutics" in a German medical journal in 1898. Largely because the building of appropriate indoor facilities within hospitals and clinics was so expensive, the idea was slow to catch on, and it was not until the 1920s and the rise in polio cases that further study was made.

### ORTHOSES AND PROSTHESES

Integral with the history of physical therapy is the evolution of prostheses, orthoses, and a host of other inventions designed to protect and assist the individual with a physical disability. The earliest prostheses were probably not too different from the crude wooden peg-leg and bucket-and-stump devices worn into the twentieth century by many people with amputations. The oldest extant artificial limb to which any degree of artifice was applied is a copper-and-wood leg dating from 300 B.C., unearthed a century ago on the Mediterranean island of Capri. The earliest surviving examples of artificial hands and arms date from the sixteenth century A.D., when several upper-extremity replacements were evidently devised for parts lost in jousting tournaments. One such hand weighed about three pounds and featured articulated fingers capable of grasping a sword when springs were released. However, as amputation was always a high-risk operation, with relatively few patients surviving to need limb prostheses, improvements in design were markedly slow to come along. Manufactured as an occasional sideline by armorers, cobblers, locksmiths, and harness makers, they were most often made of wood with generally clumsy and uncomfortable over-the-shoulder harnesses and sockets to hold them to their stumps.

The first real progress came when mechanic James Potts contrived a jointed leg for the Marquis of Anglesea, a British nobleman felled at the Battle of Waterloo in 1815. The Anglesea Leg featured a steel knee joint and articulated foot. William Selpho, Potts's protégé, brought the

*Turn-of-the-century hydrotherapy came in many forms. This "Gastric Douche," a variant of the contrast bath (alternating plunges in hot and cold water), was used at the Battle Creek Sanitarium to stimulate the circulation, activate the skin, and promote better digestion.*

## Polio's Unwelcome Debut

Poliomyelitis is popularly thought of as a twentieth-century disease because it was in the first half of this century that it became a global scourge. In fact, the virus that causes polio has been with us throughout human history. The contagion entered medical literature circa 1789, when British physician Michael Underwood noted an unnamed disease symptomized by acute fever, permanent paralysis, and a cruel preference for children. He recommended "blisters" to the sacrum and trochanter, "volatile and stimulating applications" to the legs and thighs, and "irons [braces] to the legs" in the instance of paralysis.

Polio's tendency to strike many simultaneously was first observed in 1834, when British physician John Badham encountered "four remarkable cases of suddenly induced paralysis, occurring in children . . ." in the village of Worksop, England. About the same time, youngsters on the British island of St. Helena in the South Atlantic were stricken, and in 1841 what was probably the first outbreak in the United States occurred in West Feliciana, Louisiana. As documented by a country doctor named George Colmer in the *American Journal of Medical Science*, the 8 to 10 "little sufferers" he examined were invariably under two years of age, hence his title "Paralysis in Teething Children."

By then the disease had a formal name — two names, in fact. In 1840 the distinguished German orthopedist Jakob Heine published a monograph on "spinal infantile paralysis" in which he attributed the paralysis to a "spinal lesion." Other medical investigators identified it as "poliomyelitis," in recognition of the gray (*polios*) anterior matter of the spinal cord (*myelos*) and associated inflammation (*itis*). But polio's cause remained elusive. It grew in virulence and frequency of incidence even as many other diseases were gradually yielding to better methods of sanitation and public health control. (A third name, Heine-Medin's disease, came into use still later. It memorialized not only Heine but Oskar Medin, a Swedish epidemiologist, who tracked the disease's first known occurrence in Stockholm in 1840.)

One polio cluster, involving 123 youngsters, erupted in 1894 in the Otter Creek Valley near Rutland, Vermont, leaving 50 permanently disabled and 10 dead. Another struck New York in 1907, going unnoticed until welfare officials the following year reported nearly 2,000 families seeking help for their recently paralyzed youngsters. A far more widespread epidemic occurred nine years later: in the five warmest months of 1916, there were 27,363 cases and 7,179 deaths identified in the 20 states then keeping extensive public health records. In New York alone, there were 9,020 cases, a quarter of whom died.

The public, particularly parents of young children, were profoundly frightened. The disease was now known to be infectious — in 1909, Simon Flexner and P. A. Lewis of the Rockefeller Institute had identified the agent as a filterable virus. It seemed to have an affinity for the more comfortable segments of society. Government health officials advised everyone to avoid crowds, even flee to the country, during polio years, but the strictures proved generally ineffective. Sparsely populated areas were not immune to contagions.

Medical treatment was generally misdirected, too, with most "cures" arising out of guesswork and luck. But there was a notable exception in Robert W. Lovett, a noted Boston orthopedist. Although scoliosis was his special field, Lovett had treated numbers of polio victims and was known throughout New England for his novel approach. In 1914, during yet another polio epidemic in Vermont, Lovett was invited by the state's director of public health to provide treatment and follow-up care to 235 victims in what became known as the "Vermont Plan." Setting up five treatment centers, Lovett quickly put together and trained teams of orthopedists, local physicians, and nurses to care for the cases. At the same time, senior assistant Wilhelmine Wright, who ran Lovett's "gymnasium" clinic at the Boston Children's Hospital and was herself a published expert on muscle training, took on the task of instructing a cadre of non-medical personnel. In a new procedure called "manual muscle testing," she showed how to rate individual muscles according to degree of disease involvement — from totally paralyzed to partially paralyzed to normal — and how to tailor-make a program of muscle reeducation to restore function. Wright's pioneering work, which she would subsequently publish as *Muscle Function*, 1928, stands as one of the true benchmarks in the history of physical therapy. It is the basis for much important work later taken up by physical therapists Miriam Sweeney, Janet Merrill, Henry and Florence Kendall, Signe Brunnström, Marjorie Dennen, Alice Lou Plastridge, Margaret O'Neill, and many others.

> **INFANTILE PARALYSIS**
>
> This Notice is Posted in Compliance with Law
>
> "Every person who shall wilfully tear down, remove or deface any notice posted in compliance with law shall be fined not more than seven dollars."
>
> General Statutes of Connecticut, Revision of 1912, Sec. 1173
>
> **Town Health Officer.**

*As localized polio epidemics began to strike with increasing severity and frequency in the second decade of the twentieth century, health officials vainly attempted to control the disease's spread through quarantines. This notice was posted on the door of a stricken Connecticut household in 1912.*

*"Lifelike elasticity, flexibility and likeness" were among the attractions advertised by Benjamin Frank Palmer, the inventor-manufacturer of this 1855 artificial leg. Palmer, who holds the first U.S. patent for an artificial limb, included spring-activated devices by which the knee and foot could be made to flex.*

technique to New York, where he prospered until Frank Palmer, a dissatisfied customer, thought he could improve on Selpho's product. In 1846, Palmer was granted the first U.S. patent for an artificial limb, which he subsequently manufactured in Springfield, Massachusetts. A. A. Marks, another New Yorker, came along with his own competing "American Leg" in 1854. Thirty thousand Civil War wounded and a government policy of subsidizing prostheses for service-connected amputations assured a major expansion in business after 1862. The suction socket, which permitted painless attachment of lower extremity prosthesis to stump by means of closely conforming fit and atmospheric pressure, appeared in 1863. So did Oliver Wendell Holmes's stereoscopic studies of natural gaits, which provided useful data for helping patients with amputations to relearn the process of walking. With scores of new artificial leg designs flooding the market, the United States quickly took the lead in leg prostheses manufacture.

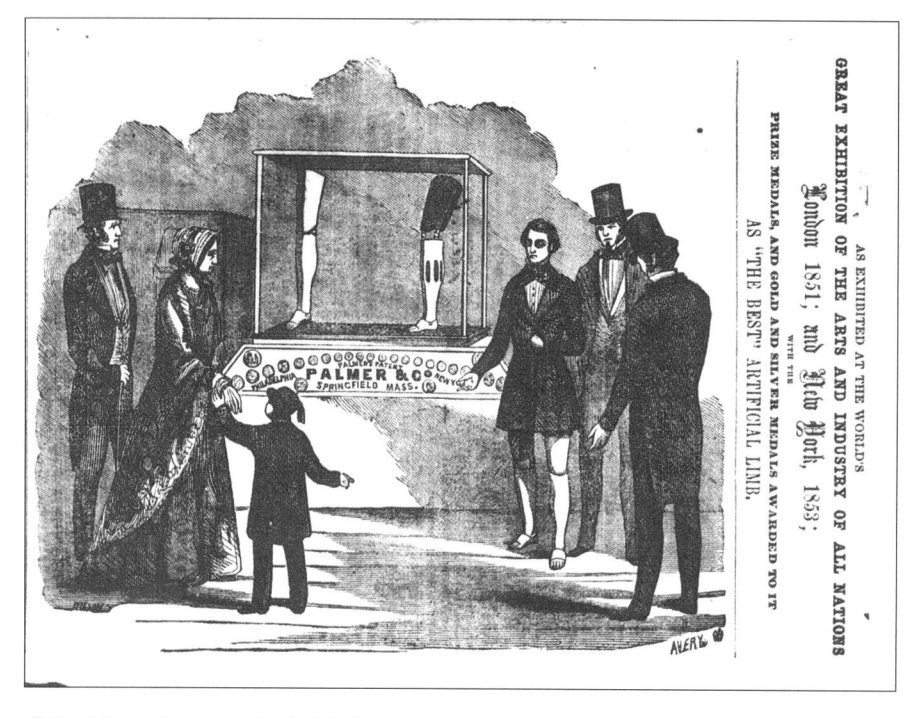

Dominance in upper extremity prostheses remained on the Continent, however, with German engineering setting the standard for making articulated joints for hands and elbows. A major refinement was added by the Italians at the turn of the century when Giuliano Vanghetti, an Italian physician, developed the concept of kineplasty, which involved the use of residual forearm muscles to power prosthetic hand or hook movements directly. Vanghetti developed the innovation after scores of Italian soldiers had their right hands mutilated during Abyssinian captivity. Vanghetti's colleagues were skeptical, and the idea did not become a surgical reality for another decade.

Casts, unjointed splints, and jointed braces, all correctives for skeletal problems, also have ancient antecedents. Even before the dawn of recorded history, leg and arm fractures almost certainly were splinted with a rigid section of wood. The first casts on record were probably those devised by medieval French doctors, who soaked bandages in a hardening agent — initially egg whites and later plaster of Paris — to encase injured parts. And mechanical bracing as an aid in treating spinal deformities can be seen in Ambroise Paré's crude breastplates of 1582. Each of these orthotic appliances has been undergoing useful modifications ever since, first by bonesetters and, after 1800, by the "strap and buckle doctors" who practiced early nonsurgical orthopedics. An important share of the improvements beginning in the last century were American-made.

It was Charles Fayette Taylor of New York, for example, who reportedly tinkered for 16 years before perfecting his so-called "spinal assistant" in the 1860s. A steel and leather appliance, it was designed to transfer the weight of the upper body to the pelvis while the spinal column was pulled into line. It is reported that Taylor regarded the manufacture and custom fitting of mechanical braces as of such importance that his clinic workrooms were as well-furnished and spacious as the rooms dedicated to seeing and treating patients. Physician Louis Sayre popularized the use of suspension in correcting scoliosis and other spinal deformities, devising among other appliances the still-current Sayre Neck Sling and the plaster-of-Paris Sayre Jacket in the 1870s. This latter apparatus was applied while the subject was slung by head and shoulders to maximize extension. Further refinements in the treatment of spinal deformities by plaster jacket came in the next two decades from a stellar group of orthopedists in and around Boston: Robert Lovett, James Sever, Edville Abbott, and Edward H. Bradford, the latter also the creator of the classic iron pipe and canvas immobilization frame that bears his name and that first came into use circa 1893.

The wheelchair is conventionally dated from the Renaissance, when it replaced the wheelbarrow and sedan chair as transport for persons with disabilities. Perhaps the first self-propelled rolling chair was designed by the inventive Prince Rupert of Bavaria around 1675. Rupert's "invalid chair" featured three small wheels, the single one in front linked to two rotary handles by which the user could pull himself around. Chairs gradually grew larger and more cumbersome, with wheels up to four feet in diameter and total weight close to 100 pounds, until 1918, when an American named Harry Jennings, Sr., devised the first light metal chair. The first commercially made motorized chair made its debut around 1915. It weighed 300 pounds and was powered by a 10-cell Edison battery.

Even ambulatory aids have a history. Canes surely began before recorded history. Rudimentary crutches

*The design of wheelchairs advanced rapidly following the Civil War. This patented 1886 model, featuring a lavishly carved wooden seatback, also incorporates a writing desk and parasol.*

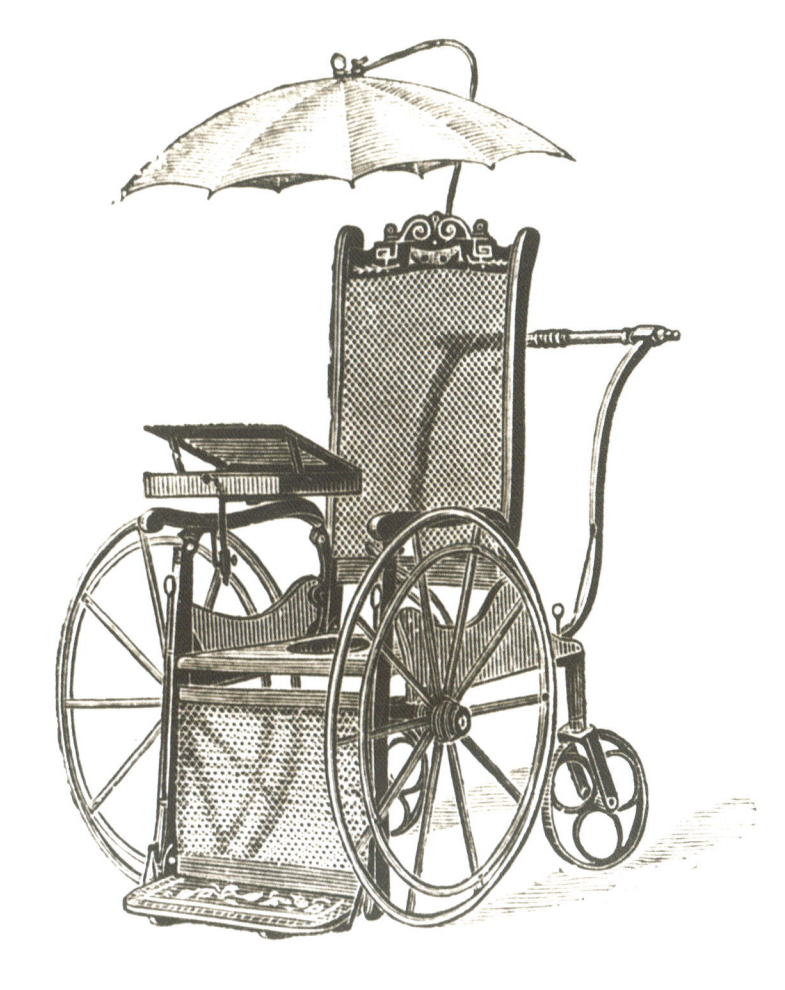

*Thanks to the efforts of E. H. Bradford and other Boston orthopedists, a specialized school for children with crippling conditions was established. Named for an early and generous trustee, The Cotting School provided an education, job training, and continuing therapeutic exercise to youngsters with disabilities. This photo shows Cotting primary schoolers circa 1911.*

came along some time later, doubtless undergoing constant homegrown tinkering and improvement over the ages. By the nineteenth century and the Industrial Revolution, with the tragic increase in injured and maimed, some manufacturers began to apply rational rules of design to crutches, and there was a burst of patented models offering adjustable height, various hand grips, underarm padding, and no-slip tips. Virtually all, however, were made of locally available hardwood, and they were relatively heavy and awkward. Not until after World War II, in fact, was there any real innovation in crutch design. The changes were reflected in the now familiar Canadian and Lofstrand crutches. The former, a single-shaft, adjustable model made of aluminum, featured two upper arm cuffs and was manufactured in Canada. The latter was of German design. Originally made of chrome-plated steel with a single forearm cuff, it too was adapted by the Canadians, who substituted aluminum to lessen the weight. Both aids became available in the United States around 1953.

### A New Social Climate

It is one of history's great ironies that even as medicine and physical therapeutics were gaining the capacity to truly ease the physical/medical side of human suffering, society was devising ever more injurious conditions in which to live. Far more than the battlefield, the industrial workplace was becoming a high-risk environment. When the total calculations of industrial accidents in the United States were initially compiled in 1913, annual fatalities were toted at a horrifying 25,000, and injuries involving more than four weeks' disability were estimated at 700,000. Few of the injured could hope to be compensated for lost income or treated for their injuries at company expense, because in contrast to social legislation in Europe, employers in the United States were not legally responsible for their workers' safety. The hordes of people who were crippled and disabled simply disappeared from public view, to be cared for by their hard-pressed families, if they were lucky, for the rest of their lives. Before the turn of the twentieth century, children who were disabled at birth or in early childhood were also without a social net other than that provided by their families; the chances of being educated or otherwise included in the community mainstream were meager indeed.

Recognition of America's growing problems with disease and disablement gradually captured the attention of reform-minded citizens and legislators. In 1887, the forerunner of the National Institutes of Health, or NIH, was born in a one-room "Laboratory of Hygiene" at the Marine Hospital, Staten Island, New York. In 1893, a group of orthopedists in Boston sponsored America's first free day school for children with disabilities, The Cotting School, where physical therapeutics and training in both independent living and a suitable trade were included as part of the daily curriculum. In 1899, public-spirited leaders in Ohio founded the Cleveland Rehabilitation Center, followed in 1917 by the establishment of the Red Cross Institute for the Crippled and Disabled in New York. The U.S. Public Health Service, an outgrowth of the smaller and more narrowly defined Marine Hospital Service, was launched by Congress in 1902, after which federal and state public health activities were bound together under the overall leadership of the U.S. Surgeon General. The first state workers' compensation laws were enacted in 1908.

All in all, these events signaled a new spirit of social responsibility gaining ground, particularly as it applied to the health of America's citizens. The events of the next few decades would test just how strong that resolve was.

*Constructed sometime between 1800 and 1825, this below-the-elbow arm prosthesis features a movable hook "hand." The ingenious metal lever that runs the length of the prosthesis rests next to the body; when the lever is pressed to the torso, the hook is made to open and grasp objects.*

CHAPTER 2

# Mary McMillan And Wartime "Reconstruction" 1914 – 1919

*Mollie McMillan enjoys a rare moment of relaxation at Reed College, Portland, Oregon. She was sent to the school in the summer of 1918 to set up a War Emergency Training Course in physical therapy. Some 200 young women eventually graduated from Reed's program, serving the war effort as reconstruction aides (or "re-aides") and carrying McMillan's methods and teachings far and wide.*

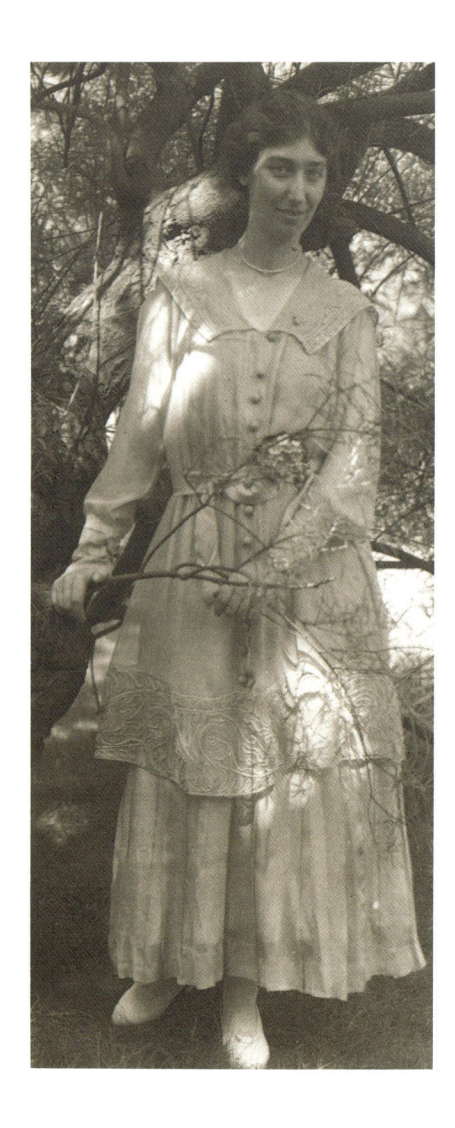

Physical therapy as a recognized medical art had its true beginnings in the second decade of this century and the carnage of World War I. Prior to the war, physical disability, particularly disability or deformity occurring as the result of birth defect or injury, was regarded by most Americans as irreversible. If those with disabilities could be made a little more comfortable, that was certainly to the good, but there was little expectation that medical intervention would make any real difference in the outcome. And the kind of extended care required to make even small improvements was not available to any but the very rich, which the disabled rarely were. The thousands born yearly with disabilities or crippled through degenerative disease were, more often than not, consigned to their homes and families or sentenced to institutional storage. Those injured in industrial accidents, or through military service, might be given pensions or other sorts of financial recompense, but little else was offered to improve their lot. And thus they remained for the rest of their lives — out of sight, out of mind, so far as the general public was concerned.

As we have seen, there had been scattered attempts at various forms of rehabilitative therapy in the United States, particularly for youngsters with polio. So, too, the idea of exercise and massage as conducive to good health was traceable in the growing influence of physical education programs in American life. But it took a crisis as immense as an international war and the disablement of millions of soldiers to demonstrate to the American medical establishment the value of physical therapy in treating a broad range of medical conditions.

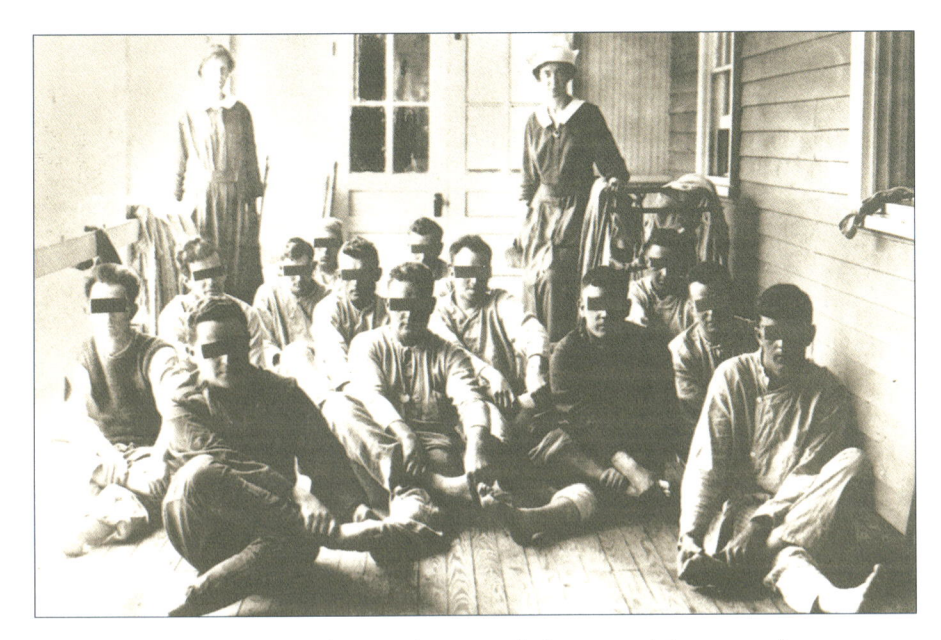

To begin with, World War I proved a powerful force in educating the American public about the social aspects of disease and disability. In a report written for the Carnegie Endowment for International Peace on the eve of America's entry into the war, Columbia University Professor Edward Devine wrote, "In civil life accidents which leave men crippled or mutilated or blind or deaf happen individually. Their victims are not concentrated in institutions devoted exclusively to their care, and they come from many different groups, not a single gigantic organization which is literally the whole nation in arms. . . . Now for the first time these everyday problems of physical disability assume such proportions and present such an appealing aspect that they command attention from the entire nation." The public would no longer be satisfied to send their wounded home with a disability check and a letter of gratitude.

The war also showed, to an alarming degree, that the so-called cream of American young manhood was, despite all the recent interest in physical education in the schools, still in surprisingly poor physical condition. One Army orthopedist, recalling the first waves of American doughboys arriving in France in 1918, would later say that all too many proved to be unfit for service even before reaching the battlefield. At one basic training camp, more than 60 percent of the men were unable to march because of foot trouble. And overseas hospitals were "soon filled with flat-footed, lame-backed, weak-kneed men," according to one harried physician. It thus became a responsibility of the army's medical service to correct the physical shortcomings of thousands of otherwise healthy men.

A third influence for change was prolonged exposure to European rehabilitation techniques, which were far ahead of American practices. American doctors who had doubted the practicality of restoring the injured to productive lives had only to look to the successes of the Allies, who had nearly a three-year lead on dealing with war wounded. Particularly notable was the example of the British. By 1917 some 1,000 members of the Incorporated Society of Trained Masseuses

*Because of the large numbers of casualties under their care, the reconstruction aides often instructed the injured to self-administer certain therapies. Here on a porch at Walter Reed General Hospital, McMillan oversees a group of doughboys engaged in resistive exercise for lower limb disorders. As was customary at the time, faces are partially masked in the photo to maintain the soldiers' privacy.*

*McMillan poses for her formal portrait in the reconstruction aide uniform. She wears the dashing broad-brimmed black velour sailor, maroon cockade, dark grey "ulster," and insignia that were part of a reconstruction aide's street wear.*

(precursor of the Chartered Society of Physiotherapy) had volunteered for the privately funded Almeric Paget Military Massage Corps, and many more would join them in the months to come. Not only were many of their wounded able to go back into battle after a brief convalescence, but those who could not often were able to resume lives as productive, wage-earning citizens, thanks to skilled physiotherapeutic intervention at an early stage.

The speed with which this social and medical change came about in America must be credited in part to the progressive leadership of the United States Army Medical Corps. But in a larger sense, it belongs to a handful of orthopedists and some 1,200 young reconstruction aides who, under difficult circumstances, threw themselves into the work with an energy, inventiveness, and good humor that had no precedent. These latter pioneers, from every part of the country and myriad different life experiences, would, within months of war's end, form the professional organization known today as the American Physical Therapy Association.

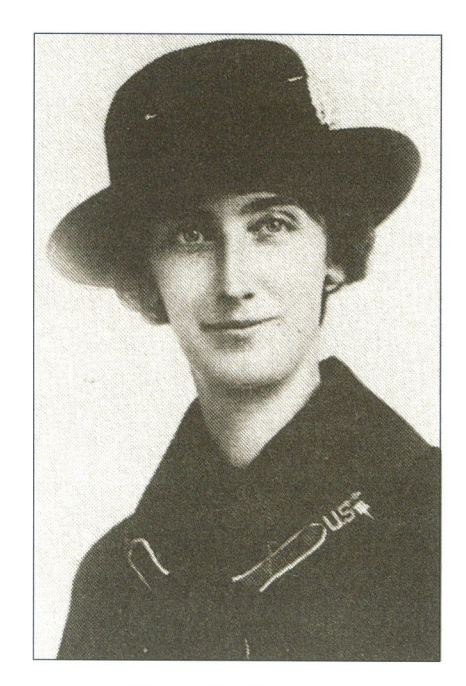

**MARY MCMILLAN: FIRST AMONG MANY**

Although it can be fairly said that every one of the reconstruction aides brought honor to the practice of reconstruction therapy in those years, one individual surely stands above all others: Mary McMillan. A key figure in the history of the American Physical Therapy Association, McMillan was both the principal conduit of British physical therapy techniques in America in the early years of the twentieth century and an influential educator in her own right. Because her contributions run so wide and so deep, her early life deserves telling in some detail.

Mary Livingston McMillan was born on November 28, 1880, in Hyde Park, Massachusetts, the sixth child of Archibald and Catherine McMillan. The McMillans were of modest means, having emigrated from Scotland just four years before Mary's birth, and although Archibald managed to establish a tailoring business in nearby Boston, life in those first years was far from secure. When consumption took both Mary's older sister Katie and her mother in 1885, young Mary was sent back across the Atlantic to be raised by McKechnie cousins in Liverpool, England.

The McKechnies proved to be loving surrogates and England to be a supportive home away from home. Mary — or Mollie, as she would ever after be known to her friends — was enrolled in a fine private school in Liverpool, and because she was a very good student, the McKechnies sent her on to preparatory work at Liverpool College for Girls and then to Liverpool University. Graduating in 1905 with training in English literature, French, domestic science, and hygiene,

Mollie went against her family's wishes and decided to make a career in the new science of corrective exercise.

Choosing to have a career at all was, in itself, somewhat daring for well-bred young English women in the Edwardian Age, as it was in the United States. But for Mollie, who always saw life as an opportunity to do good, the choice was a natural fit. On a practical scale, she was built for the work, being what the British called a "hearty girl," with remarkable stamina, broad shoulders, and, at 5 feet 7 inches, taller-than-average stature. Her fair features, wide-set blue eyes, curly crown of chestnut hair, and athletic grace turned many heads. Mollie's personality was also well-tuned to attract notice. With a fine sense of humor, quick intelligence, boundless enthusiasm, a gift of words, and a take-charge manner, she inspired the confidence and trust of everyone who knew her.

After a year of travel to the Continent, Egypt, and the Holy Land — the first of many world tours Mollie McMillan would take during her lifetime — she returned to Liverpool in 1906 to enroll in the two-year graduate course in "physical culture and corrective exercises" at the Liverpool Gymnasium College, one of several British institutions devoted to teaching Swedish or Ling gymnastics. Now 28 years old, McMillan could certainly have gone directly from this training to employment as a hands-on remedial exercise assistant with one of England's more progressive orthopedists. But she still was not satisfied. She wanted to understand the underlying pathological causes and effects that the exercises were designed to correct.

With that goal in mind, McMillan went down to London to take two more years of lectures and clinical training at the Royal College of Surgeons, at Queens Square Hospital for Nervous Diseases, and at St. George's Hospital. At the latter, she studied with Sir William Bennett, a noted surgeon and patron of the Incorporated Society of Masseuses, whose use of massage in enhancing bony unions revolutionized the treatments of fractures in England. McMillan's studies during these years included neuroanatomy, neurology, psychology, massage, electrotherapy, aftercare of fractures, and, under the tutelage of the renowned Walter Fletcher, the dynamics of scoliosis.

In 1910, with her certificates of professional competence in hand, she finally felt ready to begin her first real job. Returning to Liverpool, she was put in charge of massage therapy at the city's Southern Hospital, working principally with industrial accident victims from the Liverpool docks, and at the Greenbank Home for Crippled Children, a place of refuge for youngsters with polio, scoliosis, and a host of developmental deformities.

Both institutions were under the direction of Sir Robert Jones, nephew and professional heir of the great orthopedist Hugh Owen Thomas, who was himself the first medical member of a dynasty of Welsh bonesetters. For McMillan and Jones it was a mutually beneficial association: McMillan was an excellent assistant, and Jones was doing some of the most advanced clinical work in orthopedics anywhere. (Among the many advances for which he is remembered, Jones was chiefly responsible for popularizing the Thomas splint, invented a full 40 years earlier by his uncle but long ignored.

Jones was also a conduit for the progressive massage and manipulation theories of French orthopedist Lucas-Championnière and of British surgeon James B. Mennell, all of which McMillan absorbed.)

Shortly after Britain entered World War I in 1914, Jones became director of orthopedics for the British Military Service. Quick to grasp the value of physical rehabilitation in the treatment of men felled by compound fractures, amputations, and other wholesale horrors of war, he put out a call for women to join him in a "voluntary aide detachment," or VAD, to do reconstruction aftercare among the wounded. McMillan, who had seen comparable medical injuries among Jones's Liverpool patients, responded, and for more than two years she worked with the casualties of war. But when she tried to join a unit of VADs in France, she was turned down for medical reasons, apparently because she was near physical exhaustion. Urged to come home by her American family, she recrossed the Atlantic, her convoy dodging German U-Boats en route, and returned to Brookline, Massachusetts, to recuperate and reestablish her American roots.

McMillan did not stay down for long. After a short rest, she found work at the Children's Hospital in Portland, Maine, where from 1916 to 1918, she was Director of Massage and Medical Gymnastics, chiefly treating young orthopedic patients with scoliosis, congenital hip dislocations, clubfoot, and other childhood bone and joint abnormalities. Her director, Edville Abbott, recognized from the outset that she had "a special adaptation to this work" and forecast for her a great future in America.

### War Declared

Within a year of McMillan's return to the United States, President Woodrow Wilson declared America's intent to "make the world safe for democracy," and on April 6, 1917, the United States entered the war. Congress authorized the military draft and passed legislation making the Bureau of War-Risk Insurance financially responsible for the rehabilitation of all servicemen permanently disabled through war-related injuries. Surgeon General William Gorgas, famed for his swift eradication of yellow fever in Panama, began hasty preparations for dealing with the many thousands of casualties anticipated. On May 11, 1917, at his request, an Executive Order was signed authorizing the Civil Service Commission to employ physical therapists, occupational therapists, and dietitians as civilians within the Army Medical Department so long as the war emergency lasted. Gorgas assigned a group of physicians, including two eminent Boston orthopedists, Elliott Brackett and Joel Goldthwait, to investigate the British and French "reconstruction" programs and to make recommendations as to how the United States Army Medical Corps could implement a similar program.

In August 1917, following their report, Gorgas authorized the establishment of the Division of Special Hospitals and Physical Reconstruction. According to the plan, soldiers who were disabled overseas were to be given initial treatment at the nearest American Expeditionary Force (AEF) base hospital, most of which were in France; those men who were capable of being restored to fighting strength were to remain in the hospitals, receiving necessary "reconstruction therapy" until ready to return to combat. Nearly a dozen such facilities were set up, with special physical reconstruction units attached at Angers, Bordeaux, Brest, Nantes, Savenay, and Vichy.

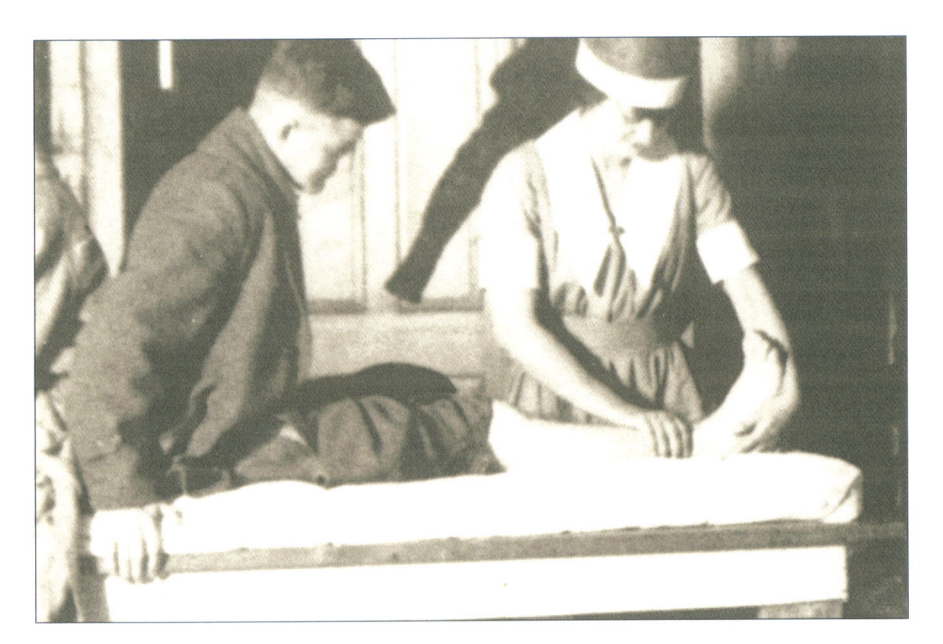

Those needing more extensive treatment were to be shipped back to the United States as soon as they could travel. Examiners were stationed at debarkation ports on Ellis Island, in New York Harbor, and at Newport News, Virginia, to classify and assign wounded returnees to the appropriate facility for rehabilitation. Sixteen of the army's general hospitals, one in each of the nation's sixteen draft districts, were initially selected to carry out the work, each having one or more designated rehabilitative specialties. Orthopedic cases, for example, were to go to Walter Reed General Hospital (WRGH) in Takoma Park, Maryland, a suburb of Washington, D.C.; Letterman General Hospital in San Francisco; General Hospital #6 in Fort McPherson, Georgia; and General Hospital #9 in Lakewood, New Jersey. Walter Reed General Hospital and Letterman were also told to prepare for the treatment and rehabilitation of returning soldiers with amputations. Altogether, the Surgeon General's Office (SGO) called for some 60,000 beds and associated services to be made ready in the United States for the newly disabled by the winter of 1918-1919. (It was estimated that for each 1,000,000 men sent overseas, there would be from 50,000 to 75,000 reconstruction cases returned to the United States.)

Each hospital was to have a "standard physical therapy unit" consisting of a U-shaped building with two wings measuring 24 by 150 feet and a center section measuring 24 by 48 feet. A gymnasium would occupy one wing, with the remaining space to be divided into a douche room, a pack room, a room for administering whirlpool arm and leg baths, a massage room, a bake room containing no less than seven electric bakers, and a mechanotherapy room with thirteen specialized apparatuses. Fitting and training rooms for recipients of artificial limbs were located in another part of the hospital. Recognizing that the reconstruction plans represented something entirely new in American medical care, Gorgas concluded his report with the wish that the new program would become

*A reconstruction aide in uniform checks resisted movement in a doughboy's injured ankle in a treatment facility at Walter Reed General Hospital, the first War Emergency Training Center set up to prepare reconstruction aides for service during World War I.*

45

*Transported by train from port debarkation sites along the East Coast, the war wounded are loaded aboard ambulances that carry them to stateside army hospitals and rehabilitation facilities. Though physical therapy was used to treat many different conditions, care of patients with orthopedic problems, such as amputations, bone and muscle atrophy, massive scar tissue, edema, and peripheral nerve lesions, accounted for the largest share of physical therapy treatments.*

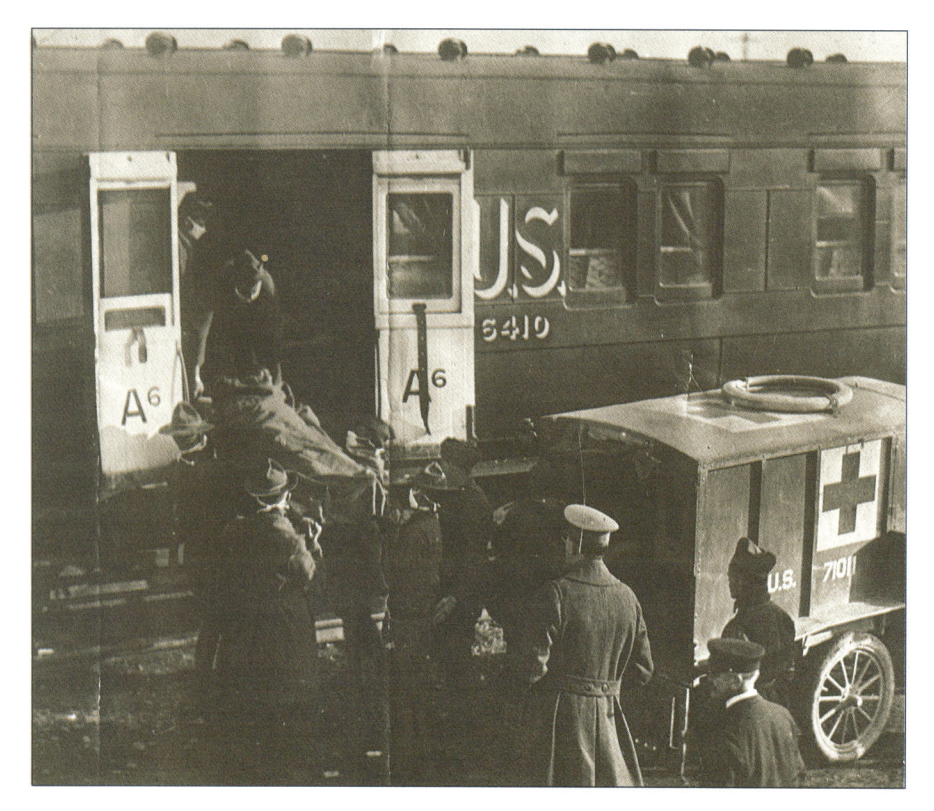

the basis for peacetime care of civilian workers with disabilities once the war emergency was over. (In actual practice, however, few of the special units were actually built. The majority of hospitals found it more practical to adapt existing buildings to their needs, and the equipment likely to be found in them varied somewhat from the theoretical specifications, probably in response to actual needs.)

The ambitious goal of the Division of Special Hospitals was to rehabilitate every one of the injured and disabled servicemen in their care (sailors and marines included) to "as near normal as possible." Inasmuch as the treatment of diseases and injuries was seen to embrace not only anatomical but also functional restoration of injured bodies, the Surgeon General's Office declared that "continued treatment requires the use of physiotherapy." This was defined as "hydrotherapy, electrotherapy, active physical exercises of all kinds, including military or other drill or modified Swedish movements, and passive exercises such as massage, etc."

Following physical therapy, many of the servicemen with disabilities were also treated with occupational therapy, which at the time consisted of handicraft activities, curative workshops, and educational and vocational instruction designed to assist veterans in taking up new careers and activities when their disability rendered them unable to resume their prewar life. (Like physical therapy, occupational therapy had no real standing with the medical profession up to that time. Rarely offered in the hospital setting, its benefits prior to the war had been available chiefly to the indigent patients of almshouses and insane asylums, for whom occupational therapy was regarded more as a social distraction than a medical good. World War I would prove a watershed event for the profession of occupational therapy as well.)

Within the organizational structure of the Division of Special Hospitals, Elliott Brackett was commissioned colonel and chief surgeon of domestic military hospitals; Joel Goldthwait, a personal friend of General "Jack" Pershing, was given similar command of overseas hospitals for the American Expeditionary Force. Ranked under them as captain and assigned as chief of the Physical Therapy Section, Division of Physical Reconstruction, in the Surgeon General's Office was yet another Bostonian, Frank B. Granger. The 43-year-old Granger was an assistant professor of physical therapeutics at Harvard Medical School and president of the American Electro-Therapeutic Association. He was one of the first figures within the American medical community to grasp the full potential of physical therapy as a medical treatment.

As neither the army nor any civilian hospitals had a ready-made cadre of skilled masseurs, electro-therapeutists, or any other sort of physical aides to carry out the prospective work, Granger laid out a plan for the recruitment and training of such a group. "Reconstruction aides," as they soon came to be called, were to be unmarried women between the ages of 25 and 40. (Not until the war ended were men given the opportunity to work as reconstruction aides, or "re-aides.") To Granger's gratification, many responded; war service was, as one woman put it, an opportunity "to come into the labor and festival of life on equal terms with men."

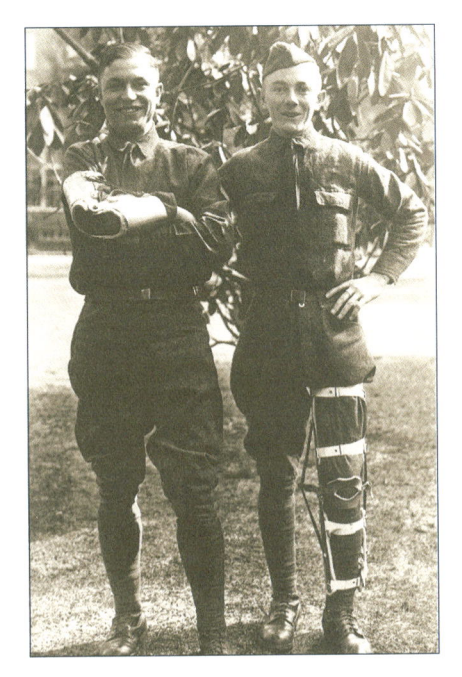

Applicants who could present a certificate showing that they had pursued a program of practical and theoretical work of not less than four months in any two of the basic modalities of reconstruction — hydrotherapy, electrotherapy, mechanotherapy, and massage — would be accepted first. Graduates of schools of physical education, skilled nurses, and persons who had been individually trained to assist in aftercare in the offices of a recognized orthopedist were also given serious consideration on the reasonable premise that they already had some knowledge of anatomy and exercise techniques. But as there was still much additional knowledge required to make most of them competent in the full range of physical therapy modalities, persons falling within this description were expected to go back to school for additional training.

Seven civilian "War Emergency Training Centers" initially won contracts to provide this service. They included three institutes in Boston — the American School of Physical Education, the Boston School of Physical Education, and Prose Normal School of Gymnastics; the New Haven Normal School of Gymnastics, in Connecticut; Teachers College, Columbia University, in New York; and Kellogg's Normal School of Physical Education, in Michigan. The only institution designated to provide emergency training on the west coast was Oregon's Reed College, in Portland. (A somewhat different set of experiential

*Proudly wearing their braces, two recovering cavalry soldiers pose for one of many snapshots that document the scores of cases physical therapists treated in World War I. At the start of the war, the Surgeon General's Office predicted that 5 to 7 men of every 100 sent overseas would return in need of physical therapy treatment.*

*A soldier undergoes diathermy at Fort Sam Houston Station Hospital. The static charge is generated by a static machine (kept at a distance) and delivered to the affected hand and forearm via the ball electrode in his hand, producing vigorous muscle contractions.*

prerequisites and training schools were listed in the prospectus for occupational therapy reconstruction aides.)

To be considered for the training program and ultimately for work in physical therapy or occupational therapy, candidates had to be citizens of the United States or in the process of becoming naturalized. They also had to pass physical fitness standards, which included standing between 60" and 70" tall and weighing between 100 and 195 pounds, with no "marked disproportion" between the two. Cheerful demeanor, coupled with "powers of personal subordination, able to cooperate generally and capable of demonstrating team play," were also deemed essential. Because the army was particularly sensitive to the potential strains of bringing men and women together in the highly charged atmosphere of wartime hospitals, candidates also were expected to be able "to associate with young men on a friendly footing without encouraging undue familiarity." To assure that this ladylike quality was observed at all times, candidates were chaperoned closely during training.

The reconstruction aides' military status was an invention of the time and one that would cause much grief in years to come. Technically civil service employees, they were accorded none of the privileges or benefits authorized for military personnel — particularly no war-risk insurance or retirement pay for service-connected illness or disability. They were nonetheless subject to the orders and disciplines of the military command structure as to where and when they would serve. And as for the rehabilitation therapies they provided each patient, reconstruction aides theoretically had to take their instructions from the orthopedists and general surgeons. (For that matter, so did the physicians in Granger's new specialty of "electro-therapeutics," who were still considered to be the mechanics of the medical field, but as there were relatively few of them in army service, conflicts rarely surfaced.)

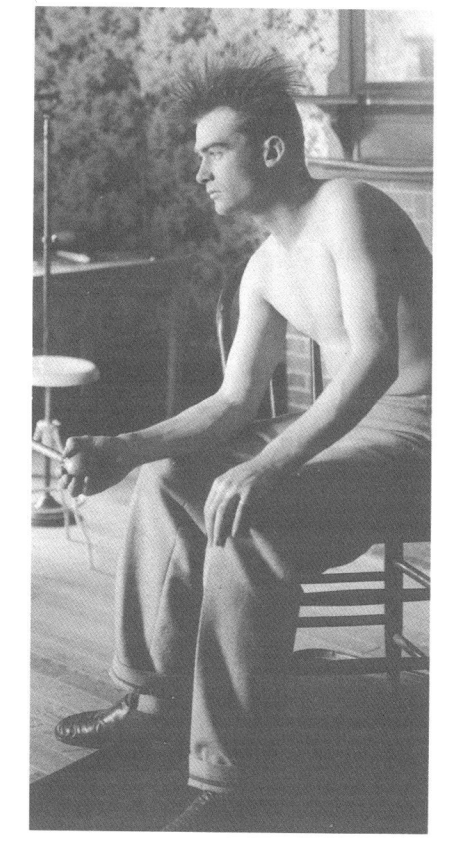

Diagnosing doctors filled out prescription forms on which were printed seven special types of functional treatment (abduction, adduction, flexion, extension, pronation, supination, and circumduction) together with the parts of the body to which treatment was to be applied. It should be noted that even among the more progressive ranks of medical men in these years and for decades to come, the physical therapeutics prescribed were based primarily on empirical knowledge and confined to well-recognized and limited techniques. In this, the Army Medical Corps' exercise regimens were typical. Devised primarily from an anatomical understanding of injuries, they consisted of formal regimens for the ankle, the shoulder, and so on. No matter what was wrong with the part, the patient was put through the same fixed list of movements, one or two of which might actually help. In the same way, the duration of specific procedures such as a diathermy treatment or a light bath seems to have had more to do with a particular clinic's work schedule than evidence of efficacy, and the selection of a particular machine was based more on anecdotal reports of satisfaction than on scientific measurements of its curative effects.

In theory, the reconstruction aides "filled" the prescriptions as specified. In actual practice, physicians were so shorthanded that many cases came down without instructions, leaving the young women to manage as best they saw fit, which tended to be more appropriate treatment than what the medical men would have directed had they found the time. The therapists' only external guidance in those circumstances was a "head aide," promoted from their number on the basis of demonstrated leadership qualities and, one presumes, a good dose of common sense. Each head aide was responsible for 10 reconstruction aides.

In taking the oath of office, a preliminary requisite of joining, every reconstruction aide was committed to serve however long the Surgeon General might need her services, just as members of the military were. "Re-aides," however, were expected to remain on duty well beyond the duration of the war. Remuneration was initially set at $50 per month base pay plus room and board, with travel expenses of $4 per diem. Persons on active duty received an additional $10 per month. Head aides earned a $10 supplement. In each instance, their pay and benefits were substantially lower than those of civilian dietitians and nurses working for the army, a point of no small matter to the therapists.

Duty uniforms were provided free of charge by the Red Cross, which picked up the tab when the army declined. The basic costume, shared by physical therapy and occupational therapy branches alike, was a calf-length, belted blue chambray dress, and each therapist was given three. With the dress came three blue-and-white organdy caps, a dozen buckram-stiffened stand-up collars and cuffs, two pairs of cuff links, four suits of woolen underwear, three pairs of flannel pajamas, two pairs of woolen tights, a gray sweater, six pairs of merino wool stockings and six pairs of cotton stockings, a pair of gloves, three pairs of sturdy shoes, and for those countless cold, rainy days and nights in the field they were given rubber boots, a raincoat, and a waterproof sou'wester for the head. Collar insignia pins (with the bronze letters "U.S." and the gilt letters "R.A." imposed on a caduceus), a steamer blanket, a sleeping bag, and a "hold-all" for small personal items completed the physical therapy aide's kit.

Occupational therapists had, in addition to the collar pin "O.T.," several white "butcher's" aprons. Street uniforms,

*In World War I, physical therapy reconstruction aides wore bronze caducei that bore the letters "R.A." on the lapels of their one-piece blue hospital duty uniforms, on their hospital dresses, and on the Norfolk jackets or capes of their street uniforms. The insignia from 1947, below, retained the caduceus but incorporated the letters "P.T.," as the official designation of their wearers changed from reconstruction aide to physical therapist by World War II.*

*Mia Donner, a former physical education teacher, was one of a handful of reconstruction aides trained and ready to go overseas. With her new War Department passport, Donner joined the first hand-picked contingent of women who shipped out in early summer 1918.*

which were to be worn in public whenever the reconstruction aide was not working in the wards, were the individual's purchasing responsibility. They included a bulky blue serge Norfolk suit, two wide-brimmed hats — one of black velour and the other of summer straw — to be worn with a maroon cockade, three cotton shirt-waists plus one of silk, a voluminous overcoat or "ulster," and a cape with no fewer than 136 buttons on its front, pockets, sleeves, and side vents. In theory, the cape was optional, but few chose to go without. Dark gray and lined with maroon silk, it gave an otherwise dour costume a touch of dash, particularly during fast-stepping parades when the cape was likely to "fly." The total out-of-purse cost to the applicant was roughly $100, or two months' salary.

Granger also laid down the basic outlines for standardizing facilities and treatments. A booklet described the seven types of cases reconstruction aides most frequently would treat by massage and medical gymnastics:

"1. Wounds — (a) Preventing the scar from interfering with function of limb; (b) preventing vicious healings when nerve gets caught in scar; (c) avoiding the stiffness of the joint of the wounded limb; (d) keeping up muscular tone of region.
2. Simple and compound fractures.
3. Ankylosis.
4. Paralysis.
5. Certain excisions (bone).
6. Motor or nervous disorders (wounds of head and spinal cord).
7. Stumps from amputation — (a) Besides the treatment of the stump by various kinds of Physiotherapy (local baths, massage, etc.) progressive physical re-education is necessary to re-establish the function of the stump and help its adaptation to its new motor activity."

## "WITH A TINGE OF RECKLESSNESS": THE FIRST RECONSTRUCTION AIDES

To supervise the reconstruction aides who, it was hoped, would soon be volunteering, Granger appointed Marguerite Sanderson, a therapist in Goldthwait's office and a 1903 graduate of the Boston Normal School of Gymnastics. At the time of her appointment, Sanderson was the 38-year-old president and instructor of corrective exercises at the Boston School of Physical Education. (One of the designated "War Emergency Training Centers," the BSPE was the brainchild of Sanderson and her schoolmates Marjorie Bouvé and Mary Florence Stratton, who had opened it with Goldthwait's financial backing in 1914.)

Sanderson was, by all accounts, a woman of great presence. Variously described as "ahead of her times," "a great organizer and disciplinarian," "a fighter," she was also characterized as having "unsurpassed personal integrity and insight." Her remarkable gift for bringing out the best in others was nicely balanced with a zesty sense of humor. As it would soon become apparent, she would need all these skills and more.

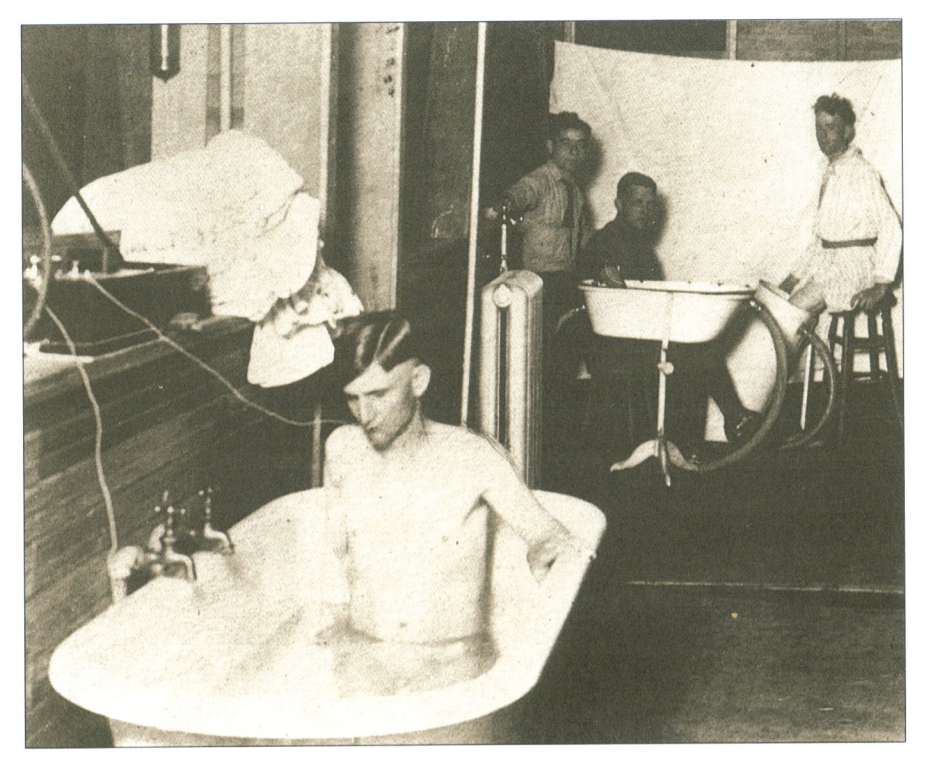

"Sandy" Sanderson reported for duty in the Surgeon General's Office in Washington, D.C., in December 1917, more or less coincident with the SGO's call for volunteers. A month after her arrival, the very first applicant appeared at her door. True to character, it was Mary McMillan.

At Sir Robert Jones's recommendation, Brackett, one of the chief organizers of the army's reconstruction program, had personally written to ask McMillan if she would consider service with the United States Army. This appeal was followed by a telegram from Surgeon General Gorgas: "Two pioneer aides needed Walter Reed Hospital immediately. Start work, do some teaching — am anxious to get best person. Wire yes or no immediately." Without hesitation, McMillan said good-bye to her colleagues at the Portland Children's Hospital and headed for Washington to be sworn in late in February 1918 as the first "buck private" in the new service.

Despite all of Granger's efforts to elevate the status of physical reconstruction among members of the medical profession, McMillan's reception at Walter Reed General Hospital was less than welcoming. As McMillan later recalled, "The United States Army Medical Corps knew nothing about physical therapy, and I knew nothing about the United States Army Medical Corps." By the time Mary arrived, several months had passed since Gorgas's administrative orders had been issued; however, nothing at all had been done to create the promised facilities. Aside from a couple of rarely used hydrotherapy tanks and some electrical apparatuses in the basement of the administration building, Walter Reed General Hospital still had no provisions for delivering to patients even the most rudimentary physical therapeutics.

After a few days of making personal calls on department heads, "selling" the concept of physical ther-

*Immediately after the war, veterans still in need of rehabilitation were dispersed to the few remaining military hospitals where physical therapy continued to be offered. This 1919 photograph was taken in the hydrotherapy room at what was then known as Fort Sam Houston Station Hospital, later Brooke General Hospital, San Antonio, Texas.*

Mary McMillan And Wartime "Reconstruction" 1914 - 1919    51

*Marguerite Sanderson, a 1903 graduate of Wellesley College's physical education department, was an early specialist in corrective exercises. After several years of working with orthopedic patients at Joel Goldthwait's medical gymnasium in Boston, Sanderson was appointed by the U.S. Army Surgeon General to plan and organize the World War I reconstruction aide program.*

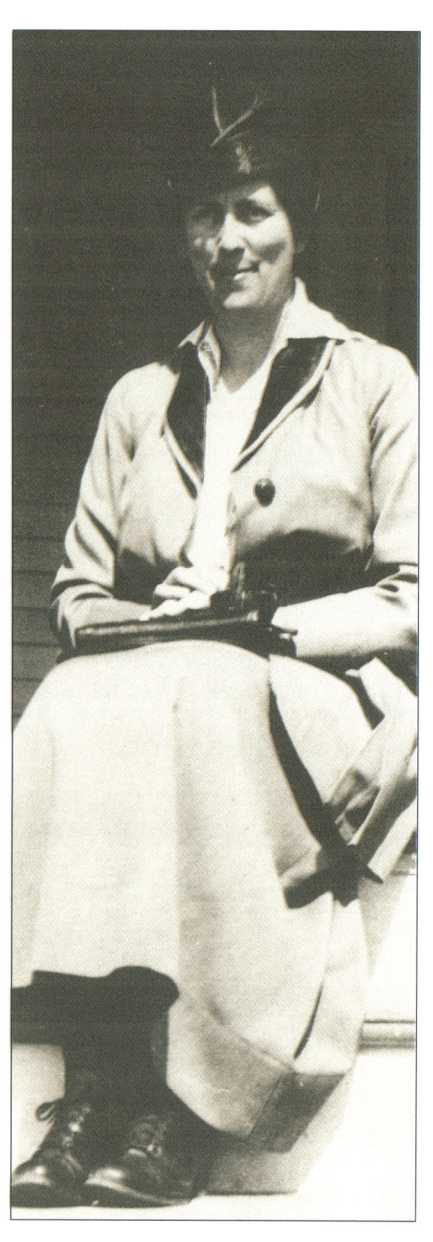

apy and her own competence, McMillan was grudgingly allowed a sun porch and a linen closet in one of the wards in Building #56. To give the business a little more professional polish, she had some prescription forms printed at her own expense. Most of the physicians she met were reluctant to entrust to her any but their most hopeless patients, presuming that she could do no further damage. (Perhaps it was for this reason that her first patient was an individual with a double amputation.) But within a week, McMillan's ingratiating manner, warmth, and enthusiasm began to soften opinion. And when word of positive, even miraculous, improvements began circulating through the hospital, the medical community was forced to look again. Perhaps there was more to McMillan's therapeutic massage than met the eye.

Meanwhile, additional young women recruits began appearing at WRGH. As former reconstruction aide Mary J. Wrinn would write after the war, "The same impulse that had sent the soldier to face death, now sent [these volunteers in reconstruction] to help him live again." Although the women came from every corner of the country and from every imaginable background, "Like purpose, likenesses of temperament, made them kin." Common to all was "an imagination that could visualize some effectiveness of a service hitherto untried; an adventurous turn that made for willingness to go wherever needed; a tinge of recklessness perhaps that would brave the unprotected risk of service overseas." They were also unusually well-educated by the standards of the day.

First to arrive was Inge Lohne, a 31-year-old Norwegian immigrant. Lohne's claim to practical experience was, like Sanderson's and McMillan's, substantial. Lohne had studied physical training in her homeland, after which she had come to America to attend New York's School of Medical Gymnastics and Teachers College, Columbia University. She had also managed massage clinics at Bellevue, Presbyterian, and New York Hospitals. Lohne was followed quickly by Helen Sheddon, Margery Rickok, Josephine Bell, and Louisa Lippitt, all of them having had some prior training that qualified them to begin providing physical therapy immediately. (Bell and McMillan would be thrown together again in 1942, when they met at Sternberg

Hospital in Manila, the Philippines, and were taken prisoners of war.)

Fortunately for the newcomers to Walter Reed General Hospital, McMillan had managed by this time to commandeer an additional room or two for the work. But as the case load continued to grow, this space also proved insufficient, and the army speeded up plans to construct Building #76, located to the rear of the Red Cross Building and connected to the hospital wards by a long corridor. Walter Reed's new facility, which would not be fully ready until the spring of 1919, featured a swimming pool, a well-appointed gymnasium, and spacious treatment rooms containing no fewer than 30 exercise and massage plinths, or tables, plus a substantial collection of heat and electrotherapeutic devices.

### BACK TO SCHOOL

If McMillan thought she would be around long enough to preside over the army's new therapy center, she was soon disabused of the notion. Based on Granger's formula that there should be two physical therapy aides and two occupational therapy aides for every 50 hospital beds, and on the War Department's projections of future casualties, the Surgeon General's Office stepped up its reconstruction aide recruitment efforts in the Spring of 1918. It called for 1,000 trained aides by September 1918, with perhaps 200 going overseas to treat acute cases and the remainder being dispersed to stateside base hospitals to handle extended aftercare. This meant that the War Emergency Training Centers had to move into high gear, turning out many more trained reconstruction aides than had initially been envisioned.

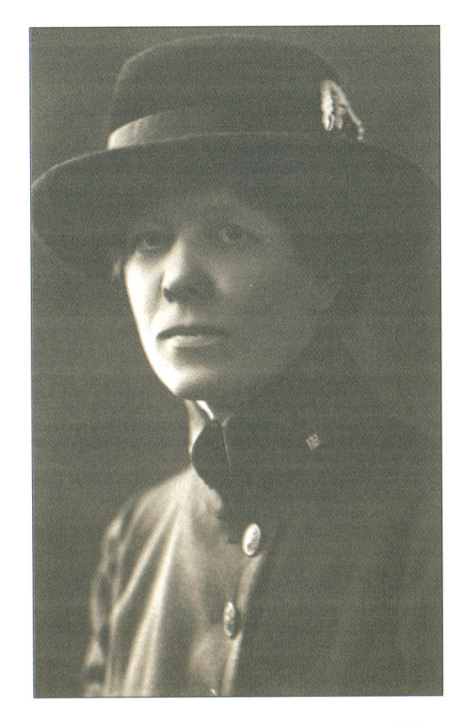

Reed College's president, William Foster, told the Surgeon General that he had more than 200 young women ready to train immediately if only he had the faculty to teach them. Foster made a special plea to borrow Mollie McMillan, whose talents he had come to know when he toured British army hospitals as a field inspector for the Red Cross. He wanted her to run the practical "hands-on" portion of his program, including the extensive course on massage. With Gorgas's reluctant approval, McMillan went to Oregon in June 1918, expecting to return in September. As it turned out, she stayed longer; the task before her was more rewarding than anything she had dared to imagine. Her students, representing 72 colleges and universities and 31 states, were of exceptionally high caliber and esprit, more than equal to the task before them.

Foster was also enormously pleased, and he wrote her a letter, imploring her to stay on for a second session: "Everybody . . . trusts your leadership. We are disposed to adopt every feasible suggestion you may make. . . . We believe that . . . there is

*Inga Lohne, who would go on to be McMillan's successor as Association president, posed in her brand new reconstruction aide uniform. Posted overseas, she was placed in charge of 13 reconstruction aides at the Third Army's evacuation hospital, Coblenz, Germany, where several hundred surgical and orthopedic patients were being readied for their return stateside.*

*McMillan, center foreground, relaxes with uniformed students and several fellow-instructors on Portland, Oregon's Reed College campus. Graduates from Reed College's physical therapy training program, called "Reedites," were greatly respected and valued in the budding physical therapy profession. Reed College, like Mollie herself, was the model for other physical therapy education programs.*

no other woman in the entire west with your professional preparation, your position of leadership is unique. . . . Knowing your attitude toward your work, I have held out to you as an inducement nothing but the opportunity for service. . . . My hope is that you will see the work with us for the present as your largest field for doing good." McMillan was apparently persuaded, for she remained on the Reed faculty until the end of the year, training another 60 or so "Reedites" before going down to the University of California at Berkeley to consult briefly with the director of the Department of Physical Education there about setting up another satellite War Emergency Training Course.

The Reed College physical therapy curriculum became the standard by which all other "emergency" programs were measured. It consisted of 457 hours of classroom work, including 112 in massage, 99 in anatomy using cadavers borrowed from the local medical school, 66 in remedial exercise, 32 in physiology, 10 in hydrotherapy and electrotherapy combined, 23 in the theory and practice of bandaging, 6 in kinesiology, and 2 in ethics. Ten hours were devoted to the psychological effects of injury and recovery, with students being taught "cheerfulness against adversity and mental training to assist the badly wounded to 'forget' lost functions and cultivate new ones." Trainees also received 163 hours of practical experience in the treatment of patients at a local "reconstruction clinic" at the Portland Hospital, also under McMillan's supervision. French language courses were provided as an optional elective.

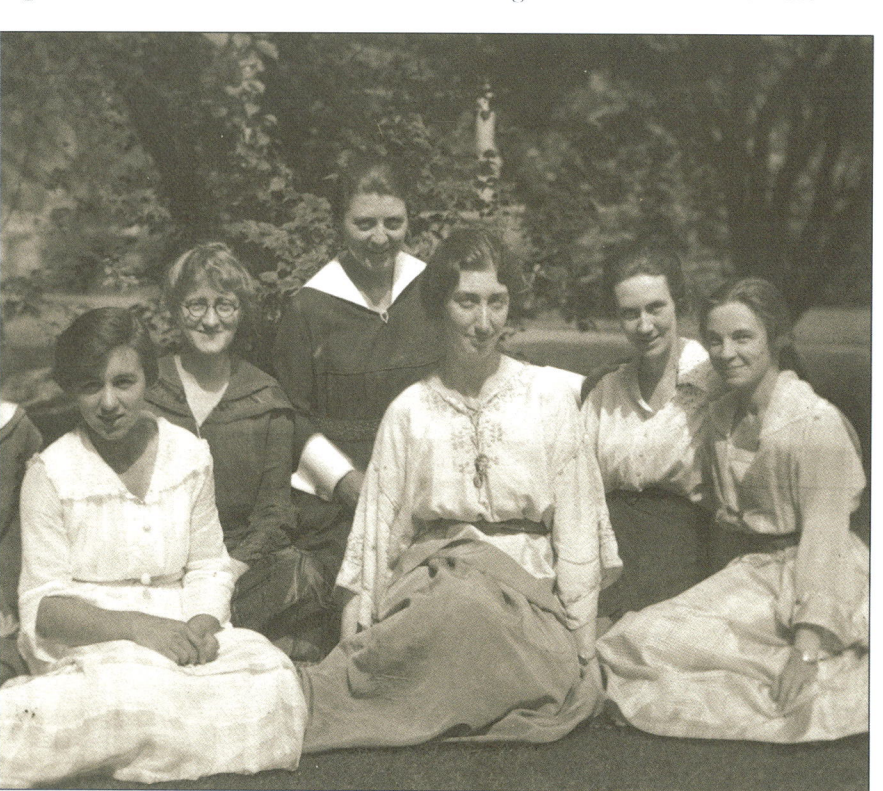

During the three-month program, the Reed "girls" were put through their paces. Future APTA President Marguerite Irvine, who was in McMillan's first class of students, recalls that the summer was so hot that the students took sleeping bags out onto the lawn to get a good night's rest. Before morning classes, the women had to join in an hour of calisthenics, do 10 pull-ups on the chinning bar, run

*Healing The Generations*

around the track, and swim the lake. But for Irvine and the rest there was little complaining. Camaraderie ruled the day. "We all loved Miss McMillan very much. She was a warm person, easy to approach.... Always ready and willing to listen to you and your troubles and always able to enter into our fun times without losing her dignity as our 'Head Instructress.' A lovable and loving person." If there was anything for McMillan's adoring students to find fault with, it was her British way of speaking and her choice of medical terms, which sometimes left students scrambling for an interpreter.

### OVER THERE

In May 1918, well before any "Reedites" had completed their training, the first 24-woman unit of reconstruction aides to be sent overseas gathered at one of the Nurses' Mobilization Stations at the Holley Hotel on New York's Washington Square. There they received passports, immunization shots, and last-minute lessons in army regulations and military drill at a nearby armory. (They were told that drilling prepared them to respond quickly should they need to evacuate their hospital during a bombing raid.) Louisa Lippitt, ever so briefly stationed at WRGH, was promoted to head aide of Unit #1. More experienced than anyone else in the group, she had recently left a job as director of the Corrective Department for Girls at the University of Wisconsin. The others were Juliet Bell, Matilda Beniman, Bertha Bowles, Florence Burrell, Minerva Crowell, Dorothea Davis, Ruth Earl, Jane Feinman, Rena Fiske, Sarah Fletcher, Ethel Gray, Myrna Howe, Elizabeth Huntington, Anne Larned, Blanche Marvin, Harriet McDonald, Juanita Metherall, Magna Nashe, Mabel Penfield, Frances Philo, Eunice Taylor, Anna Voris, and Dorothy Wellington. All were posted to Base Hospital #114, which was a special orthopedic center set up at Beau Desert, near Bordeaux.

On June 6, Marguerite Sanderson came to see her "girls" off. One of the assembled warmly recalled the occasion. "We were certainly ripe for a visit of inspiration, for we had been putting in some hard time... an endless hodgepodge of rules, cautions, rumor, prophecies, call-downs, regulations, and contradictions." The writer continued, "With the first word that Miss Sanderson spoke... the clouds and cobwebs blew away, and the wholesome sun of clear purpose came out.... She [reminded us] of our good fortune in being the first to set sail in the high adventure [and] of what our work in the war should mean to post-war physiotherapy. And then she came down to the brass tacks — the conditions we should have to face and the situations we should have to meet."

Sanderson concluded her pep talk with some homely advice on getting enough sleep, dressing warmly, and wearing the "influenza masks" issued each therapist and soldier for their protection while packed in the close quarters of shipboard. This last seemed like particularly good advice. The second and more virulent strain

*With this pocket-sized brochure, Reed College announced a novel three-month-long intensive program to prepare women for war service. Reed had to its great credit the services of Mollie McMillan. Asked to define "reconstruction," this great teacher said simply, "It is a new word for a new work."*

of the great influenza pandemic was abroad that summer and would, by the following spring, fell some 734,000 soldiers and staff of the United States military, adding immeasurably to the case load of the overseas hospitals. Lest any reconstruction aide still retain some romantic notion of what lay ahead, the director of the Nurses' Mobilization Station, Miss Lang, gave some practical tips. "You are Pioneers," she told them. "Very few people 'Over There' know what you're for. Still fewer want you around. Don't get in the nurses' and doctors' way. Make yourselves scarce . . . until you have made such a place for yourselves . . . that no ward will be complete without you."

Lang's predictions turned out to be unpleasantly apt. No sooner had Anna Voris and several others arrived in France than they were separated from the rest of the unit and deployed to Base Hospital #6, Bordeaux. Arriving "weary and bedraggled" after a long train ride, they were greeted contemptuously by the officer in charge: "Reconstruction aides! What do you expect to do? I didn't ask for you, we don't need you, I don't know where to put you." Ignoring his words, the doughty group found makeshift accommodations for the night and, after a fitful sleep, set about making themselves useful in the care of several score of influenza patients who had come off the ship with them.

If any of the young women in the early units had second thoughts about the work ahead, the various diaries and letters that have survived this period give little indication. Indeed, the more arduous or frightening circumstances became, the greater the adventure seemed. Lena Hitchcock, a therapist attached to the 27-woman Unit #2, described her group's last days in New York as they awaited orders to sail. Day after steamy hot July day, they marched up and down the armory to the cadence of their marching songs, "suffocating under our felt hats, our madras waists wrinkled and clinging, our new boots heavy and uncomfortable." Their drill major despaired of getting his charges to conform to army regulations. "Some of us are a terrible trial because of the shape, size and parts of the female figure. The major explains the 'At Attention' position. 'Feet at an angle of forty degrees, head up, chin in, stomach in, eyes front, thumbs at the seams of trousers — e-rr-pants-no-no-drawers-no-I-er mean skirts,' he stutters."

Esprit, which was high to begin with, soared when the reconstruction aides were invited to participate in New York's 1918 Fourth of July parade. Hitchcock recorded, "We swing into line behind the Army Nurses. Here we go 'Company Front' two files, thirteen abreast, with our head aide Susan Hills marching alone in the center six paces ahead. When we turn into Fifth Avenue a band strikes up 'Onward Christian Soldiers.' Flags of the Allies flutter from every window. My heart stirs, thrills—we are off to the Crusades."

When Hitchcock's unit finally got its sailing orders, it was divided into six squads; each squad was given a different route by which to walk and ride "inconspicuously" to the Cunard Pier and the transport ship. Multiple movements, they were told, would help them elude the German spies thought to be lurking around the city. Hitchcock went on to report, "On the pier itself, although crowded with

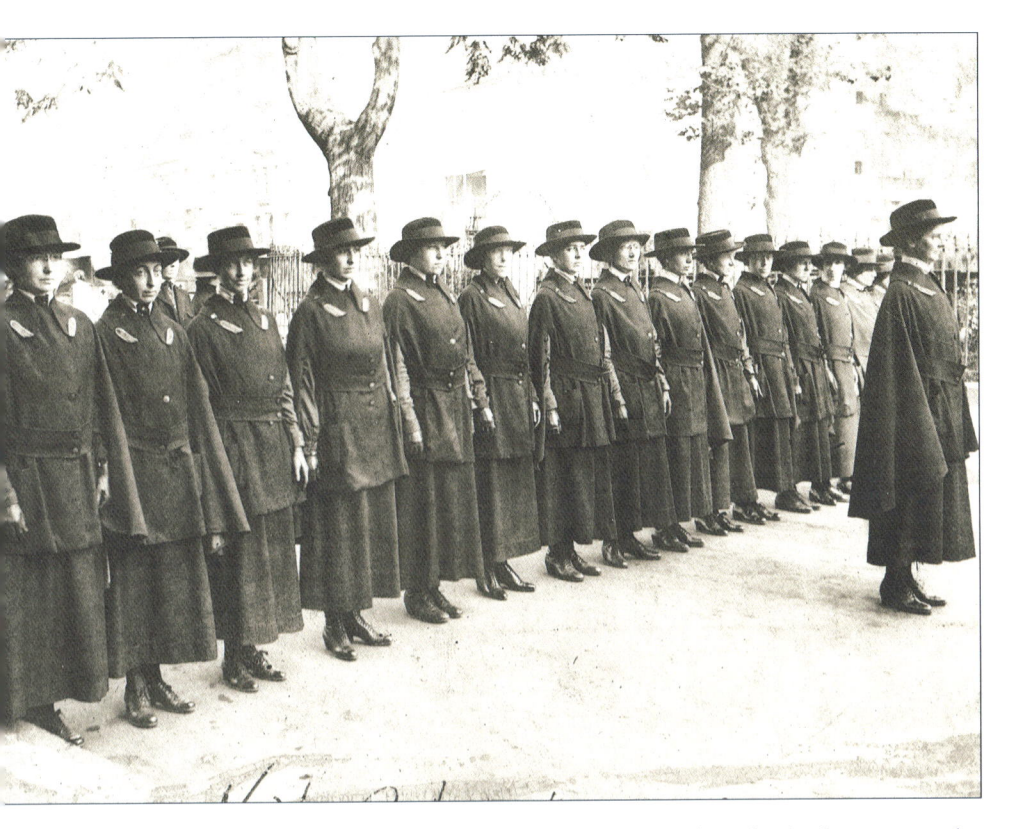

*Reconstruction aides, awaiting transport overseas to U.S. Army hospitals, typically spent two weeks in the New York staging area learning military drills. Here, on July 4, 1918, a group in wool suits and capes, no less, prepares to swing onto Fifth Avenue as a band strikes up the chords of "Onward Christian Soldiers."*

people, the silence is unnatural. Here are no sad or gay farewells, no joyous bustle; only the shiff-shiff-shiff of marching feet. . . . We finally reach our gangway. An officer stops us. We write the name of our nearest relative and whom to inform in case of death upon a card."

As Hitchcock's ship pulled out into the open channel, they learned they were part of a huge convoy of 27 camouflaged ships. Portholes were sealed and blackened, life jackets distributed, submarine look-outs posted, and "drowning drills" rehearsed. Once across the Atlantic, the reconstruction aides transferred from their larger ship to a smaller, less conspicuous channel boat and crossed to France under a moonless sky. No one was allowed below decks in case the ship should be sunk; cigarettes were extinguished, whispering forbidden.

Hitchcock's group finally reached its destination, Base Hospital #9, Chateauroux, only to find a reception no better than the one that greeted Voris and her colleagues. The commanding officer told the exhausted group that he wasn't "running a boarding house, but if we are useful, we may stay until they can arrange our transportation home." The head nurse then showed them to "unfinished barracks with a dirt floor and no glass in the windows."

Maude Cook, part of Unit #3 that shipped out in September, recalled arriving at Base Hospital #105, Camp Kerhuon, Brest, France, in a drenching downpour, their transport an open army truck so crowded that everyone had to ride standing. Before the ship-weary reconstruction aides had a chance to stow their belongings, they were called to help the nurses get ready for the imminent arrival of a thousand patients. Many were fresh influenza cases right off the transport ships; others were the first contingent of a long line of casualties from Pershing's late-September Meuse-Argonne offensive in the north. Cook spent her first days improvising. "We heated water for bathing the wounded over salmon cans with alcohol-soaked

57

cotton for fuel. We turned and re-turned soiled pillow slips, washed towels and carried drinks for long days — dressed always in our rubber boots and rain clothes. We carried our canteens to bed with us to have warm water for bath and laundry the next morning. Our spirits rose in proportion to our hardships, and we were a happy unit."

Another reconstruction aide described being pressed into service with "hardly the status of scrub women." For several weeks, she and her sister aides mopped floors, sterilized instruments, made plaster bandages, washed rubber gloves, and kept four dressing carts in order; all the time, the military staff let it be known that their official line of work was "unnecessary, even frivolous." She was posted to a "double-decker building with about 70 ambulatory cases billeted in two long rooms upstairs . . . 90 men occupy the beds downstairs. . . . The men are trussed up in fracture frames with sandbags, ropes and pulleys keeping their poor legs in the desired position. They are in great pain most of the time, but so patient and gay. Many have complicated systems of Dakin tubes and bottles irrigating the hideous gaping wounds." Another described her status in a poem:

*Versatility, Thy name is Physio!*
*What detail did they put you on?*
*Nurses aide*
*Butter-spreading*
*Card-filing*
*Night duty*
*Hash detail*
*O.T.*
*Surgical Dressing*
*Lemon-squeezing*
*Premiere danseuse*
*Typewriting*
*General Goat.*

As was all too apparent, no preparations had been made to house or employ the arriving reconstruction aides; in truth, the nurses who had arrived several months earlier had not fared much better. Many of them found that the physical therapy equipment promised had not arrived, having been bumped in transit in favor of more urgently needed combat supplies. And the simple matter of their own personal hygiene was often totally confounding: although the hospitals had water and laundry facilities to maintain adequate standards of cleanliness among their patients and doctors, there had been few if any provisions made for the reconstruction aides. A bedside bucket of cold water was often their only washing facility. Laundry was left to drip between the bunks.

By the Armistice in November 1918, however, working conditions in the American Expeditionary Force (AEF) hospitals had improved substantially and so had the status of the overseas reconstruction aides. Physicians and surgeons begged for additional people, and thanks to the successful efforts of the War Emergency Training Centers, the Army Medical Corps was able to distribute some 200 aides among 20 overseas base hospitals. As far as their patients were concerned, there could not be too many. The AEF reconstruction aides were a bright spot in otherwise dreary surroundings. Easily recognized by their blue uniforms and the "U.S." and "R.A." insignias on their collars, they earned such affectionate nicknames as "Blue Bird," "Poor Thing," "Pretty Tough," "Rubbing Angel," and "Real American."

Their housing in Europe, however, never improved. Marguerite Sanderson, who arrived in September 1918 to supervise the growing number of overseas therapists, reported living in barracks in which floors were continuously under water, with only enough heat in the fireplace "to warm the andirons," and where one had to wear gloves while writing letters to make frozen fingers work at all. Isabel Noble, describing housing at Base Hospital #114, Bordeaux, recalled barracks "of pestiferous memory" in which an unmeditated slam of a door was apt to bring "a semi-frozen mouse . . . on to one's head; where the temperature, day in and day out, was somewhere in the genial neighborhood of 0 above; where the prudent composed themselves for slumber with umbrellas spread over their heads to catch the chilly drip-drip-drip from the roof; and where the stoves were only moved in as the occupants were moved out."

Ironically, the November Armistice created new difficulties for the reconstruction aides. As fresh battlefield casualties ceased, the majority of the hospitals' medical officers packed up to return to the United States, but civilian staff could not leave until the wounded were evacuated. The PTs, who were left to carry on, could not help but feel abandoned by their superiors in the Medical Corps. Sanderson wrote Lohne, "The care of the poor old P.T.s here doesn't seem to concern anyone. . . . [But] I am proud to say that there is but one R.A. who wants to go home, and I think all of us whose work it has always been to care for the chronic cases, realize our great opportunity is here and now, and not something we can consider finished as the surgeons (not all) do." In closing, Sanderson added gamely, "It's been a real battle from start to finish to establish our standards, but it's been fun to do it together." (The one reconstruction aide who did ask to be sent home was Harriet MacDonald, part of Unit #1. Injured during an air raid on her hospital, she had postponed necessary surgery on her leg to remain at her post as long as needed. She subsequently underwent three operations back in the United States, but too late. She spent the rest of her life on crutches or in a wheelchair and was finally awarded modest "compensation" by an act of Congress in 1931.)

Representative of the postwar work done at all the AEF hospitals is the example of Base Hospital #8, a 20,000-bed hospital complex located in the little village of Savenay, near Nantes. Here 30 PTs put in 14-hour days, six and seven days a week, as wave after wave of orthopedic cases were brought in from distant hospital field stations to be stabilized before being sent home. In November 1918, Savenay reconstruction aides clocked

*The camaraderie inspired by hard work and a sense of purpose was something every reconstruction aide cherished. This scrap of an invitation — to attend a pancake party — came to Mollie McMillan during her months as a physical therapy instructor at Reed College, Oregon*

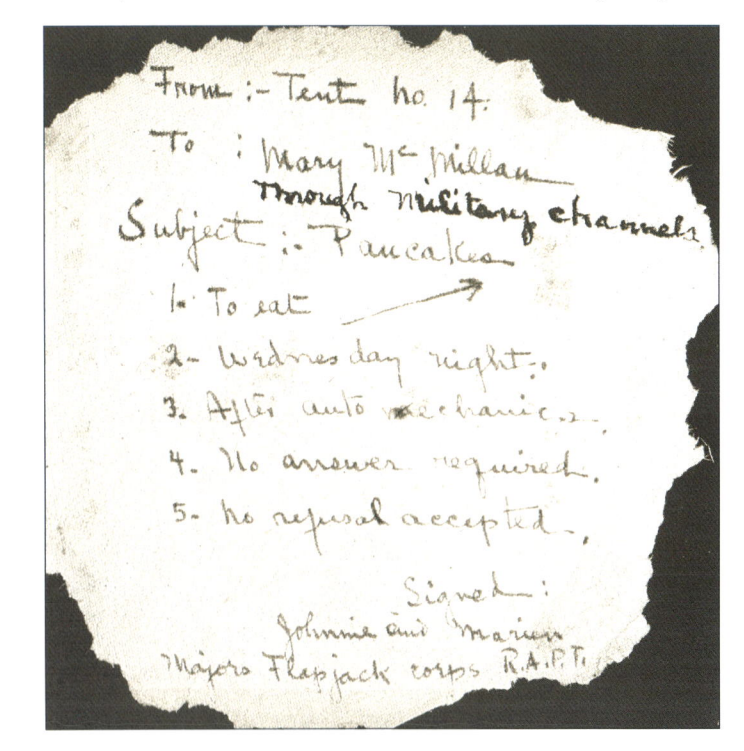

*Their classroom training over, a large group of graduate reconstruction aides stand together for a group shot. Soon to be deployed overseas or sent to one of the nearly 60 U.S. treatment centers operating during the height of the war emergency, they muster as a unit one last time.*

3,440 treatments; in December, 5,251 treatments. The heavy work load continued to grow as 1919 began. In January PTs delivered care to 6,568 patients; in February, 6,528; in March, 4,333; and in April, 4,218.

Much of the work carried on in the overseas hospitals was "massage of fractures," according to PT and head aide Susan Hills, who, like Sanderson, had worked with Goldthwait before the war. Writing in the summary account of the Medical Department's work in World War I, Hills said that army orthopedists had come to see that in the case of remobilizing many kinds of fractures "an ounce of prevention is worth a pound of cure." Prior to the war and the widespread acceptance of Mennell's and Lucas-Championnière's "early movement" principles, the general practice had been to splint and otherwise immobilize an injured limb so long as inflammation was present. Contracture deformities, requiring additional follow-up surgery, were a common result. "It has been found, however," Hills continued, "that careful manipulation around a draining wound instead of checking actually hastens the recovery." She added, "Of secondary importance to final results, but of primary importance to the patients, is the comfort and relief that follows a little massage given to men who have laid, strapped and tied, for months in most uncomfortable positions."

When the Third Army, United States Army of Occupation, established its headquarters in Germany in January 1919, the remaining surgical and orthopedic patients were moved to two evacuation hospitals at Trier and Coblenz, to which 13 physical therapists were assigned. After seeing to a relatively smooth transition of services, Marguerite Sanderson sent a final note to Inga Lohne. "I don't think anyone could have had a finer, pluckier, more loyal lot of people do a job. . . . I really feel that I am the luckiest person in the A.E.F. to have known you all." Sanderson returned to the United States and to civilian life in July 1919. Granger, who retired at the rank of lieutenant colonel, left at about the same time, although he maintained his connection with "reconstruction" as medical counselor to the United States Veterans' Bureau.

Meanwhile, Mary McMillan returned to Washington, D.C., in January 1919 to work in the Surgeon General's Office. On March 15, 1919, she was promoted to chief head aide in the Department of Physiotherapy at Walter Reed General Hospital. Then, following Sanderson's retirement, McMillan took on the additional duty of supervisor of reconstruction aides, with another "Reedite," Emma "Emmy Lou" Vogel, succeeding her at Walter Reed. As the wounded continued to come home from the war, filling up wards in stateside army hospitals, McMillan oversaw the deployment of PTs wherever needed. Although her staff was shrinking, there was much still to be done.

## POST-WAR CARE

While the overseas physical therapy reconstruction aides had rendered important service behind the battle lines, it was only when the bulk of orthopedic cases were brought home and distributed to specialized hospital centers that the Physiotherapy Division of the Reconstruction Department came into its own. In the two years following the Armistice, stateside reconstruction aides gave some 86,000 disabled soldiers more than 3.5 million treatments.

Try as the SGO administrators did to make demobilization an orderly process, the reconstruction aides found themselves constantly having to pack up and move on a few hours notice from one army hospital facility to another as patient loads ebbed and flowed. Helen Bradley and Laura Plunkett were part of a group of nine "Reedites" who had expected to go overseas but were redeployed at the last moment to Fort Sam Houston, Texas, in January 1919. When they arrived, they discovered that the medical staff thought they were there to teach "the boys to make little baskets." Bradley later recalled, "The idea was so fixed in the doctors' minds that they were most disappointed and felt that these [physical therapy] girls should at least try to do the O.T.'s work." Undaunted, "the Holy Nine," as they came to be known, unpacked their few belongings and settled in. "Work was our keenest pleasure. To see the dear brave boys getting better under our care, the satisfaction of the growing department until there were 60 PTs with our 'Plunkie' Chief of them all.... New machines and new methods arrived daily." Slowly the medical staff came around. "The boys themselves helped most in this, for from the beginning, they were anxious for their treatments and loud in their praise of the benefits received. Gunshot wounds healed, stiff joints loosened, and paralyzed muscles functioned again."

Ruby Decker, a fresh young graduate of the Normal School in Battle Creek, Michigan, was also part of the Fort Sam Houston physiotherapy staff, but only after she had spent her first five months as a raw recruit at Camp Sherman, in Chillicothe, Ohio. Decker recalled how anxious she felt as she toured the Ohio site: "A parachutist on his first jump couldn't have been more scared. All I could see was ward after ward of patients with terrible wounds and deformities, all of the men lying on rubber sheets with irrigation bottles dangling over them." With scarcely any time for orientation, Decker was put to work. Her first assignment was to treat a patient with a diagnosis of "ankylosis of the wrist." The prescription called for hot arm

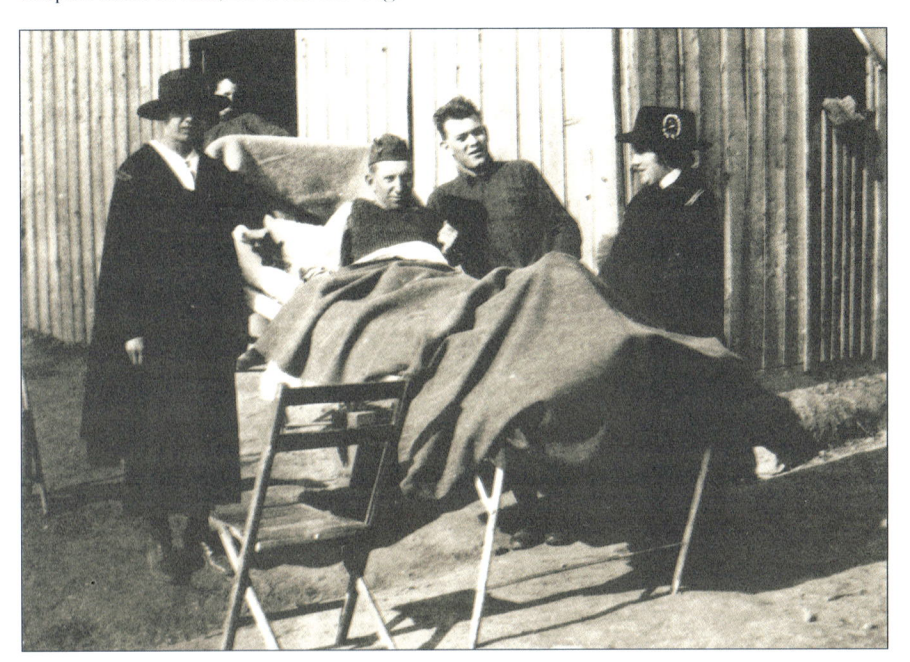

*At Base Hospital #8, Savenay, France, reconstruction aides join two of their recovering patients for a bit of sunshine shortly after the Armistice. Constance Greene, one of the first reconstruction aides to arrive in Savenay, would later describe the hospital as "miles of brown prefabricated buildings, surrounded by mud." The crowded wards in which she worked presented "forests of wood traction frames."*

baths, massage, and exercise, "which made sense since I could see that the man had a stiff wrist. But I couldn't figure out where his 'ankle' came into the act. I also didn't know what to make of the next line on the prescription which said 'Where Wounded: Verdun Front.' I had never heard about either the back or the front of 'the verdun' in my anatomy class!"

With the help of a good medical dictionary and some common sense, Decker survived her first day. The next day, she discovered that the only electrotherapy machine at Sherman with which she was familiar— a static electricity device — was already considered outmoded; she scrambled to read all the documentation on the newfangled machines. In-service training sessions, a regular feature of the reconstruction aides' routine at stateside hospitals, also contributed to her growing skills. Decker recalled a ditty she and her "sisters" sang on the way to lectures: "In this amphitheater drear/ We turn hot and cold with fear/ Nurse bring in that swollen knee,/ Now, young women, what do you see?/ Synovitis, by gosh!"

The work loads for all reconstruction aides were often very heavy. Grace Green kept score during her Fort Sam Houston stint. "Some days I gave over 50 [massage] treatments, besides six or seven electrics (kept one ward man and two nurses busy preparing the patients for me), until my hands were so sore I could not close them."

### THE WORK TO BE DONE

The men receiving extended care in United States hospitals had a broad range of diseases and disabilities, including shell shock, tuberculosis, and trenchfoot, but it was amputations and gunshot fractures with underlying pathologies of osteomyelitis, contracted soft tissues, and paralyzed muscles that were the chief concern of the orthopedic service and the physical therapy reconstruction aides. Neurosurgical cases involving peripheral nerve lesions, while less numerous, were also treated with often surprisingly favorable outcomes. As had been true overseas, the specific treatment plan was technically left to the ward surgeon, whose familiarity with the new modalities was understandably limited.

For guidance, however, he had a set of directives worked out by division heads Brackett and Granger. And as a second fail-safe he had the reconstruction aides, who knew their patients best and were not afraid to speak up when they thought a case was being mismanaged.

As a class, the amputations were given the least physiotherapeutic treatment on the theory that a substantial part of the involved structures had been removed in the process of amputation. Here, the prescribed treatment consisted primarily of applying radiant heat and light to the amputation site, massaging it to mobilize adherent scars and to prevent edema, and exercising neighboring joints to prevent contractures. Once the patient had been fitted for a temporary prosthesis, which was made in an adjoining hospital shop, he moved on to one of the curative workshops designed to teach him how to use it. (Permanent prostheses were purchased upon discharge by the individual patient. Given a subsidy for the purpose by the War-Risk Insurance Bureau, the veteran could presumably "shop around" among the burgeoning independent prostheses shops for the design he liked best.)

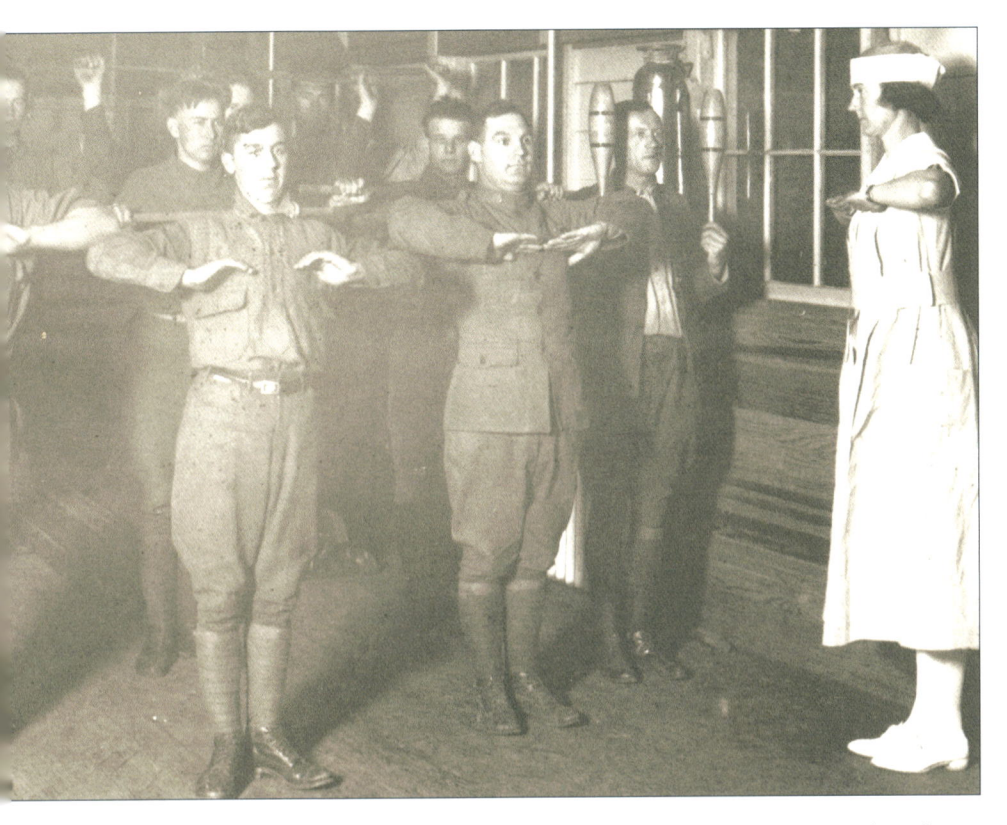

According to army hospital protocol, individuals with upper extremity amputations were typically the final responsibility of the OT reconstruction aides, on the theory that these patients' principal challenges in civilian life would be in managing occupational and vocational tasks which, in most cases, involved good manual skills. Patients with lower extremity amputations, by contrast, needed more extensive assistance in physical reconstruction, first in accustoming the amputation site to receiving the appliance and bearing body weight and then in learning the range of balance and locomotion skills necessary to attain a successful gait. Patients with foot and leg amputations, therefore, were retrained by physical therapy reconstruction aides. Because there were so many men in need of help, reconstruction aides often ran classes with a dozen or more men working simultaneously at a single task.

The fractures presented a different kind of challenge in that they were frequently associated with acute osteomyelitis, probably because of the difficulties associated with battlefield surgery and the lack of antibiotics. Follow-up operations, chronic inflammation, and disuse commonly triggered a vicious cycle of ulceration and scar tissue formation, muscle atrophy, poor circulation, pain, and more inflammation and disuse. Where medicine previously had little success in reversing such pathologies, physical therapy now proved to be invaluable. Virtually all of the therapeutic modalities — conductive heat, conversive heat, or diathermy, electrotherapy, light or radiation, hydrotherapy, massage, and active exercise — were called into play in restoring these patients to maximum function.

The neurosurgical cases came under physiotherapeutic care almost by chance. Most medical men had traditionally approached this category of disability as all but hopeless of improvement, and patients were no less discouraged. By the time the neurosurgical patients reached the United

*Fort Sam Houston, one of the principal reconstruction centers after the war, began its rehabilitation department in January 1919 with nine reconstruction aides. The "Holy Nine" soon made daily exercise treatments like the class shown here a regular part of the program.*

*McMillan's personal scrapbooks archive not only the birth of American physical therapy but also her love of flowers and gardening.*

States, their conditions were further complicated by contractions and deformities requiring additional corrective surgery before a formal regimen of therapy could begin. But coincident with the application of such physical therapy treatments as massage and hydrotherapy, prescribed merely to make patients more comfortable, it was noted that unexpected improvements often occurred in the secondary neuropathies. Indeed, many atrophied muscles responded with renewed movement, and this led surgeons and PTs to undertake more extensive and purposeful experimentation with all of the standard therapies and a few not-so-standard as well. (Some of the best work in this area had been pioneered in England by the American R. Tait McKenzie. McKenzie, who had volunteered to work with the British medical service prior to America's entry into the war, was not a physician but a professor of physical education at the University of Pennsylvania. He is said to have carried out his novel therapeutic program in England with a team of 20 masseurs, masseuses, and gymnasts!)

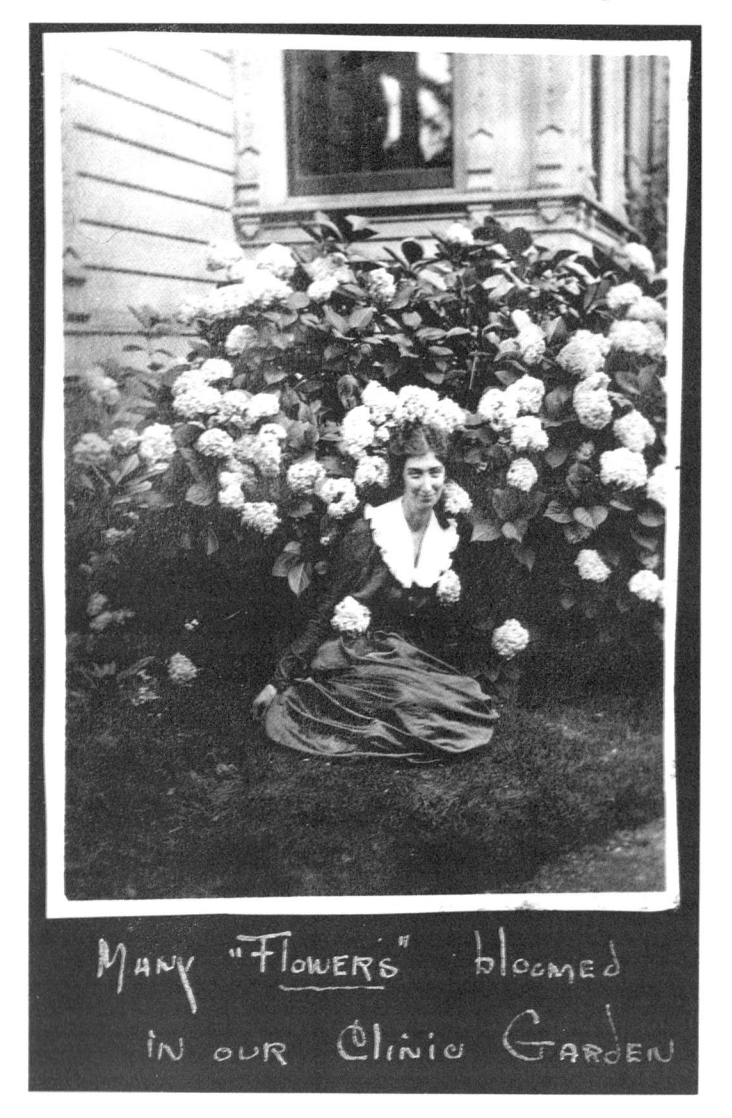

Of the more conventional treatments, massage and passive movements continued to be the most commonly administered for all classes of disability. Reconstruction Aide Harriet Forest, who served at Camp Gordon, Georgia, in 1919, recalled working with a young soldier who had been wounded in a close encounter with an exploding artillery shell. "One of his legs, from the knee down, was so full of shrapnel bits. We worked and worked on that leg, massaging very gently, and eventually removed more than 100 pieces of metal." Trenchfoot, a major syndrome developing out of prolonged periods of exposure in trench warfare, was also treated with massage in the acute phase in the hopes of staving off gangrene and ultimate amputation of the affected limb. According to the records of the Surgeon General's Office, massage constituted about 40 percent of the total number of treatments in most hospitals. There are few data to document the specific techniques used, but it is likely that the majority of physical therapists followed principles brought over from England and taught by Mary McMillan.

Active or corrective exercises, also known as muscle reeducation, constituted another 25 percent of therapeutics managed by reconstruction aides. Suitable for patients who had voluntary control of movement, the exercises combined some of the meth-

*Many "Flowers" bloomed in our Clinic Garden*

odology of physical education with the systematic work carried out by Wilhelmine Wright and others in the treatment of infantile paralysis.

### THE RECONSTRUCTION AIDE'S ARSENAL OF EQUIPMENT

Exercise rooms in United States-based army hospitals were typically equipped with primitive joint mobility gauges and various Zanderlike mechanical apparatuses, although the cost and elaborateness of the commercial units often prompted reconstruction aides to devise homegrown substitutes. Along with simple pulley-and-weight systems, crude trolleys on ball-bearing wheels were manufactured in hospital workshops for use in retraining. The trolley made it possible for patients to practice the early stages of muscle abduction or retraction with minimum resistance, and the psychological rewards of seeing results, however small, often made the difference between a soldier's continued effort at movement and giving up.

To make some of the repetitive exercises more enjoyable, the therapists also devised targeted games and sports. Where muscles in the forearm and hand were so stiffened as to prevent the hand from closing, the wounded soldier might be given a pair of lightweight boxing gloves and a punching bag and thereby induced to retrain muscles. Where a shoulder and upper arm needed work, a sledge-and-bellringer device similar to the carnival "strong man" game might be used. Reconstruction aides measured their patients for the extent, strength, and speed of movement every two weeks, tacking the charted results at bedside where everyone could see the progress. It was a blatant form of competition, but for many it seemed to provide the necessary incentive to continue the hard work of rehabilitation.

Of the various forms of hydrotherapy, whirlpool baths quickly became the most widely used. Developed during the war by the British as a variant of the French army's "current bath," the whirlpool bath featured a motor-driven propeller that aerated the water stream. It was used chiefly to treat ankylosed and edematous limbs as well as peripheral nerve injuries. Not only did it prove to be very effective in increasing mobility in joints and

*Friendships born during intensive War Emergency Training Courses were nourished by frequent exchanges of letters among scattered reconstruction aides. Shown are notes to Mia Donner, who was stationed overseas for many months.*

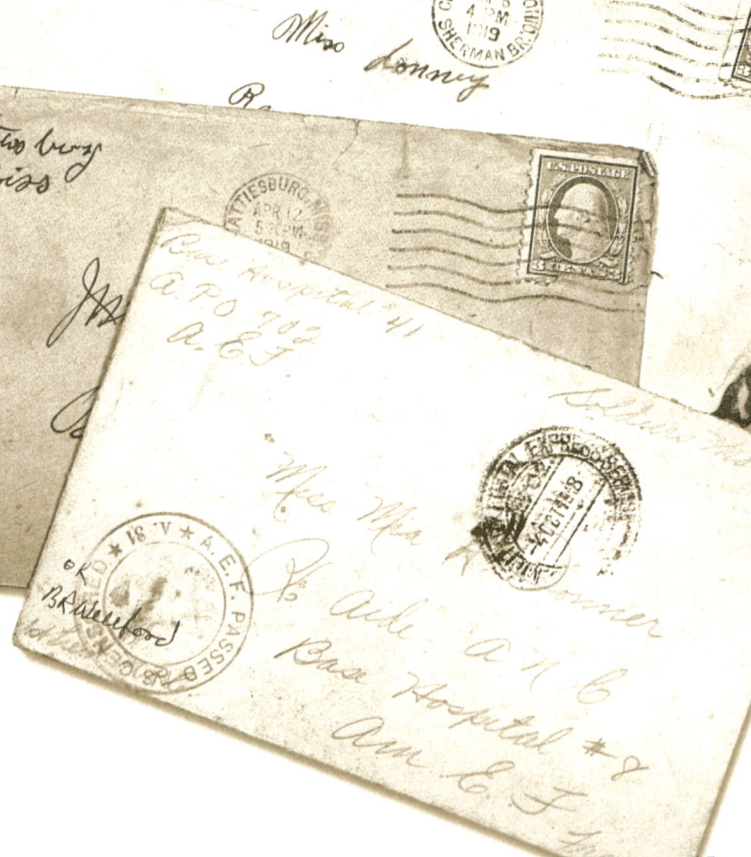

*En route to France, Mia Donner's group stopped briefly in Liverpool, England, where each one received the note of thanks from Britain's King George V, right. The majority of therapists who served in World War I were released in droves after the war ended; the army, in an effort to regain the needed physical therapists, sent out form letters such as the letter addressed to Janet Merrill, far right, offering better terms of employment. Merrill chose, rather, to find civilian employment teaching at one of the War Emergency Training Courses in Boston.*

softening limbs, but it reduced pain and apprehension in patients and allowed overworked PTs to administer follow-up massage and passive manipulations more efficiently. After a 10- to 20-minute immersion in a whirlpool tank, most patients' daily massage time could be effectively reduced from 30 minutes to 10.

Contrast baths, employing alternating two-minute submersions in hot (110°) and cold (60°) water for an effect sometimes referred to as "circulatory gymnastics," were used whenever an increase in blood flow was desired. The so-called cabinet bath and general hydropathy were chosen for their overall tonic effect. Patients were first exposed to the dry heat of 50 overhead electric lamps for 4 to 10 minutes, after which they were showered with rapidly alternating jets of hot and cold water at pressures ranging from 10 to 30 pounds.

Paraffin wax baths were another new hydrotherapeutic technique in limited use. The wax bath traced its

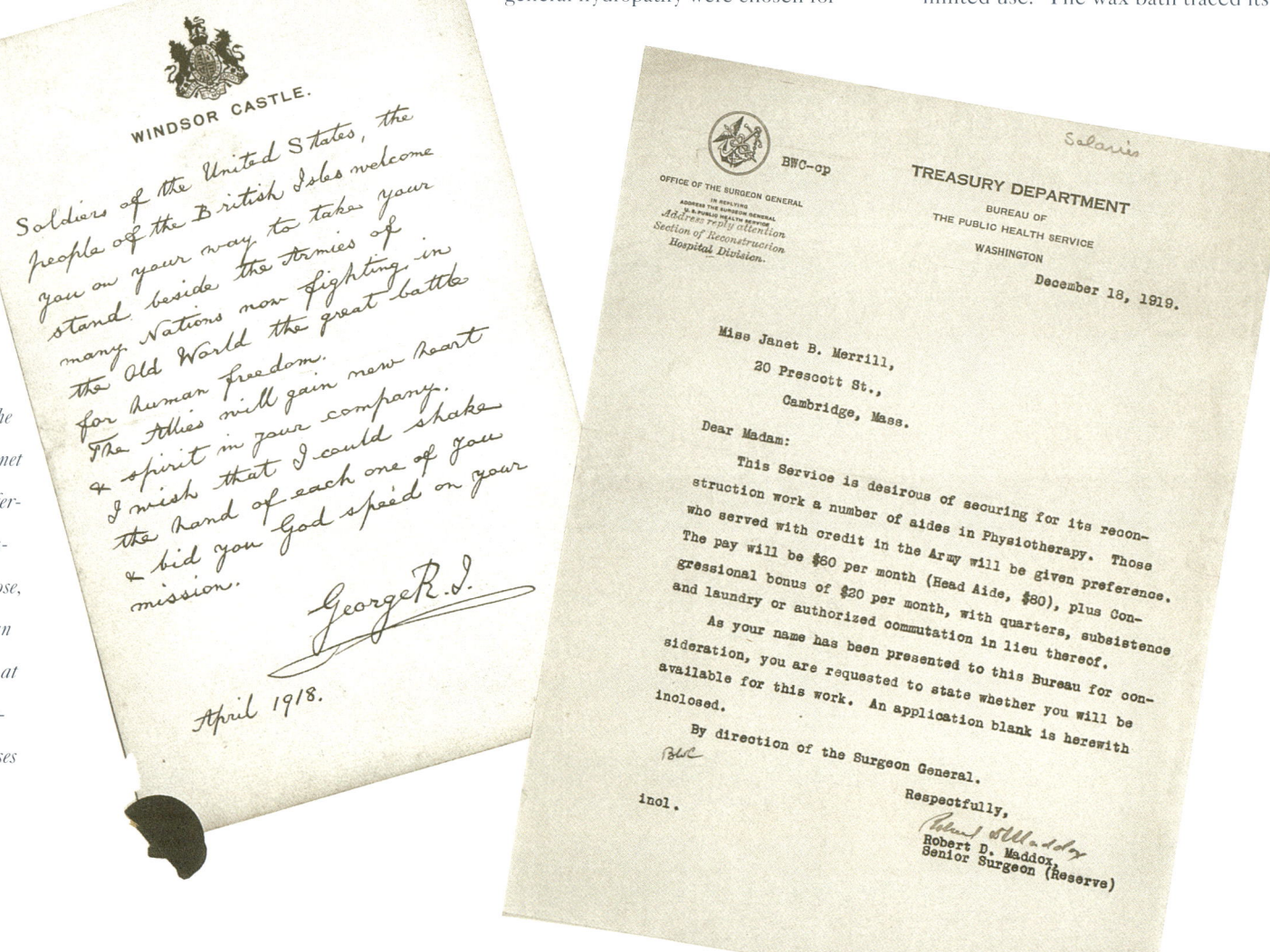

---

WINDSOR CASTLE.

Soldiers of the United States, the people of the British Isles welcome you on your way to take your stand beside the armies of many Nations now fighting in the Old World the great battle for human freedom.

The Allies will gain new heart & spirit in your company. I wish that I could shake the hand of each one of you & bid you God speed on your mission.

George R.I.

April 1918.

---

BWC-cp

OFFICE OF THE SURGEON GENERAL
Section of Reconstruction
Hospital Division

TREASURY DEPARTMENT
BUREAU OF
THE PUBLIC HEALTH SERVICE
WASHINGTON

December 18, 1919.

Miss Janet B. Merrill,
20 Prescott St.,
Cambridge, Mass.

Dear Madam:

This Service is desirous of securing for its reconstruction work a number of aides in Physiotherapy. Those who served with credit in the Army will be given preference. The pay will be $60 per month (Head Aide, $80), plus Congressional bonus of $20 per month, with quarters, subsistence and laundry or authorized commutation in lieu thereof.

As your name has been presented to this Bureau for consideration, you are requested to state whether you will be available for this work. An application blank is herewith inclosed.

By direction of the Surgeon General.

Respectfully,

Robert D. Maddox,
Senior Surgeon (Reserve)

incl.

66  *Healing The Generations*

origins to France and Edmond Barthe de Sandifort, who used molten paraffin or beeswax to heat arthritic hands in France in 1913. A British army surgeon at Leeds Hospital had subsequently noted that tannery workers sometimes dipped tired hands in wax vats with restorative effects, and he introduced the wax treatment to his own patients. From there it was widely taken up on both sides of the Atlantic, usually as a substitute for the whirlpool bath, although no one was as yet certain as to its genuine value.

A favorite modality when water baths could not be used, as in the case of open wounds, was the radiant heat and light bath, commonly referred to as a "baker." The typical army hospital physiotherapy clinic was equipped with several adjustable portable units designed to treat localized pathologies and a large, nonportable unit with a 1,500-watt tungsten-filament lamp to provide deep heat to nerve injuries in shoulder, back, buttock, or thigh.

For the first time in medical history, it would appear, electrotherapy — in the various forms of galvanic, sinusoidal, and faradic currents — was employed systematically as a means of stimulating muscular movement when voluntary movement was not possible.

Perhaps because treatment of neurosurgical cases was always an excruciatingly slow process, with progress measured in the most subtle terms, surgeons and physical therapy reconstruction aides made it routine practice to keep precise medical records of each neurosurgical patient's condition. This, too, was a relatively new idea. Recorded were a description of muscle groups impaired, degree of atrophy, vasomotor changes, DTP (distal tingling on percussion), and measurements of limb girth, joint mobility, and electric responsiveness. (Applying galvanic current to muscle areas and charting the response became a key tool for tracking progress.)

Diathermy — in these years strictly of the high-frequency type — was used broadly as a follow-up to bone grafting, as a means to diminish pain and improve heart action in pneumonia, and as a treatment for acute bursitis, hypertrophic arthritis, and for other conditions in which deep heating was thought to assist healing. The machines tended to be both large and noisy, with crackles and thunderclaps constantly being produced by the arcing sparks and spinning static wheels. Another vivid feature was the effect on patients' hair, which was likely to stand on end. A diathermy clinic looked like nothing so much as Dr. Caligari's Cabinet of Horrors.

### WINDING DOWN

Between 1919 and 1920, the ranks of the physical therapy reconstruction aides shrank from their top strength of 748 in 49 hospitals at home and overseas to a mere 175 in 11 stateside hospitals. Deciding that her work with the SGO was essentially completed, McMillan resigned in June 1920 to return to Boston and civilian life.

The army's commitment to maintaining physical therapy as an important part of its medical services was firmly established. Summing up the success of the reconstruction aide program, Joel Goldthwait declared,

*Helen Bradley, one of the "Holy Nine" at Fort Sam Houston, kept a scrapbook of her service. This cartoon and scrap of poetry confirm her recollections of the "brave, joyous, and appreciative boys" for whom her high-spirited group cared.*

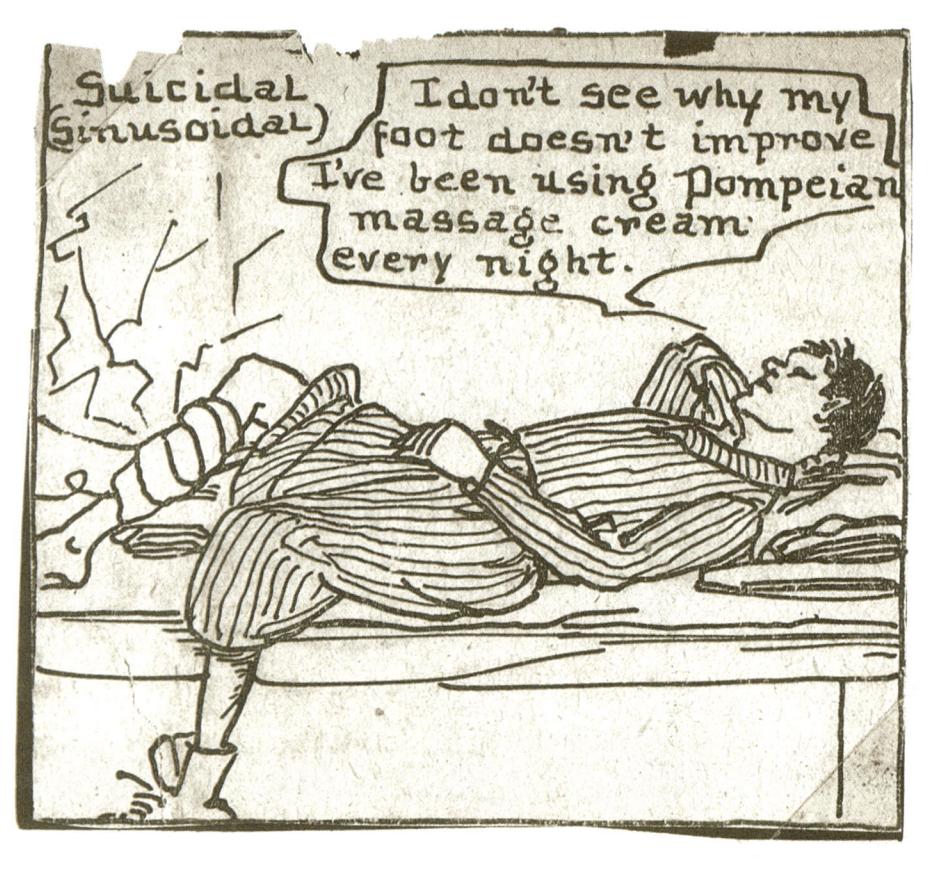

"The war demonstrated, in a manner that probably nothing else could, that even severe injury need not lead to serious disability, provided suitable treatment following the care of the wounds can be given. Good primary surgery and good nursing, of themselves, do not yield results which can be considered satisfactory. . . . With the coming of the first group of Aides to France a new era opened for the hospitals of the AEF. . . . Not only were many men saved to useful lives, who would otherwise have been crippled, but the principle of physiotherapy and occupational therapy was so definitely established that civilian hospitals must [now] provide a staff of such workers."

To ensure that the army would also be able to staff its own peacetime hospitals, the army sent one of its career medical officers, Major James B. Montgomery, to train with Frank Granger in Boston for several months. Montgomery subsequently returned to Walter Reed, where he reorganized the physical therapy service. All army hospitals constructed during the next two decades were required to include adequate space for physical therapy facilities.

Ironically, economic pressures on the military to cut down its medical personnel after the Armistice had prompted the SGO to release its PTs too quickly and in too great numbers. When the army let it be known that it would welcome some of them back to staff the permanent facilities, most of the former reconstruction aides wanted no part of the offer. Many had taken jobs with the United States Public Health Service, to which responsibility for post-war care of those with long-term disabilities had passed. (After 1921 these same veterans' hospitals

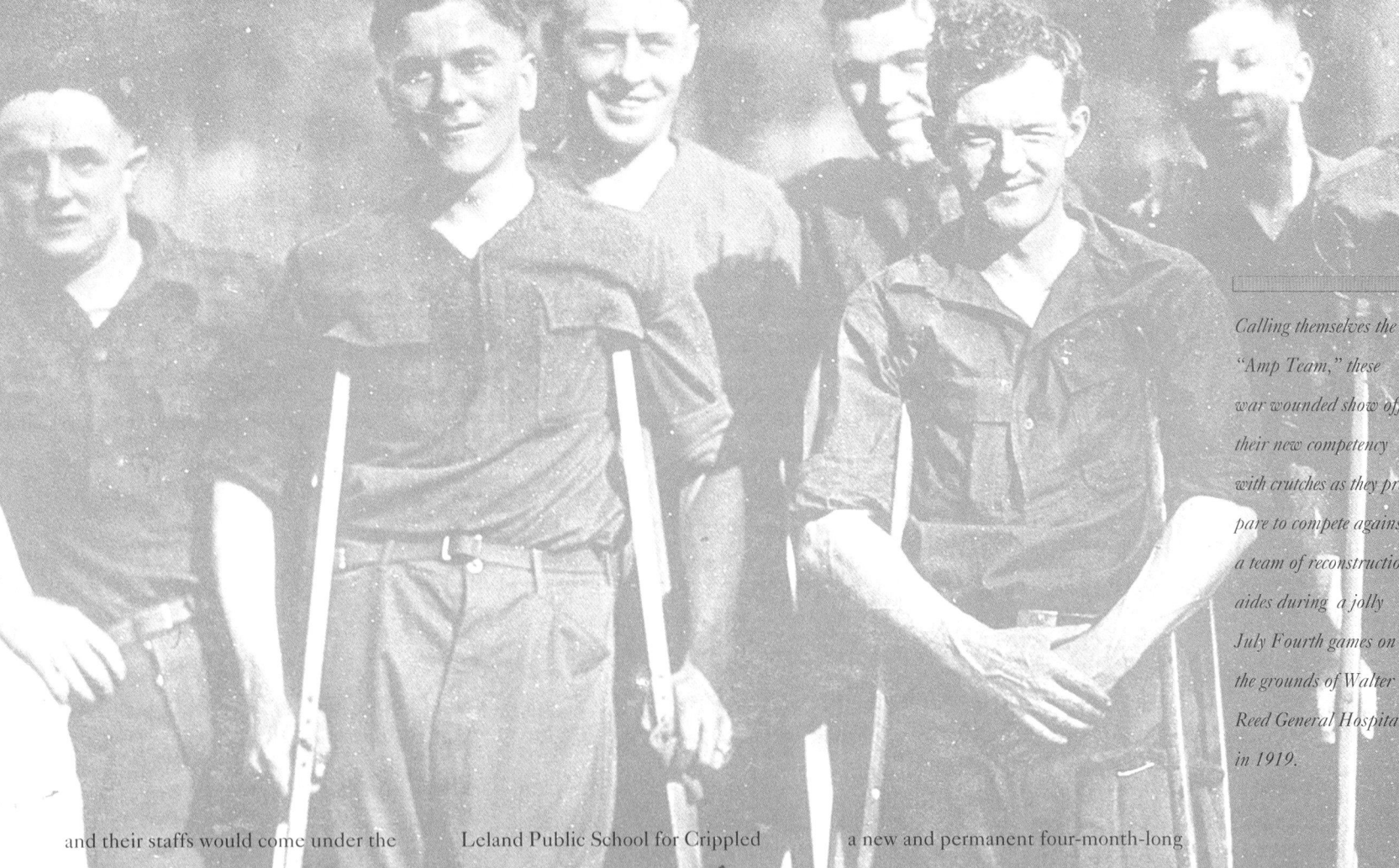

*Calling themselves the "Amp Team," these war wounded show off their new competency with crutches as they prepare to compete against a team of reconstruction aides during a jolly July Fourth games on the grounds of Walter Reed General Hospital in 1919.*

and their staffs would come under the control of the newly created Veterans' Bureau.) Other former reconstruction aides had found positions in civilian hospitals, in the private practices of orthopedists, in industry-based clinics, or in facilities for children with disabilities. (Detroit's pioneering Nellie Leland Public School for Crippled Children and Gates Hospital in Elyria, Ohio, sponsored by the Ohio Society for Crippled Children, were just two of many such institutions for these children.)

Consequently, in 1922, Montgomery named Emma Vogel to direct a new and permanent four-month-long training program for physical therapists at Walter Reed General Hospital in order to assure the army of an ongoing force of well-trained physical therapists. As Goldthwait had predicted, physical therapy — both as a "principle" and as a profession — was here to stay.

## CHAPTER 3

# With Vision, Faith, And Courage
# 1920 – 1939

*In a small "clubroom" for reconstruction aides set aside at Walter Reed General Hospital, Superintendent Mollie McMillan snatches a few leisure hours in the spring of 1920 to work on her manuscript for* Massage and Therapeutic Exercise, *published the following year. In this same room, the first informal discussions concerning formation of a professional association took place.*

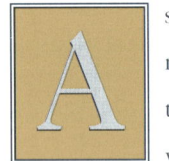

Asked to give her assessment of what it takes to be a successful innovator, Mary McMillan once described three essentials: "The first is Vision — without vision there can be no forward movement. . . . The second is Faith in the purpose . . . keen, alive, kindled with enthusiasm. The third . . . is Courage, courage to overcome all odds and difficulties." McMillan was speaking at the time of Amy Homans, one of America's pioneer educators in women's physical education, but she might just as well have been describing the shared characteristics of the women who set about organizing what would become the American Physical Therapy Association.

It all began when McMillan and the Surgeon General's Office were engaged in shutting down the army's reconstruction aide program. Convinced more than ever that physical therapy had a major role to play in the future of America's health and concerned that the nucleus of people equipped to carry on such a program had to be maintained, McMillan and several colleagues at Walter Reed General Hospital talked about the possibility of forming a national professional organization. (A national organization was also the goal of a group of reconstruction aides stationed at Chicago's Fort Sheridan, who formed the World War Reconstruction Aides Assembly about this time. But the WWRAA's purposes were considerably narrower. Welcoming both PTs and OTs, practicing or retired, this society concerned itself principally with gaining official military status for all former reconstruction aides while maintaining lively social ties among old friends. The group disbanded in 1949 on the occasion of its 30th reunion, when advancing age and the intrusion of World War II inclined survivors to turn their energies elsewhere.)

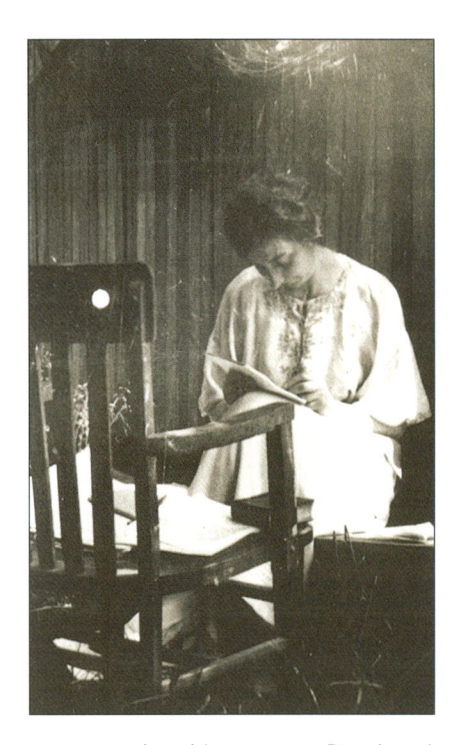

Supporting McMillan and her co-workers in their organizational efforts were several of the doctors who had served in the army's Division of Reconstruction during the war. Elliott Brackett favored whatever means it took "to preserve the resources developed [during the war] that they may be turned to the relief of the industrial reconstruction, which problem we shall always have with us." And shortly after his return to civilian life, Harold Corbusier wrote to say that such an organization was needed "to advertise to the physicians of the country the importance of the various methods of treatment by physical means." Corbusier also thought such a group could set rigorous standards for physical therapy practitioners, a necessary next step if their work was to gain a full measure of respect.

McMillan contacted former colleague Frank Granger to ask if he would serve as temporary chairman of such a drive, and when Granger gave his enthusiastic support, the effort was launched in earnest. In January of 1920 the nucleus at Walter Reed drew up the prospectus of an organization, tentatively named the American Women's Physical Therapeutic Association, or AWPTA, and sent more than 300 letters to former reconstruction aides. But as McMillan would later declare, the time was not yet ripe and the responses were rather tepid. By late 1920, however, circumstances had changed markedly. Practically all the emergency hospitals that had employed physical therapy reconstruction aides either had closed or were in the process of closing. McMillan, her work in the Surgeon General's Office completed, had resigned in June to return to Boston as staff therapist in Brackett's orthopedic practice. And as she had anticipated, the ex-reconstruction aides were finding working conditions out in the real world capricious and sometimes lonely. It was also true that women were gaining self-confidence in the political and organizational arena: with the passage of the Nineteenth Amendment in August, women had finally won the Constitutional right to vote.

### "THE PULL-TOGETHER FEELING"

McMillan and her committee decided to try again, contacting some 800 candidates both within and outside the military service. Respondents who wished to participate in the enterprise were asked to send annual dues of $2 and to fill out a primary ballot on which they could nominate for one-year terms a president, two vice-presidents, a treasurer, and two members-at-large to complete the Executive Committee.

This time some 120 enthusiastic responses were returned. Many letters and contributions came from Los Angeles, San Francisco, Portland (Oregon), Washington, New York, New Haven, Chicago and Boston, where loosely organized groups of active PTs, many of them working in the Public Health Service or in veterans' hospitals, seized on the idea of a national association as a way to give greater impetus to their own local struggles for recognition. The nominations were tabulated, a formal ballot was drawn up, and in February 1921, a second round of mailings was sent out to dues-paying members only. Voters were told to have their ballots returned to Granger's office no later than March 24, 1921. Meanwhile, the core of national activists decided it was time to hold a face-to-face organizational meeting. New York was chosen

*At the 6,600-bed hospital at Fort Sheridan, located just outside of Chicago, the patient load immediately following the Armistice was enormous. For a time, reconstruction aides were scheduled to work day and night shifts in Ward 45, shown, in order to deliver the much needed rehabilitation treatments.*

*Fitzsimons General Hospital, Denver, Colorado, was one of the six military hospitals to remain in operation following demobilization. Shown here is a treatment room devoted to electro-therapeutic treatments.*

as the most convenient middle ground for the scattered contingents of East Coast reconstruction aides. On January 15, 1921, some 30 women gathered at an old midtown Manhattan eatery called Keen's Chop House. Granger, Corbusier, and five other physicians and surgeons also attended.

Although there are only scanty records of the meeting, it appears that much of the discussion revolved around membership qualifications. Was the group open only to former reconstruction aides, or could others with similar training in civilian life be considered? Was the proposed name of the organization too exclusionary? For instance, were men unwelcome? What about Canadians? Or people with conventional nurses' training or degrees in physical education? The consensus was that the society should consist of any woman whose physical therapy training and experience equaled or surpassed that required of wartime physical therapy reconstruction aides, regardless of actual service. A six-member committee, headed by Gertrude Healy, former head aide at the army's Fox Hills General Hospital, Staten Island, New York, was given the task of drafting a Constitution and Bylaws. A month later the committee met with McMillan and several others for a second time in New York. Various compromises in wording were worked out and a final version was prepared and sent to the 30-woman Boston organization which, for purposes of efficiency, had been designated a kind of pro tempore legislative body. McMillan wrote to a colleague that she was spending so much time during evenings and weekends thinking and talking about the "Association" that she feared a letdown when the goal was reached.

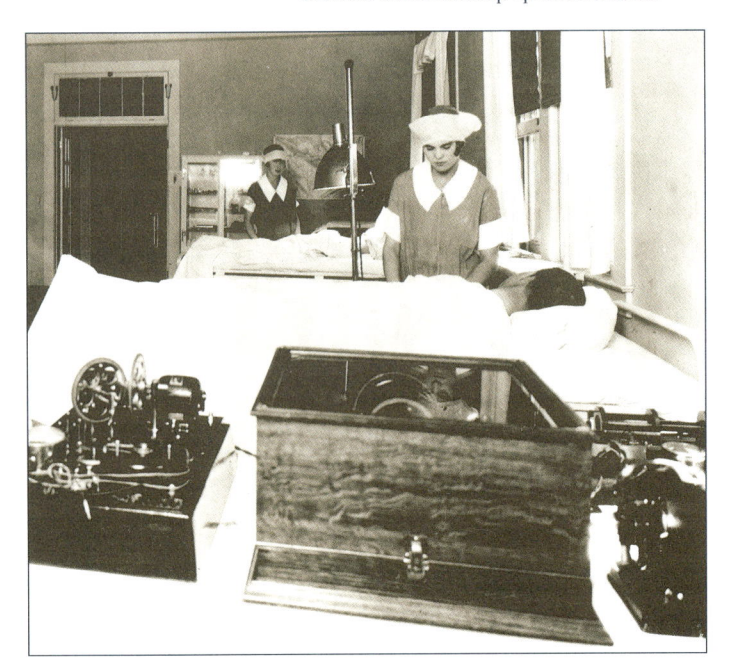

McMillan need not have worried, for when the final mail ballots were counted on March 24, 1921, she found herself more engaged than ever. To no one's surprise except her own, voters had chosen Mollie McMillan as their first president. Her Executive Committee represented a highly competent, geographically diverse collection of wartime associates. Vice-presidents were Beulah Rader, then serving at Whipple Barracks, Prescott, Arizona; and Emma Heilman, director of physical education at Reed College, Portland. Members-at-large on the seven-woman Executive Committee were Hazel Furscott, formerly at the army's Letterman Hospital in San Francisco, and in 1921, director of the new Physical Therapy Department at Hahnemann Hospital, University of California, in the same city; and Marion Swezey, formerly at Walter Reed General Hospital, who was working in the new Physiotherapy Department at the Gary Hospital, Gary, Indiana.

Significantly, the group's treasurer, Janet Merrill, was technically an "outsider," albeit undoubtedly well known to all either personally or by pro-

*Healing The Generations*

fessional reputation. Although Merrill had not enlisted as a reconstruction aide during the war, preferring to remain in the Public Health Service, she had been closely involved in training scores of women who had, having directed the army's War Emergency Training Course for reconstruction aides at Boston Children's Hospital/Harvard Medical School in the fall of 1918. Still at Boston Children's Hospital, Merrill had been named director of physical therapy in 1921, when Arthur T. Legg had succeeded Lovett as head of the orthopedic service. Merrill also held prestigious posts as chief of the Physical Therapy Service of the Harvard Infantile Paralysis Commission and technical director of Harvard's eight-week postgraduate Course 441 in physical therapy. Until a secretary could be appointed by the fledgling Executive Committee, Merrill served as interim secretary of the Association, too. (As would continue to be the policy for many years, the choice of secretary was heavily influenced by geography; the closer she lived to the elected president, the better, for efficiency's sake.) Records indicate that first-year membership stood at 274, representing 32 states.

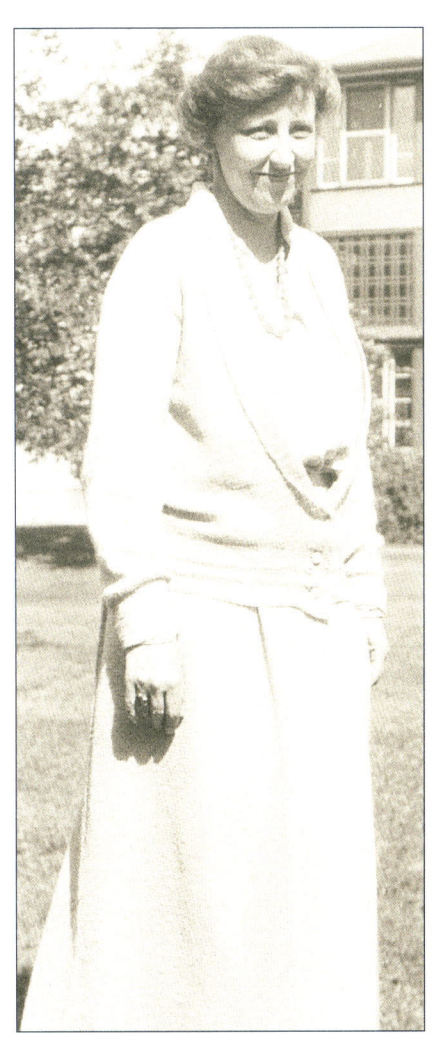

### P.T. REVIEW

The results of the election appeared shortly afterward in the *P.T. Review*, the official organ of the Association, which published its maiden issue in late March 1921. The *Review* was by any measure a modest offering. Published quarterly and distributed free to every member, it was 16 pages long, 7 1/2 x 5 1/2 inches in size, and dressed in a blue jacket whose color was reminiscent of their World War I uniforms. But like the proverbial dancing dog, whose footwork is not to be watched too closely, those responsible for the *Review*'s publication were amazed that it "danced" at all. Its masthead listed just two contributors, and "temporary" ones at that: Editor-in-Chief Isabel Noble, who had taken on this labor of love shortly after moving to Boston to work in the office of Dr. Lovett; and Business Manager and Assistant Editor Elizabeth Wells, another retired reconstruction aide and newcomer to Boston looking for a full-time paying job. Precisely how the work was divided up we do not know, but McMillan personally delivered the final copy, admittedly a few days beyond deadline, to a Brookline printer with whom she had bargained hard for a price within the Association's meager budget. The cost of publishing and mailing this first issue was $73.66.

*Janet Merrill, a charter member of the Association, was elected as the first treasurer and served also as interim secretary in 1921. Here, she stands in the courtyard of Boston Children's Hospital, where she served for many years as director of physical therapy.*

*The inaugural 16-page issue of the* P.T. Review, *below, carried a letter from Joel Goldthwait predicting that "the publication . . . will do much to preserve the standards and advance the science of the profession." McMillan's* Massage and Therapeutic Exercise, *first published in 1921, was in such demand that a second edition was needed in 1925, shown below right. The preface to the McMillan classic contained a prophetic statement by Harvey Cushing, a renowned Boston neurosurgeon. He told his peers in 1919 that "mayhap a new profession for women as important as the nursing profession may arise" from the (continued opposite)*

Editor Noble greeted her new readers with a plea for forbearance: "We trust our readers will be lenient about any sins of omission and commission. . . . We hope to improve as time goes on." The first issue contained greetings from Marguerite Sanderson and a rousing half-page article by Joel Goldthwait on "The Value of Physiotherapy as Proved by the War." (Goldthwait's influence on physical therapy would continue. In 1935 he wrote *Body Mechanics*, which became a standard reference for a generation of therapists.) Also reported were brief news notes from local organizations, a summary of the events that had brought the organization into being, a directory of charter members, and a six-line review of a new 274-page, illustrated book by Mary McMillan, entitled *Massage and Therapeutic Exercise*. The reviewer pronounced the "little book . . . of great value" to former reconstruction aides and physicians, an understatement by any measure. McMillan's book, the first textbook written by an American physical therapist, became an overnight standard in the treatment of musculoskeletal disorders as practiced between the wars. It went into three editions, the last published in 1932.

Under the *Review*'s "S.O.S." headline appeared eight separate classified advertisements for job openings. Among the opportunities listed in the first issue were work with crippled children in Maryland and with patients with cerebral palsy in Kansas, as well as several openings in the expanding field of "industrial work" in New York and Illinois. One particularly demanding job listing called for "a bright, cheerful aide in a private hospital for mostly nervous patients . . . able to teach folk dancing, calisthenics, sports, and take charge of hydrotherapy." The "S.O.S." column would soon grow into an informal vocational bureau along the lines of the English Chartered Society's "Appointment Bureau." In addition to printing employment opportunities, "S.O.S." volunteer manager Dorothea Beck actively sought placements for members through her network of professional connections. She also advertised the service in medical journals, prompting solicitations for physical therapists from as far away as South Africa.

### ARTICLES OF FAITH

The *Review*'s maiden issue included the full text of the Constitution and Bylaws of the Association. Article II of the Constitution was particularly instructive in that it set forth the new Association's basic reasons for existence, which were: "To establish and maintain a professional and scientific standard for those engaged in the profession of Physical Therapeutics; to increase efficiency among its members by encouraging them in advanced study; to disseminate information by the distribution of medical literature and articles of professional interest; to assist in securing positions for its members; to make available efficiently trained women to the medical profession; and to sustain social fellowship and intercourse upon grounds of mutual interest." It is noteworthy that in the wording of this statement, the Constitution specifically perpetuated the concept of physical therapists as supportive aides or assistants to physicians and surgeons. The principle, which would come up again and again over the years, would not only cloud the relationship between these two groups of professionals but also call into question their respective occupational titles.

The Bylaws defined the three categories of membership: "Charter members shall be the reconstruction aides in Physiotherapy who have served satisfactorily with the United States Army and Navy or with those of the Allies, whose training and experience must total one year and who apply for membership in the Association within one year of the ratification of the Constitution. Active members shall be graduates of recognized Schools of Physiotherapy or Physical Education, who have had training and experience in Massage and Therapeutic Exercises, with some knowledge of either Electrotherapy or Hydrotherapy, and whose character and personality are definitely suited to this work. The Executive Committee shall have power to formulate such rules as will maintain a standard for eligibility and to institute such entrance examinations as they deem advisable." Honorary members, who could be proposed by any member and were to be elected by the Executive Committee, were required to be "graduates of Medical Schools conforming to the standard of the American Medical Association."

In June 1921, a second issue of the *P.T. Review* appeared, this time looking and sounding considerably more self-assured. Freshly dressed in the gray that would become its familiar wrap for 24 years, and partially subsidized by advertisements, the quarterly boasted an imposing array of 11 staff members, with Elizabeth Huntington as editor-in-chief. Huntington was a former reconstruction aide with the American Expeditionary Force. Her paying job as an editorial assistant at the *Youth's Companion* gave her a certain journalistic panache, and Noble and Wells happily accepted demotions to assistant posts on the *Review*. Josephine Bell, head reconstruction aide at the Army of Occupation's facility in Coblenz, Germany, was listed under the title of "foreign correspon-

*efforts of former reconstruction aides who served in World War I. Shown below is the third and final edition of McMillan's book, published in 1932.*

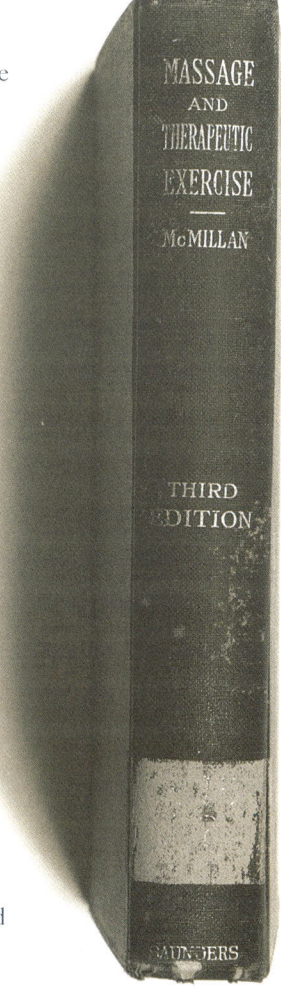

dent." The *Review*'s paper was of better quality, too. Within its pages were an article by Elliott Brackett on physiotherapy's role in treating industrial accidents, a cartoon drawn by an anonymous reconstruction aide, and an impressive article by member Margaret Blake on exercise treatment as practiced at Rochester Clinic in Rochester, New York.

Perhaps the most significant offering in the issue, however, was the inaugural message from President Mollie McMillan. McMillan promised to do everything in her power "to live up to the trust and confidence" bestowed upon her by her friends and fellow workers, for as she explained, "There is no cause dearer to my heart, no group . . . for whom I have greater affection. . . . Although we are scattered," she declared, "the separation only serves to bind us closer together." She went on to tell members that initial plans to hold the first conference in June 1921 had been overly optimistic. "Since our first Convention must be a big success, it seemed wiser to the Executive Committee to postpone it for a year." She urged everyone to set aside time for the following summer, when a conference "worthy of our profession" would be held, perhaps in conjunction with that of the American Medical Association, whose official recognition the AWPTA was seeking.

McMillan continued her "intimate talk with dear friends" with some motherly counsel. "There are eight or nine local associations, with from 10 to 40 members in each. In addition, there is in our National Association a considerable percentage of members . . . who live in small cities or towns." She called upon the stronger, urban groups to assist those in isolated locations to share whatever they might have in the way of professional interest or educational value, so that all parts of the organization might grow stronger together.

Lastly, President McMillan wrote of the need to set a firm standard for the profession, following the example of Britain's Chartered Society of Trained Masseuses, whose certification process was growing more rigorous with each passing year. The AWPTA, said McMillan, still had "many bridges to cross" before it could consider itself on a par with its British sister organization, but each and every member could make a personal contribution through her own pursuit of post-graduate studies in physiotherapy. "It is up to you and me to see that our foundation is laid on sound principles that will endure."

As if to drive the point home, the second issue of the *P.T. Review* concluded with the announcement of another summer graduate course in physiotherapy at Harvard Medical School. Course 442, which was offered coincident with Course 441, included lectures on electrotherapy by Granger, on hip and back strain by Brackett, and on pre- and postoperative curative exercise by physician Frederick J. Cotton, plus daily clinics at several hospitals — all for a tuition fee of $50. Mollie McMillan was listed as instructor in The Theory and Practice of Massage, a course she would continue to give for the next 10 summers.

As circumstances soon proved, McMillan and the AWPTA had good reason to be concerned about standards, even maintaining the ones with which they began. The September issue of the quarterly *Review* devoted considerable space to "the Letterman Tangle." The commanding officer at the army's San Francisco-based General Hospital, in a cost-cutting effort, had attempted to put a nurse with two weeks' "training" in charge of physical therapy treatments. The reconstruction aides there, seeing a dangerous precedent in the making, had asked the AWPTA to intercede. McMillan and the Executive Committee had instantly telegraphed a protest to the Surgeon General, and after some official clearing of throats, the offending Letterman plan was withdrawn.

The *Review*'s editors, however, were not content to end the matter there. "Whoever has functioned as a government employee has learned to expect stupid orders," wrote Editor Huntington indignantly. "But this order is not only brainless; it is harmful. First, it injures the patients. . . . Second, it harms physiotherapy, because it spreads the idea that the work is a kind of pleasant handicraft that can be picked up in a few spare hours. . . . Third, it harms the nursing professions, because it takes the nurses . . . away from their chosen work and places them in an uncomfortable and undignified position. They are required to stroll in some fine morning and ask for two weeks' worth of boiled down P.T., much as if it were a box of concentrated food tablets." In a clear sign that the Association's value as a political pressure group was appreciated, three more of Letterman's therapy staff coincidentally applied for membership.

Hammering away once again on the subject of improving educational standards, McMillan urged members to encourage and support the offering of postgraduate physiotherapeutic courses in their part of the country. "We have so much valuable material for further study," she told them, "Why not . . . increase our possibilities for forging ahead in our profession? Capable and efficient women are more and more in demand."

With the start of 1922, the AWPTA raised dues to $3 and mailed ballots for its second election of officers. Mary McMillan was returned for a second term, receiving 64 votes to Marguerite Sanderson's 40. (Sanderson married shortly after, and aside from occasional letters to her old friends, she ceased to be involved in activities of the organization.) Rader, Merrill, Furscott, and Swezey were also reelected; new faces on the Executive Committee were Inga Lohne of Boston and Lillian Drew of New York. Of greater consequence, the membership was polled on changing their organization's name. The "American Physiotherapy Association" won out over three other choices, none of which included the proscriptive word "women." Of more immediate concern, membership in the fledgling organization slipped back to 182.

The March 1922 issue of the *Review* carried the election returns as well as news of the ongoing effort to get Congress to extend military benefits retroactively to reconstruction aides, particularly those who had served overseas. "If there was emergency work to be done . . . if there were rules of conduct and dress to be observed, if there were hours to be kept . . . we were, to all intents and purposes, as drastically military in status as hobnails and hardtack," wrote the editor with

*Emma Vogel, one of McMillan's "Reedites," went on to establish the first post-war course for civilian physical therapists at Walter Reed General Hospital. In 1923 she and her students were guests at a White House garden reception given by President Calvin Coolidge.*

more than a touch of sarcasm. "But if the question was one of life insurance, or of a new issue of clothes, or the dozen and one minor benefits that accrued to established military standing, nothing could have been more civilly civilian than we." The editor concluded with the remark that reform was not likely to come soon, based on the confused state of the army's own records, but that "if we all pull together" in pressing for recognition, "a satisfying conclusion" might be won someday. The March 1922 issue also brought the second article by a physiotherapist member, this time by Eleanor Fisher on "Heliotherapy as Given at United States Public Health Hospital No. 45, Biltmore, N.C."

The *Review* provided more news and discussions about the acute shortage of reconstruction aides in the physiotherapy wards of the United States Army hospitals due to hasty demobilization. To generate new candidates the army initiated a formalized four-month-long training program at Walter Reed General Hospital. Its director, Major James Montgomery, who had trained briefly with Granger, was assisted in teaching the course by Emma Vogel, a McMillan protégé still serving as a civilian at Walter Reed. Candidates, who had to have attended an approved school of physical education for at least two years and present proof of good character, would receive $15 a month plus room, board, and uniforms. In exchange they signed a one-year service contract with the army. (Eleven students completed the first program, which within a year was lengthened to six months, then to nine months, and finally to twelve months in 1934.)

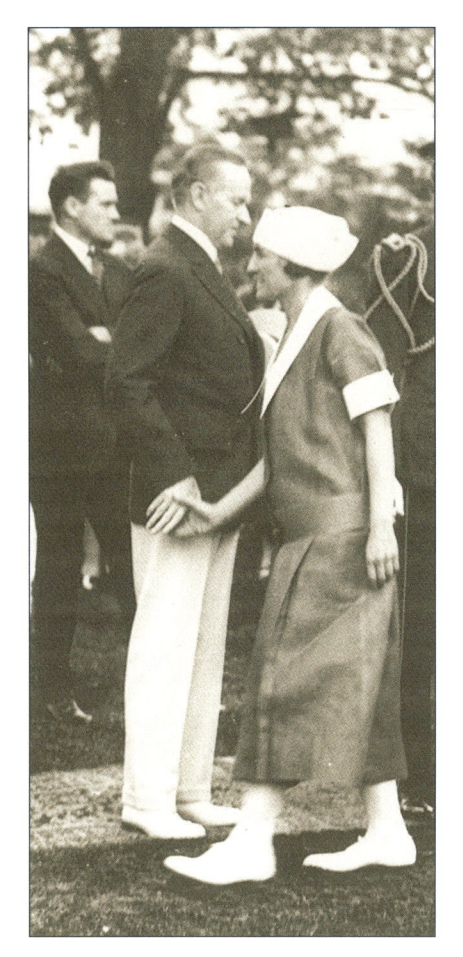

Announced under "Educational News" were two new private schools offering certificates in physiotherapy. The New York School of Physiotherapy had no specified entrance requirements and offered instruction in "hygienic gymnastics by non-medical Swedish and American instructors." The New Haven School of Physiotherapy offered a six-week course, under the direction of former army reconstruction physician Harry Eaton Stewart, to individuals with a high school diploma and two or more years of advanced training in nursing or physical education. Stewart, who had been assistant director, Section of Physiotherapy, Surgeon General's Office, during the war, was author of the influential textbook *Physical Reconstruction and Orthopedics*, published in 1920.

Just how critical an issue the standardization of training was becoming was underscored in a *Review* article by J. F. Krasnye, former chief of neuropsychiatric services at one of the army's base hospitals. Writing on "The Status of Physiotherapy Aides, As It Is and As It Should Be," he observed that the rising demand for physiotherapists had brought many impostors into the field. "In some places most of the Physiotherapy work is in the hands of either inferior attendants, graduates in massage, or people who rank with the manicure or beauty parlor help." What was needed to change the situation, he said, were better schools and "proper recognition" of those who attend them. "Students should be granted a diploma declaring him or her to be a Graduate in Physiotherapy with the letters P.T. following the constituent's name. . . . These Graduates . . . should be under the control or recognition of some central examining board or committee with authority to pass upon the qualifications and examinations and give a certificate of merit to those who deserve it." Only in this way, Krasnye said, would physiotherapy aides "be on a sound foundation and their relations to medical science and the general medical profession be conspicuously and officially established." The idea, which many applauded in theory, seemed well beyond the little group's reach.

### A "Worthy" First Conference

Another absorbing topic in 1922 was the first Annual Conference, which ran for three days beginning Wednesday, September 13, at the Boston School of Physical Education. Subjects discussed included how substantive matters were to be voted on in the future — by chapters or by individuals; whether qualified men could become members now that the organization had changed its name; whether the much-debated minimum standards for education and training ought to be spelled out in a constitutional amendment; what additional efforts might be made to further the status of physical therapy within the medical establishment; and how to bring in more of "the kind of members of whom we shall be proud." Finances were also of concern. Treasurer Merrill reported that there was just $295.46 on hand, and although most of the Association's needs were met by volunteers, the *Review*'s printing and mailing costs had to be paid. She urged everyone to pay next year's dues early, lest the treasury find itself with nothing but "good will" on the balance sheet.

The conference was a great success. Sixty-three women from 14 states, nearly a quarter of APA's membership, attended, including delegates from several midwestern and western states. (Remarkably, the conference provided Executive Committee member Hazel Furscott with her first opportunity to meet McMillan and some of the other officers.) The reunion of so many old friends was enormously gratifying. McMillan told members, "We shall endeavor to be as informal and homelike in our meetings as possible, in order that we shall be able to get close to one another in understanding." Everyone was urged to speak up about the difficulties encountered in her professional life, in the hope that colleagues might have workable solutions.

One of several papers delivered was that by President McMillan on "Exercise Therapy," particularly as applied to two neurological conditions — spastic paralysis and locomotor ataxia — which she said often went untreated for lack of scientific application. Also on the program were talks on hydrotherapy, muscle reeducation, infantile paralysis, posture training, and physiotherapy in relation to industrial accident cases, this latter a theme frequently explored in the early years. Joel Goldthwait turned up to give a speech about the promising future of physical therapy, and Frank Granger conducted a tour and demonstration of his electrotherapy unit at Boston City Hospital. The conference ended with the Boston-based Massachusetts Chapter hosting a convivial dinner followed by entertainment. Marion "Mamie" Dawson sang, Susie Pierce played instrumental selections, and finally, Minerva Crowell performed "nonsensities."

By APA's third year, membership had risen again to 240. It was time for McMillan to step aside, taking the role of "elder stateswoman." Always interested in the professional and organizational issues of the Association, she continued to participate through her activities with the Massachusetts Chapter, of which she became president in 1924. At the same time she continued to provide physiotherapy in Brackett's office, to co-direct Course 442 at Harvard, and to write occasionally for the *P.T. Review* and other professional journals.

In the spring of 1923 Norwegian-born Inga Lohne succeeded her as second president of APA. Lohne had been among the first group of reconstruction aides to go overseas in 1918, and when she was mustered out in August 1919, she took a teaching position at Sanderson's Boston School of Physical Education. Joining the Lohne team were charter members Dorothea Beck of New Jersey and Lily Graham of Los Angeles, who were elected the new co-vice-presidents. Three other Bostonians — Merrill, who was returned for a third stint as treasurer, Winifred Tougas, who became secretary, and Elizabeth Wells, who succeeded Huntington as editor of the *P.T. Review* — continued the dominance of the Massachusetts Chapter.

Lohne's one-year term was relatively quiet, leading her to declare somewhat prematurely upon handing over the gavel to her successor, "I am sure the Association has passed through its most troublesome years." Lohne presided over APA's tentative effort at forging a professional union with the powerful American Medical Association, a bid that was politely turned down at the AMA's next meeting. She and her Executive Committee worked to clarify the somewhat murky issue of the relationship between the national organization and the local groups, the bedrock on which APA was founded. As reported in the *P.T. Review*, the Committee felt that the local associations — which currently included five regularly constituted locals, Pennsylvania, Massachusetts, New York, Cleveland, and Chicago, as well as several more informal groups — should be "incorporated with the National body and become chapters of it" with chapter constitutions that conformed to the national organization's regulations. Only members qualified to join the national group could be accepted within the local chapters.

Wells, responding to complaints that the *Review* was not serious enough, did her best to deliver more news, book reviews, and scientific articles, while still giving space to "PT humor," social notes, and the occasional cartoon in issues that sometimes ran to 32 pages. The June 1924 issue included the first bibliography on physical therapy literature, provided by the independent Hospital Library and Service Bureau. PT's working in rural areas without access to a well-stocked hospital library could borrow from the Bureau's free "Package Library," consisting of topical collections of excerpted works from current medical journals on subjects relating to physical therapy. The bibliography would become a permanent fixture of the *Review*, although its selection would later pass to the *Review*'s own editorial board.

Dorothea Beck followed Lohne into the APA presidency in 1924. Beck's professional background included a two-year program in Hygiene and Physical Training at Wellesley College (the curriculum that of Amy Homans's Boston Normal School of Gymnastics, transplanted to Wellesley). Beck had gone from there to take the Emergency Course in Reconstruction at Columbia Teachers College in 1918 and had served for more than a year as head aide at the army's Camp Travis, Texas, and Fort McPherson, Georgia. Briefly in private practice in Montvale, New Jersey, after the war, Beck had distinguished herself as one of APA's most effective early organizers.

During Beck's two-term presidency, the Association began to settle into a degree of comfortable routine. Once again the Executive Committee represented some of APA's best and brightest, and Frances Philo Moreaux, a former reconstruction aide in the First Overseas Unit, took over as unpaid editor of the *Review*.

Although the AMA had rejected the idea of taking APA under its wing as an affiliate organization, it had shown a certain interest in playing a minor mentoring role. Consequently, APA scheduled its annual conferences coincident with the AMA's conferences and invited leading physicians and surgeons to appear in roundtable discussions, to read papers, and to act as toastmasters at banquets. (At one early gathering, the featured speaker, E. W. Ryerson, appeared on the podium to read a paper on "Ancient Methods in Chinese Physiotherapy." Discovering that he had left his notes at home, Ryerson recovered nicely with happy recollections of Fort Sheridan and his work with the reconstruction aides, always a crowd-pleaser.) APA members were also extended a reciprocal welcome at AMA presentations of particular interest to them.

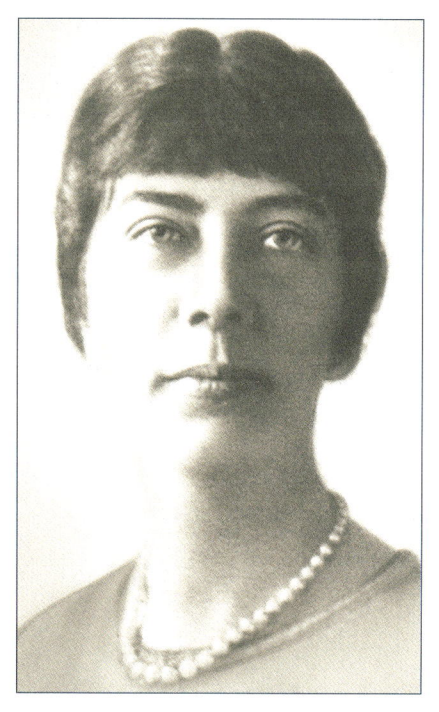

AMA President Ray Lyman Wilbur of Stanford University, set the tone of this conditional relationship in 1924, when he took time out from his own conference in Chicago to deliver the keynote address at the APA

*Dorothea Beck of New Jersey, the Association's third president, called on members to engage in a nationwide effort of "educational propaganda." "People," Beck said in her inaugural address, "still say, 'Physiotherapy? What in the world is that?'"*

*With Vision, Faith, And Courage 1920 – 1939*

*Male reconstruction aides were extremely rare in the early years. Notable exceptions were the two shown here, Carroll McAllister, left, and Eselle Terry, right. Both joined the war effort in 1919 and served together at Fort Sheridan, Illinois. Carroll McAllister was the first man to join APA and, along with his wife, worked at the physical therapy department at Letterman Hospital in San Francisco.*

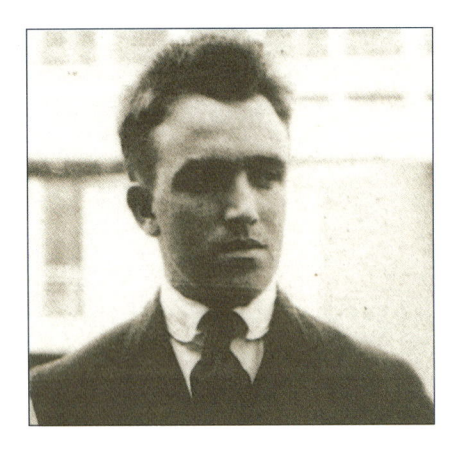

meeting next door. Wilbur made very clear the terms on which the AMA saw their working relationship. "The great opportunity of [APA] lies in studying closely its field, and keeping itself well in harness so that it does not run after extravagant claims but maintains itself on a basis that can always be defended. The future of physiotherapy is going to depend upon the confidence shown it by the medical profession."

President Beck told conference attendees that the best way to assure that confidence was for APA to make a concerted effort to get the states to institute a licensing procedure. She asked the chapters to lay the groundwork by surveying the background and training of the scores of amateur "physiotherapists" currently working in their territory. With this information, Beck said, APA could begin a program of "educational propaganda . . . to show what a quack is and warn against them."

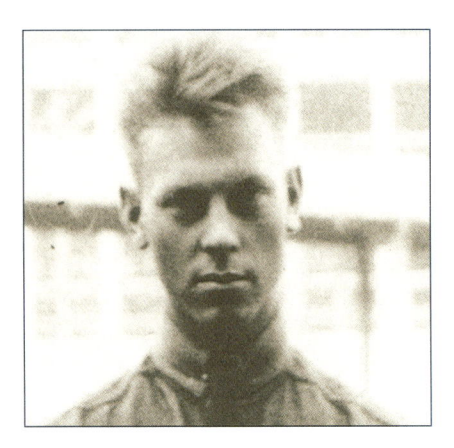

### THE AMA AS WATCHDOG

In rooting out "quacks" and raising public and professional perception of what highly skilled physical therapists had to offer in their stead, the AMA was glad to lend a hand. In 1925 it formed the Council on Physical Therapy, with Harry Mock, a former officer in the army's reconstruction service, as chairman. The council's initial charter was to be a watchdog in the marketplace of therapeutic equipment, educating general practitioners in making rational choices when confronted with a wealth of costly and mystifying appliances. (The editor of the *Journal of the American Medical Association* estimated that at least 100 different companies manufactured electro-therapeutic devices alone and claimed that doctors were inundated with salesmen making false claims.) But the council soon expanded its mandate to address the practice environment as well. In its first official report, issued in 1926, the council noted that there were growing numbers of osteopaths and chiropractors, as well as profit-hungry "charlatans" and "cultists," operating out of barber shops and athletic clubs, who, in the guise of being physical therapists, were prescribing treatments and claiming cures for imaginary diseases. The council also warned that unscrupulous practitioners often used physical therapy to satisfy the "treatment habit" of undesirable and incurable patients whose bills were paid under state industrial compensation laws. Unethical and unscientific practices like these, the council said, not only tarnished reputable PTs but undoubtedly took business away from mainstream physicians and surgeons. The council promised to keep everyone apprised of the worrisome situation.

### Schooling And Curricula

From APA's vantage, the strongest weapon in maintaining professional standards was educational training. The original APA Constitution limited membership to graduates of "recognized schools of physiotherapy." But nothing was said at the time concerning who should give recognition or on what basis. The army's War Emergency Training Courses had received de facto recognition, but these programs had been discontinued in peacetime. In their wake had come a jumble of good and bad post-war programs and apprenticeships, with predictably unstandardized results.

Miles Breuer, a physician practicing in Lincoln, Nebraska, represented the quintessence of the problem. He wrote in the January 1926 issue of the *American Journal of Physical Therapy* that while the ideal person to do the hands-on "messing and puttering" of physical therapy might be a "nurse" with special training, they were too expensive for the typical physician.

Not to worry, he said, "Making connections, applying electrodes, waiting around for patients to dress and undress, and watching the clock . . . requires no high degree of skill." He advised his colleagues to take a girl "fresh from clerical office work, without any knowledge whatever of medical work," and teach her "something new each day" under close supervision, after which she would be quite capable of carrying out any physician's prescription unattended. Breuer's only reservation was that the newly minted "technicians" not be given "any ideas of what specific diseases are treated by the different modalities" for fear that they might try diagnosing and treating on their own. These paragons of medical assistance, he noted in closing, could be had for about $12 a week, which was one-third to one-fifth the cost of their school-trained counterparts!

APA members, by contrast, thought that the oncoming generations of physical therapists should be required to have at least two years of physical education or nursing training, to which was added successful completion of a specialized course in the various modalities of physical therapy. It was not enough to require it for their members, of course. They needed hospitals, government agencies, and individual physicians to make such standards a requisite of employment. Lacking the necessary clout to make this happen on their own, they asked the AMA Council on Physical Therapy for help both in accrediting physical therapy training programs and in educating physicians to be more selective in the physiotherapists they brought into their practice.

To get things rolling, the APA Executive Committee named a Committee on Education and Publicity in late 1926 to draw up a minimum standard curriculum for schools offering a complete course in physical therapy. The report, which would not be completed until 1928, recommended a course length of nine months, consisting of 33 hours of physical therapy-related instruction per week for a total of 1,200 hours. The entrance requirement for the specialized course was graduation from a recognized school of physical education or nursing.

Coincident with the work of the Committee on Education and Publicity, physiotherapist Lucile Grunewald, assistant director of the Department of Physical Education for Women at the University of California, Los Angeles, undertook her own extensive "Study of Physiotherapy as a Vocation." Presented as "the first [thesis], as far as we know, on Physiotherapy as a profession," the work was designed to provide a rational basis by which UCLA could develop its own program leading to a bachelor's degree in physiotherapy. The editorial board of the *Review* was so impressed with the content of Grunewald's study that it published the work in three parts, beginning in October 1928.

Like the committee, Grunewald was looking for an ideal standard for educational requirements, but unlike the volunteers who worked at the task in their spare time, Grunewald had the facilities and support to carry out the task in impressive detail. Her approach was to send questionnaires to 236 "successful" physiotherapists throughout the United States to ask them what their educational backgrounds were, what subjects they regarded as absolutely essential to their work, and where, in their view, their own educational training had fallen short. She also included a series of questions to assess her respondents' subsequent professional development, including the nature of their practice and what sort of modus vivendi they had worked out with physicians regarding who determined the specific treatments for patients. Grunewald also interviewed numbers of physicians as to how they worked with physiotherapists. And she surveyed those states and cities in which legislation controlled in any way the practice of physiotherapy. In each category of investigation the answers added up to the same conclusion. The phrase that best described the profession of physical therapy in the United States in 1928 was "anything goes."

Based on her studies, Grunewald was in accord with the APA committee's minimum curriculum standards, but she disagreed on the matter of where those courses could best be taken. She argued that current schools of physical education and nursing consistently fell short in one or more particulars — they failed to attract fully qualified instructors, they taught the management of apparatuses but not their underlying actions, or they treated the physiotherapy parts of their curriculum almost as an afterthought, scheduling classes late in the day for students already fatigued by stints of nursing duty. She proposed that a far more favorable environment would be a university offering a four-year course of study that included liberal arts, fundamental science courses, and specialized physiotherapy education. Not only would the extended course provide the student with the necessary scientific background, she suggested, but it would allow the student to develop "mature judgment, vision, imagination, and other qualities which come only with time and a liberal education." She concluded that in the very process of requiring students to meet the highest educational standards, only the best candidates would survive. "If a generous admixture of literature and social sciences are necessary to humanize a doctor, they are also necessary for a physiotherapist."

The *Review*'s editors, in presenting Grunewald's proposal, called it "an encouragement and inspiration to all," but for the moment they found its prescriptions unrealistic. Physical therapy was still too young to demand a university degree of all who practiced. They held out the hope that such standards might apply in the future. Meanwhile, the Committee on Education and Publicity sent a draft of its own curriculum plan for review to schools from which large numbers of members had graduated. Copies were also sent to the AMA's Council on Physical Therapy and to its Council on Medical Education and Hospitals. And to further validate its work, early in 1930 the committee sent some of its members on a three-month tour of all the schools whose current or planned curricula seemed to meet or exceed its standards.

Reporting to the ninth Annual Conference in Detroit that summer, the committee had found 11 schools that met or exceeded its minimum standards: the New Haven School of Physiotherapy, the Philadelphia Orthopedic Hospital, the Los Angeles Children's Hospital, Northwestern Medical School, Battle Creek Sanitarium, Harvard Medical School Courses 441 and 442, Walter Reed General Hospital, Tacoma General Hospital, the hospital schools of the Universities of Michigan and Wisconsin, and the Boston School of Physical Education.

Approved essentially as written, the curriculum and the list of qualified schools were subsequently published in the *Journal of the American Medical Association* with the urgent request that AMA members follow its recommendations in hiring. As APA found itself in the uncomfortable position of being both judge and jury in approving schools, and as some of the schools objected to the Association assuming responsibilities ordinarily vested in "a more authoritative body," the AMA's Council on Medical Education and Hospitals was eventually persuaded to step into the role. When an updated list of 14 approved schools appeared in 1934, it was over the signature of the AMA. APA, while recognizing that the subject of an acceptable educational standard would never be finished, was very pleased finally to have set a baseline. Approved at this time were Stanford University Hospital; the Hospital for Ruptured and Crippled, New York; and the College of William and Mary, Williamsburg, Virginia.

### "What's In A Name?"

Another issue that arose in the 1920s and that would continue to vex the Association for years to come was what members should call themselves professionally. To factions inside and, more importantly, factions outside, the terms "Physiotherapist," "Physiotherapeutist," "Physical Therapist," and "Physical Therapy Technician" were all fighting words.

The debate was fueled principally by a relatively small group of physician specialists who treated acute and chronic diseases using physical modes of treatment such as electro-therapeutics, ultraviolet light, and diathermy. Searching about for a sector and mode of practice that would clearly distinguish them from competing medical specialties, and most especially from orthopedists, with whom they crossed most often, the so-called "electro-therapeutists" formally laid claim to the term "physiotherapist."

With the newly formed American Congress of Physical Therapy as their parent organization, the physicians began a campaign to persuade members of APA to give up their current name on the grounds that the term could apply only to persons with medical school education. The public, they said, was accustomed to any professional title ending in "ist" belonging to a physician, as in "radiologist" and "neurologist." The congress suggested as preferable for members of APA the designation "physiotherapy technician."

Members of APA, feeling a practical necessity to get along with the physiotherapist-physicians, gave the sensitive subject a fair hearing. The Executive Committee consulted medical dictionaries and also queried the AMA Council on Physical Therapy for an opinion; in addition, APA asked a number of orthopedist friends if the physicians' complaint had validity. Not surprisingly, most respondents recommended that APA go along with the request, if only because the former electro-therapeutists outranked them. One of the few physicians to urge the APA to stand its ground was Rochester orthopedist Ralph Fitch, who commented that APA already had a perfectly good name and should keep it. He added mischievously, "If all physicians were as meticulous in their work as they are in their criticisms, humanity would be much better off."

A special advisory committee of APA convened to consider a suitable response to the medical men. Jessie Wright, on the faculty of the D. T. Watson School in Pennsylvania, spoke for many when she found the designation "technician" unacceptable. "Does the word technician carry with it distinction, specific definition, dignity? . . . Does it not suggest mechanically following set technique, which is impossible? . . . Each individual case offers different problems." When all the evidence, pro and con, was in, the question was put to a vote of the membership at the Cleveland Conference in 1926. The "suggestion" was roundly defeated, and the American Physiotherapy Association's professional title was retained.

This act of solidarity was not enough to end the matter, however, and four years later we find the Executive Committee surveying members on the question again. A weary-sounding Dorothea Beck, reporting on the latest contretemps in the May-June 1930 issue of the *Review*, suggested that it was time to stop letting the medical community treat APA members like second-class citizens. "We have in the past served the medical profession with undivided allegiance; we have upheld their hands in the army, in hospital work and in private practice; we have rigorously followed the ethics of our profession and the tenets of our Constitution, and we shall continue to do so. But we also stand for the true dignity of the science of that profession in the American Physiotherapy Association." In a move that finally assured APA legal title to its own name, the American Physiotherapy Association incorporated in the state of Illinois in 1930. At the same time the official emblem — a triangle enclosing the caduceus and the letters "P.T." — was copyrighted, and pins were made up in the Association colors of blue and gold. Still up for grabs, however, was the nomenclature that would distinguish physicians specializing in physical therapy from hands-on physical therapists. Many members of APA had voluntarily decided to accede to the physicians' pressure and were calling themselves "physical therapy technicians," or "PTTs." Such tags would become fairly standardized by the 1940s, with only a handful of APA members continuing to chafe at their implications.

### SHIFTING THE CENTER OF GRAVITY

One leader who remained adamantly and vociferously opposed was Gertrude Beard, who succeeded Beck in 1926. Each of Mollie McMillan's successors had brought something new in terms of personal vision to the organization, but when Gertrude Beard took the reins as the fourth president, it was a signal that more than management style was about to change.

Although elections had been held each year and two nominees had been named to run for each office, it had become an unwritten custom that top officers served two years and that the vice-president conventionally was elected president when the changeover came. It had also been traditional that the leadership was chosen from the East Coast, where the majority of members lived and worked, but as the Association had expanded in numbers and influence and as other chapters had grown in strength, it followed that new talent should be brought into APA's inner circle. The election of Beard and several members of the Executive Committee, all of whom hailed from the Chicago area, thus marked the passing of the baton to the Midwest. And the fact that Hazel Furscott of California was named vice-president was a fairly reliable indicator that the West Coast would have its say soon.

Another sign of evolutionary change within APA was the fact that Beard had not served as a reconstruction aide. A 1909 graduate of Monmouth College of Nursing in Illinois, she had attended the first course in physical therapy at the Pennsylvania Orthopedic Institute and School of Mechanotherapy in Philadelphia in 1914. During World War I she had served as a nurse in the orthopedic section of the Army Nurse Corps, where she had an extended opportunity to observe the work of the physical therapy reconstruction aides. Beard had subsequently attended Harvard's Course 441 in 1920, studying with Janet Merrill. Thus equipped, Beard had gone on to take a position as director of Chicago's first Physical Therapy Department at Wesley Memorial Hospital and subsequently at Northwestern University Medical School. Joining APA in 1924, she demonstrated such leadership qualities that she was elected president without having first served an "apprenticeship" on the Executive Committee.

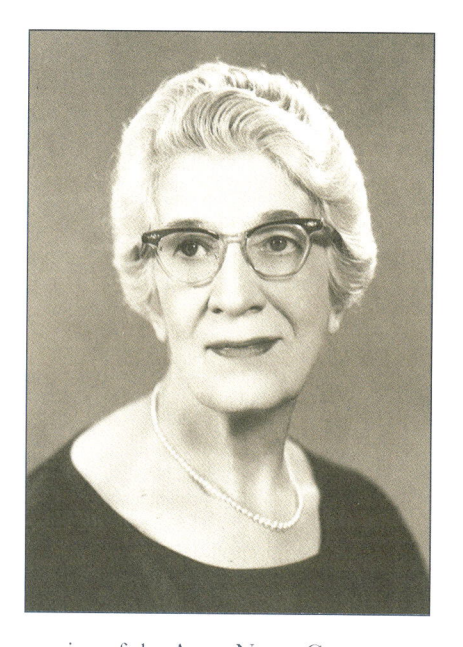

*Gertrude Beard, on the faculty of Northwestern University, began her professional career as a World War I surgical nurse, but a 1920 summer course in physical therapy made her eligible to join as a charter member of the Association. She presided over the Association from 1926 to 1928.*

*With Vision, Faith, And Courage 1920 – 1939* 87

*A 1925 issue of the Walter Reed General Hospital reconstruction aide education program's newsletter includes group photos of the four OTs, top, and 13 PTs, bottom, who graduated that spring. Following World War I, the number of PT graduates from army-sponsored programs each year remained small, creating a severe shortage of PTs at the onset of World War II.*

The Beck-to-Beard transition was anything but easy. Much of what had passed for organization under succeeding Boston regimes had been carried on informally through regular personal contacts at various members' homes, leaving only the most cryptic kinds of written documentation to pass along to the new team. Adding to the problem, retiring president Beck fell ill with pneumonia just when the new midwestern team most urgently needed her help.

Writing to Beck in October, successor Beard reported, "We . . . held a session . . . acquainting ourselves with past records as best we could, and again this afternoon, transacting what business we felt capable of doing." She went on to describe, with barely disguised impatience, the Executive Committee's difficulties in knowing where Association matters stood. "First of all, we are at a loss to know what our Constitution is. Have the proposed amendments as found in your files been adopted? We have not received the minutes of the last two conferences, you see, and it is hard to know just what has been done. On what standards are the accredited schools based? Why is the New York School not in the list? None of us know anything about it, but find many [membership] applications from its graduates. What foreign associations are given reciprocity? Are members from the Canadian Association taken without question? What schools of physical education are on the list? . . . Is the advisory committee a standing one or is it appointed by each new Executive Committee?"

Despite the early confusions, Beard and the Executive Committee soon took hold, and changes began appearing in virtually every facet of APA business. The *P.T. Review*, for example, underwent several changes during Beard's tenure: in September 1926 it took a new, more formal name as the *Physiotherapy Review*; the following March, after Frances Moreaux resigned as editor, it came under the steady hand of Dorothea Beck; and in August 1928 it became a bimonthly journal. Because the gathering of news items from chapters had always been an uncertain process — like "pulling a cat across a rug," said one frustrated editor — the Executive Committee decreed that henceforth each issue would be a collaborative affair with a specific chapter designated to oversee a portion of the content. Beard suggested that any chapter that failed to come up with a good accounting of itself when called to publish faced the ignominy of having its issue go out with the pages blank!

In step with the Association's growing professionalism, the *Physiotherapy Review*'s editorial content became

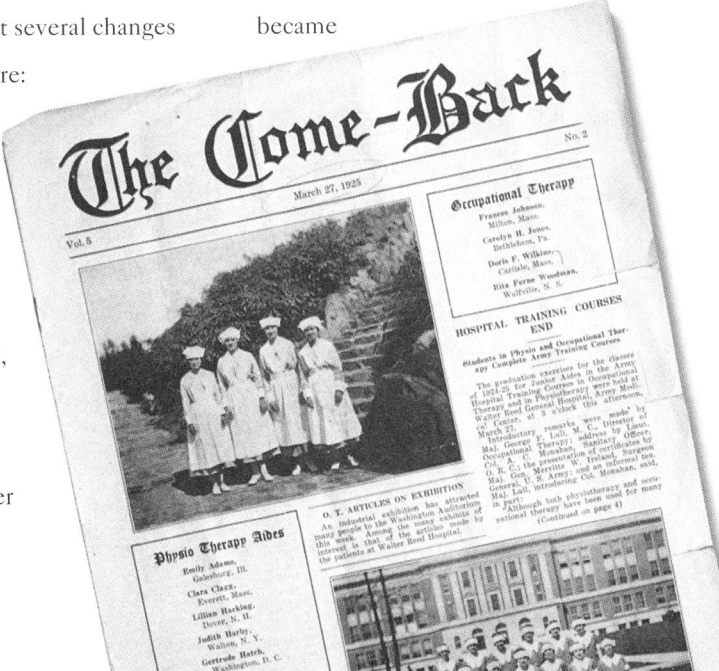

88 *Healing The Generations*

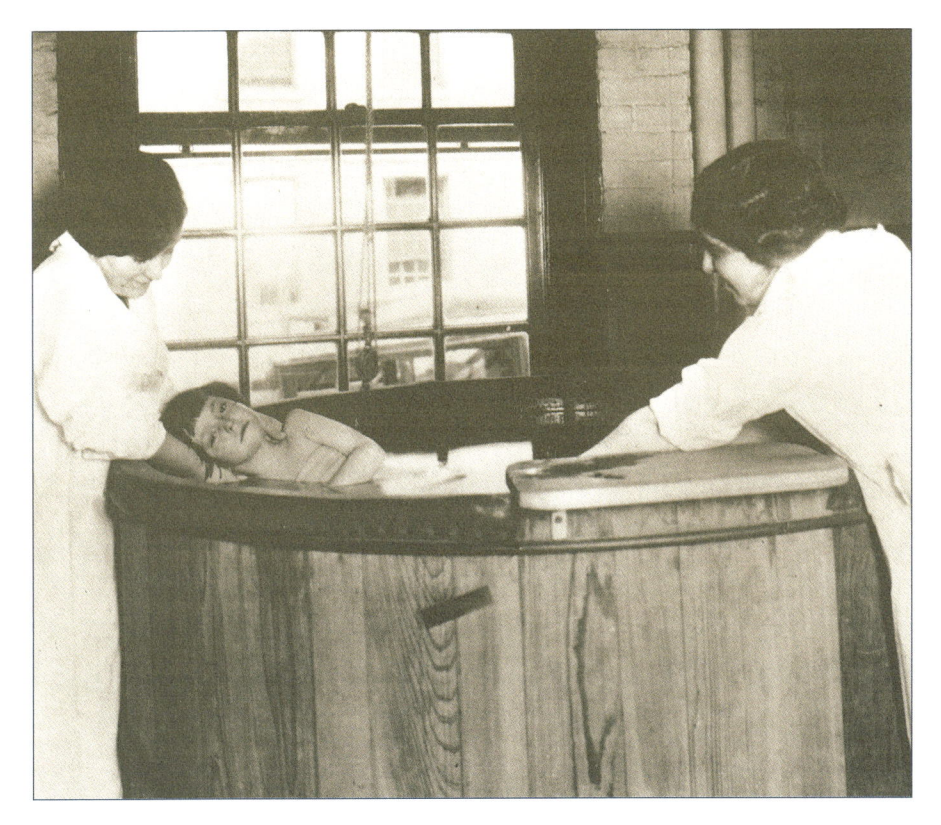

more substantive and scientific. Ida May Hazenhyer, surveying the articles between 1926 and 1930, gives us a sense of issues at the forefront of practice in those years. The most popular topics in order of frequency were: electrotherapy, with fifteen entries; physical therapy as a profession, with eleven; posture, ten; hydrotherapy, seven; "spastic" (a category that included hemiplegia and cerebral palsy), seven; poliomyelitis, six; arthritis, five; ultraviolet therapy, five. Surprisingly, fractures and massage were treated only three times each. And such topics as head and spinal cord injuries were scarcely noted at all.

That many APA members were beginning to see research and writing as part of their professional growth is indicated by the roster of contributors: between 1926 and 1930, 40 articles were member-written. Typical of the high caliber of submissions was Rosalie Donaldson's 1927 paper on "The Importance of Position in the Examination of Muscles." Not only did she footnote her sources, a rarity in the *Review* in those years even among physician-written studies, but she also went beyond clinical observation to analyze scientifically the significance of her findings. Another notable offering was Agnes Sussdorf's article on preventive physical therapy in the workplace. In explaining her work for a forward-looking industrial company, she said: "The aim here is to *keep* the employee well instead of to *get* him well." "Wellness," as the approach would come to be called, was very much a novel notion then.

Further adding to the value and authoritativeness of the *Review* in these years were the abstracts of relevant physical therapy literature from other journals. Selected and written by John Stanley Coulter, a former World War I physical therapy physician and medical director of Beard's physiotherapy program at Northwestern University, the abstracts appeared in every issue, save one, from December 1928 to Coulter's death in 1949. All told, Coulter's contributions would amount to some 183 abstracts!

*Early pool therapy at Boston Children's Hospital is demonstrated here by Director Janet Merrill, right, and her assistant, Eleanor Gillespie, left. The youngster, who had contracted polio, was tenderly lowered into warm water, after which guided muscle reeducation procedures were begun.*

# An Ideal Physical Therapy Department

*Alpine light treatment, dispensed with a floor-standing high-energy bulb, was but one of the standard pieces of equipment recommended for a modern physical therapy department by Coulter. Notably, in this photo the physical therapist is wearing protective goggles, demonstrating increasing awareness of safety procedures.*

In 1928 the *American College of Surgeons Bulletin* published John Stanley Coulter's "Minimum Standard for a Physical Therapy Department of a General Hospital." It provides a comprehensive view of the goals, if not the realities, of the PT's institutional working environment in the years before World War II. Under "location and space," for example, Coulter thought facilities should have adequate southern exposure to accommodate a sizable glass-walled sunroom and be easily accessible from hospital wards and the street. Floor covering should be linoleum or some other resilient material, as cement is tiring and apt to be damp, risking shocks around electrical equipment. Treatment rooms should have at least one electrical outlet and a call system so that the unattended patient could summon help if needed.

Under "equipment," Coulter cautioned against being swept away by appearance. Always more important than fancy appliances in determining "the value of the service rendered . . . is the knowledge of its personnel." He then produced the following basic list, costing some $3,500. He said it would equip a space of 30 x 24 feet and would enable one technician to treat 16 to 20 patients per day, and two technicians to treat as many as 50 daily.

## *Massage, Muscle Training, and Therapeutic Exercise*

4 Treatment Tables with Pads
1 Mirror on Stand for Posture Training
1 Wheel for Shoulder Exercise
1 Sayre Head Sling
1 Wrist Cone
2 Pr. Light Dumb Bells

1 Ankle Exerciser
1 Shoulder Abduction Ladder
1 Rowing Machine
1 Foot Inversion Tread
1 Table for Hand Exercise (complete)
1 Pronation and Supination Exerciser
APPROXIMATE COST. . . .$294.00

## Ultraviolet Radiation

1 Ultraviolet Radiation Combination
1 Quartz Lamp Outfit
1 Adapter
1 Prism Applicator, Medium
3 Localizers (1/2, 3/4, and 1 inch)
1 Quartz Pencil Applicator, 2 3/4 x 1/8 inches
1 Quartz Rod, 2 3/4 x 1/4 inches
2 Quartz Applicators (1 Nasal, 1 Pharyngeal)
APPROXIMATE COST. . .$1,234.00

## For High Frequency, Galvanic, and Sinusoidal Currents

1 Galvanic and Sinusoidal Machine and Mobile Cabinet Stand
2 High Frequency Machines and Mobile Cabinet Stands
2 Lamps and 1500 Watt Bulbs on Floor Stand
1 Electro-diagnostic Set
3 Metal Handle Electrodes
2 Spongio-Pilene Electrodes, Rubber Insulated, 3 inch
2 Spongio-Pilene Disc Electrodes with Stud, 1/2 inch
4 Dispersive Electrodes (2@4x6;1@6x8;1@10x12 inches)
2 Pr. 8 foot Electrode Cords
2 Threaded Adapters
2 Multiple Cord Connectors, Insulated
2 Universal Handles only
2 Interval Timers
4 Pure Gum-Rubber Bandages, 3 inches x 3 yards
5 Lbs. Electrode Foil
6 Electrode Clip Connectors
1 Complete Set Aluminum Needles with Handle
1 Large Metal Handle Electrode
1 Attachment Cord with Threaded Connection
2 Bifurcated High Frequency Cords
1 Auto-Condensation Couch Cushion
APPROXIMATE COST. . .$1,850.00

## Whirlpool Bath Room

1 Leg Whirlpool Bath
1 Arm Whirlpool Bath with Stand
APPROXIMATE COST. . .$150.00

As for personnel, Coulter reminded his readers, "Hospitals that have gone into physical therapy with the idea of only machine therapy will come out of it with a bitter feeling toward the whole subject and their machines will soon be covered with dust." He urged that the hospitals accept nothing less than the very best in trained "physical therapy technicians," and professed that the best were invariably members of APA. He also strongly recommended that the department be under the supervision of a physician, whose compensation ought to be based on an 85 percent share of the net profits, the remainder going to the hospital. "This keeps the hospital out of competitive medicine, keeps the physician interested in keeping down expenses, and gives him practically all the profit!"

**CONSTITUTION AND BYLAWS**

During the first winter, the Beard team also drafted a revised Constitution and Bylaws, the organization's third set of regulations, and they were passed the following summer. The new Constitution was longer by several articles, more exacting in language, and incorporated numerous changes in the governance of the Association. Under "Purpose," it included a very specific statement regarding the ethical relationship of physical therapists to the medical profession, namely, "to cooperate with, or under, the direction of the medical profession." PTs had always subscribed to this policy, and during the war it had been institutionalized in the military routine, but the APA leadership was concerned that in the more diverse venues of civilian physical therapy practice, the principle needed restatement.

Two-year terms were instituted for all officers, with elections to be held in even calendar years. The status of chapters was further enhanced. No longer were members polled individually when voting on policy at annual meetings. Rather, votes were taken by chapters. A chapter having 10 or fewer members was apportioned one delegate vote; 15 members earned two votes, and still larger chapters were entitled to an additional vote for every additional 10 members. Unaffiliated members-at-large, of which there were still substantial numbers, could also participate in the voting according to the same formula through caucuses formed on the floor.

Membership qualifications were tightened. "Active" members had to have worked a full year at physical therapy within two years of graduating from an approved training program. This change meant that any reconstruction aide who had taken an extended leave from practicing physical therapy after the war would no longer be accepted outright; she would have to take an approved refresher course before applying. (Leaves of absence are an old tradition with physical therapists. Former reconstruction aide Ruby Decker, for example, had tried her hand at selling books and auto parts and at raising chickens before settling down to a distinguished career as a physical therapist. Others had left the profession briefly to marry and raise children.)

New categories of membership were introduced. "Junior" members were persons who qualified for membership in every particular save a year's experience; applicants fresh out of school were thus given two years' grace to qualify fully for active status. Graduates of foreign schools were approved if they had graduated from a school or program approved by the Chartered Society in England. And the definition of "Associate" members was expanded from physicians only to include those educators and scientists who had made major contributions to the knowledge and practices of physical therapy. Perhaps as a reflection of these changes, APA's membership rolls began to increase again. Eleven more chapters were officially admitted, bringing the number to 16. Among the second generation of chapters were Minnesota, Northern California, Southern California, Oregon, Rhode Island, Wisconsin, the District of Columbia, Washington, Michigan, New Jersey, and Texas. All told, APA counted 292 members in 1927 and 394 in 1928. The Executive Committee felt confident enough of APA's stability to raise annual dues to $5.

The 1927 Constitution was also accompanied by three new Bylaws. One established standing committees, another gave its blessings to Robert's Rules of Order as parliamentary authority, and a third dealt somewhat ominously with "Discipline." Anyone found guilty of violating APA's rules of professional conduct could be "suspended at any time by a majority vote of the Executive Committee" following a "trial" held before the Executive Committee. Expulsion was possible following a unanimous vote of displeasure.

One of the new standing committees created was charged with investigating state licensure practices. Two states already had laws licensing physical therapists — Pennsylvania since 1913 and New York since 1926. A few others had provisions embedded within their general medical practice acts, but in most parts of the country there were few if any laws concerning the legal status of anyone other than physicians, surgeons, and nurses. It was not that the Association wanted to promote more legislation on its behalf. To the contrary, the Executive Committee had come to believe that state legislation governing the profession was neither attainable nor desirable. The country was simply too large, the issues too diverse, the individual legislative bodies too difficult to work with, and the Association still lacking in sufficient clout to achieve what it might wish for. "Get into politics," the Executive Committee was counseled by a member of the AMA Council on Physical Therapy, "and you will find yourself tossed into the soup with the cults, the 'paths,' and countless other drugless healers from whom you wish to separate yourselves. The consequences are likely to be unpredictable at best, and very possibly you will end up worse off than you began."

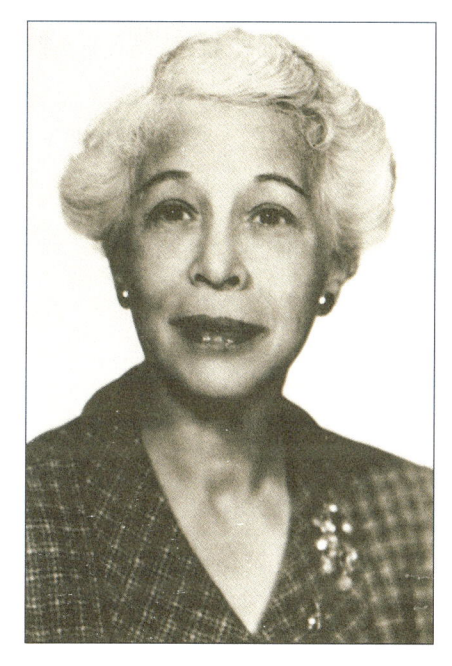

At the same time, the Association could not ignore the fact that licensing requirements were sometimes forced upon members, and being prepared to fight defensively when they were unreasonable was only prudent. Ida May Hazenhyer, in her colorful "History of the American Physical Therapy Association" written in 1946, told of one member whose city ordinances required her to be licensed in one of the existing classifications, which did not include physical therapy per se. When the member declined to be classed as either a masseuse or a barber, the exasperated city official told her that the only other choice was to be a cosmetician. Left with no recourse, the embattled member paid the fee. In doing so, she earned the right to apply make-up, give Russian baths, dress hair, apply manicures, or do anything else that might conceivably enhance her clients' condition, which in her case included using her own fine skills as a physical therapist.

*California-based Hazel Furscott, president of the Association from 1928 to 1930, was the first leader chosen from the western states. A former reconstruction aide at Letterman Hospital, Furscott had also headed the Physical Therapy Department at the University of California Hospital before going into private practice.*

*Edith Munro, the sixth president of the Association and a Bostonian, served during a somewhat fractious period for the young and growing organization. In her acceptance speech, Munro reminded members that "Nothing can grow that is continually being torn down.... We must have ready... something with which to rebuild."*

APA's mandate to the Standing Committee on Licensing was to be on the alert for pending legislation that might make the lives of members more difficult and to help state and local chapters mount effective opposition before such proposals were cast into law. During the next few years, APA had frequent reason to be glad of the committee's vigilance.

### "Second Growth"

As APA moved toward its second decade of life, members could feel flushed with the pride of accomplishment. Although the Association was still very young, enormous strides already had been made. Membership was growing in both numbers and professionalism, the *Physiotherapy Review* was widely read and admired for the quality of its articles, and virtually all of the founders' far-sighted objectives were in the process of being addressed. Most importantly, perhaps, the validity of physical therapy as an essential partner of medicine and surgery was gaining public recognition. So many achievements might have engendered smug satisfaction in another group, but for a new generation of APA leaders, they became baselines on which to set still more ambitious goals for the future.

What was not anticipated, however, was a pair of calamities that would soon bring a redirection in the structure of United States health care and consequently in the affairs of the American Physiotherapy Association. The first was the growing severity of anterior poliomyelitis and the efforts to combat its terrible aftereffects. The second was the Great Depression of 1929. In the 1930s the two circumstances became intertwined.

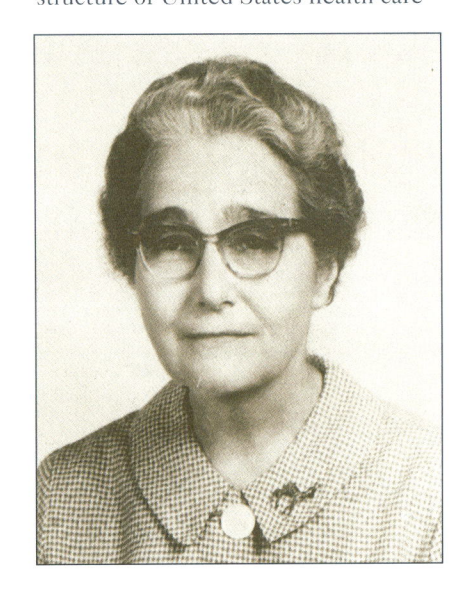

That poliomyelitis should play a significant role in the shaping of APA's history during this period was perhaps not so surprising after all. Such a role had existed earlier in the century when isolated epidemics of this infectious disease had first struck. In subsequent decades it had only become a greater scourge. Indeed, not a single year had passed since the terrible summer of 1916 that did not bring another well-publicized incidence of "infantile paralysis," as it was commonly known. While Lovett and Merrill were still considered the leading authorities on polio, there were numbers of orthopedists in other parts of the country who were coming up fast. In Los Angeles there was Charles Lowman, who studied with Lovett at Boston Children's Hospital, then founded the Los Angeles Orthopedic Hospital in 1919, and subsequently became director of the Physical Therapy Program at the University of Southern California. Lowman was a pioneer in the use of warm-water exercises, or "hydrogymnastics," as he called them. The idea seems to have been prompted by a visit to Chicago's Spaulding School for Crippled Children in 1923, where a rudimentary wooden exercise tank was in use. Soon after the visit, Lowman converted his own hospital's lily pond into two pools for the treatment of orthopedic patients. Lowman had as his resident Susan Roen, an early member of APA. She would subsequently write, with Lowman and with fellow physical therapists Ruth Aust and Helen Paull, the influential *Technique of Underwater Gymnastics* in 1937.

In Baltimore, physicians George Bennett and Robert W. Johnson of The Johns Hopkins University School of Medicine, began working with Henry Kendall of the Children's Hospital School in the early 1920s to develop pioneering techniques in examination and aftercare of poliomyelitis. (Kendall, who was partially blinded in World War I, had been trained in therapeutic massage at the Red Cross School for the Blind in Baltimore.) And in New York, Leroy Hubbard, an orthopedic surgeon in New York's State Department of Health, had become an authority on polio aftercare.

Although children remained the most vulnerable to polio, the most prominent victim in the years between the world wars was a 39-year-old adult named Franklin Delano Roosevelt. Roosevelt developed paralytic polio in his legs and lower trunk in August 1921 while vacationing at Campobello, his summer retreat off the Maine coast. First treated by Robert Lovett and subsequently by George Draper in New York, Roosevelt worked arduously for more than two years to recover his mobility. Despite experiments with hot- and cold-water exercises, electrotherapy, heliotherapy, osteopathy, and Emil Coué's course in "positive thinking," the once-vigorous politician succeeded only in gaining the use of a wheelchair. Such a life, for someone with ambitions to national political life, was unacceptable.

In 1924 Roosevelt heard that a fellow polio patient had made a substantial recovery from paralysis after treatment in the curative waters of Warm Springs, Georgia. With renewed hope, Roosevelt went there to swim and exercise for six weeks; and indeed, he did make progress, getting up onto crutches successfully for the first time. Roosevelt's spirits soared, and with the cautious encouragement of medical friends, he invested the better part of his personal fortune in the purchase of the dilapidated old Warm Springs resort. Here he planned to build a center for the hydrotherapeutic care of "polios" like himself. Roosevelt then persuaded his former law partner, Basil O'Connor, to manage the establishment, which was to be called the Georgia Warm Springs Foundation. Shortly after, Roosevelt reentered the political arena.

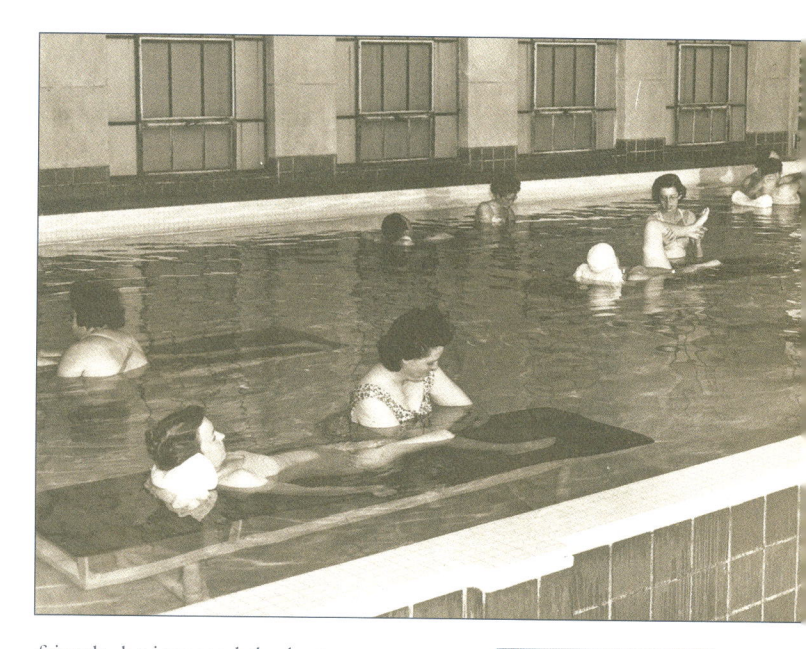

The combination of Roosevelt's charisma and O'Connor's organizational skills proved a great boon to the treatment of polio. Favorable publicity attracted financial contributors and large

*The Georgia Warm Springs Foundation, established during Franklin D. Roosevelt's presidency, treated 61 patients its first year. Like Roosevelt, patients came there "to swim the way to health" in its warm waters and beautiful surroundings. Here, several patients are treated simultaneously by therapists.*

*With Vision, Faith, And Courage 1920 – 1939*

*Alice Lou Plastridge, who had successfully treated Franklin D. Roosevelt during his rehabilitation, was invited to Warm Springs to succeed Helen Mahoney as Supervisor of Physical Therapists in 1929. She remained at the facility for more than 20 years.*

numbers of patients to the center in the early years, as many as 70 at a time. And it also drew many talented physicians and physical therapists to the work. Leroy Hubbard became the center's first medical director, bringing with him Helena Mahoney as chief of the physical therapy treatments. Mahoney was a public health nurse, but she had studied with Lovett in Boston and was trained in muscle testing. She in turn recruited several new graduates from nearby Peabody College, a leading school for physical education in the South. None of the graduates had ever treated polio before, but they were well versed in swimming, anatomy, and kinesiology, and they made a cohesive, teachable team. First came 19-year-old Mary Hudson Veeder, then 10 other Peabody graduates including Lucille Daniels, who would go on to become a major figure in the profession, earning degrees from Northwestern and Stanford and coauthoring with Catherine Worthingham the highly acclaimed textbooks *Muscle Testing* (1946) and *Therapeutic Exercise* (1957). Daniels also served in numerous leadership roles with the American Physical Therapy Association in the 1940s and 1950s.

A later arrival was Alice Lou Plastridge. Plastridge was already an experienced physical therapist in the field of polio. Born in Vermont and trained in "corrective gymnastics," she had worked for a time in Boston with Wilhelmine Wright and Robert Lovett in the care of patients with polio before going into her own private practice in Chicago in 1917. In 1926 Lovett recommended her to the Roosevelts, and she spent a month at Roosevelt's home in Hyde Park, New York, giving him intensive treatment in muscle reeducation. Returning to Chicago, she took on the polio aftercare of Margaret Pope, the adult daughter of wealthy hosiery manufacturer Henry Pope.

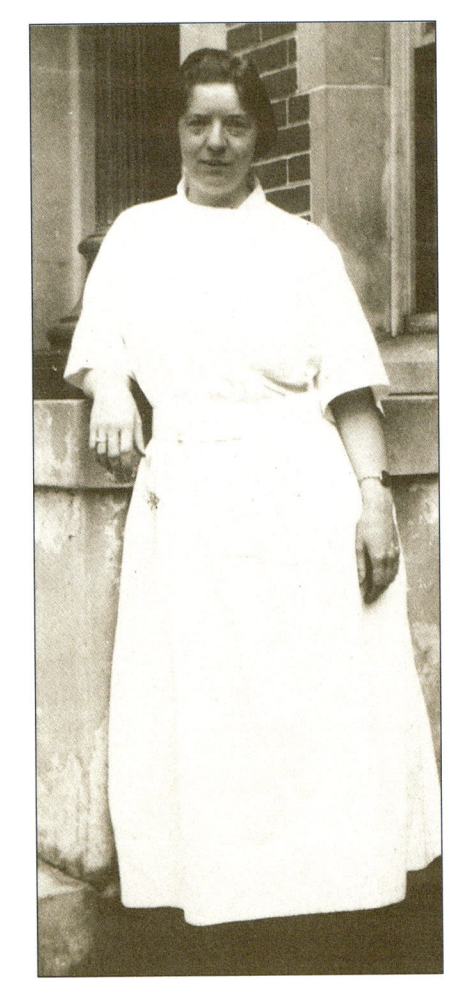

Henry Pope, through his concern for making young Peggy's life more comfortable, would have a tremendous influence not only on the course of Plastridge's career, but on several practical aspects of polio care in those years. Pope had met Roosevelt in Boston, where the future president and Margaret were both being fitted for braces. In those days, application of leg braces took three to four weeks from measurement to final fitting, with the resulting hand-forged parts being exceedingly heavy. After observing the work in Boston, Pope came away determined to see the product improved. He engaged John Klenzak, his most inventive mechanic, to study the problem. Klenzak, who worked at

*Healing The Generations*

the hosiery mill's Paramount Textile Machinery Company in Kankakee, Illinois, soon came up with a brace that substituted aircraft construction tubing for the traditional forged steel, thereby cutting the weight in half. Klenzak figured out the means to manufacture prefabricated parts to speed up the fitting and assembly process. He also devised a toe-lift feature that simulated normal gait: on the heel strike the toe went down and on the swing-through it lifted again, thereby preventing the walker from stubbing a toe or tripping. Pope never patented the Klenzak brace, and for years his Pope Foundation supplied them on a non-profit basis to individuals at a cost in the neighborhood of $50 per leg. When other brace manufacturers complained that he was putting them at a competitive disadvantage, Henry Pope formed the Pope Brace Division as a commercial subsidiary of Paramount. It was eventually bought by Parke-Davis, the pharmaceutical company, and sold off again in the 1970s.

The Pope Foundation, however, continued to be active in polio research. With its assistance, Pope ran a free orthopedic clinic one Sunday each month at the Paramount facility to which anyone could come for treatment and brace fittings. Pope also underwrote the research and production of the original Hubbard tank, which was named for Carl Hubbard, another of Paramount's engineers. (Family lore has it that the tank's distinctive keyhole shape was Margaret Pope's idea.) The first Hubbard tubs were handmade in 1928 at Paramount from the same stainless steel materials used to make hosiery machines.

Pope was a major financial contributor to Roosevelt's Warm Springs, which is how he came to take his daughter there in 1929 and how Alice Lou Plastridge found herself there as well, as an observer during Margaret's treatment. While they were there, Director Mahoney fell ill, and Plastridge was persuaded to take her place as director of physical therapy. She

*Mildred Elson, a physical therapist on the staff of Wisconsin General Hospital in Madison, had the opportunity to experiment with this first version of the Hubbard tank, made by a hosiery company machinist named Carl Hubbard for his employer Henry Pope when Pope's daughter, Margaret, contracted polio.*

97

*Margaret Campbell Winters, a member of the Illinois Chapter, served as president of the Association from 1932 to 1934.*

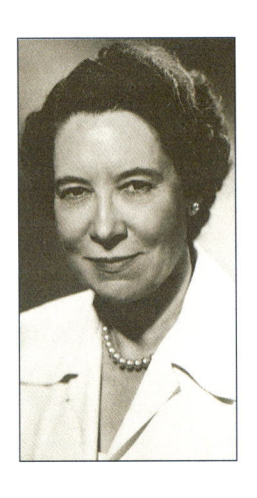

would remain at Warm Springs for 20 years, rising to become technical director of the graduate education program and a much-sought-after demonstrator of polio care in many parts of the world.

As it happened, Plastridge's arrival in Warm Springs occurred on the eve of the Great Depression, and in the dark days thereafter, it began to seem that the foundation might have to close down for lack of funds. Physical therapists elsewhere were also facing uncertain times. Beginning in 1930, diminishing budgets caused many hospitals and private medical practices to reduce or even close their physical therapy services. As the nation's financial crisis deepened, some of the training schools, unable to place their graduates for lack of employment openings, temporarily discontinued courses. Even the army was forced to curtail programs. Walter Reed General Hospital cancelled its 1933 training course and let go 12 of its 15 staff physical therapists. One of these was Florence Peterson (the future Florence P. Kendall). The remaining 34 physical therapists had to be spread among 14 other army hospitals, gamely working extended hours at diminished salaries to keep their programs running.

Not surprisingly, the financial pressures were passed along to APA as members lost jobs or had salaries trimmed. In 1933 the Executive Committee decided to give unemployed members a year's grace in paying their dues. Even so, membership the following year dropped from 774 to 745, and a year later it plummeted to 683. Then, just as the clouds of uncertainty seemed darkest, Franklin Roosevelt was elected the nation's thirty-second president in a landslide. The change in administration brought "A New Deal" both for the care of "polios" and other disabled Americans and, indirectly, for the future of physical therapy.

Most immediately, the Warm Springs Foundation won a new lease on life. In 1933 O'Connor inaugurated the annual "Birthday Ball," held on the anniversary of the president's birth. Ranging from gala affairs at the nation's most fashionable hotels to wheelchair "dances" at Warm Springs, the hugely successful parties raised more than a million dollars each year for the work at the rehabilitation center. As this was more money than the center needed, O'Connor looked for a way to extend the program's reach, and in 1937 the National Foundation for Infantile Paralysis (NFIP) was inaugurated. Still more money began rolling in, literally, via the "March of Dimes" coin collection campaign, which was launched in 1938. As a result the NFIP was able to inject sizable sums of money into hundreds of local facilities engaged in some facet of polio aftercare. It was also able to lend essential equipment to needy families and hospitals in many parts of the country. (Notably, the NFIP bought and loaned out hundreds of the body-encasing mechanical respirators familiarly known as "iron lungs." Invented in 1928 by Philip Drinker, an engineer on staff at the Harvard School of Public Health, to treat acute carbon monoxide poisoning among gas company employees, the device became a life-saver for patients with bulbar and spino-bulbar polio.)

APA member Lucy Blair, who was intimately involved in polio aftercare in these years, recalled the effect of the first Birthday Ball and NFIP fund distribution on one midwestern city: "Approximately $900 was raised to be used locally. Three facilities were providing physical therapy services for polio patients, so the money was divided in thirds; $300 was a tremendous gift in those Depression years!"

A far larger "gift" was Congress's passage in 1935 of the Social Security Act, which, along with provisions for unemployment insurance, contained sections devoted to health care and vocational rehabilitation. Of greatest significance to physical therapy was Title V, part 2, under which the Children's Bureau, United States Department of Labor, became responsible for seeing that the individual states extended broader and more consistent services to children with all kinds of crippling conditions. At the time of enactment, 12 states offered a full range of care statewide, although standards generally were ambiguous. In 23 other states, the services were token at best and concentrated in major cities. The remaining states and territories took no official position whatsoever on the care of children and the disabled. Also of enduring significance to physical therapy was the act's Title VI, which provided the United States Public Health Service with the funds and the authority to build a system of state and local health departments and to extend its informational activities.

"In the early thirties," Blair reported, "the acutely ill polio patient was isolated at home unless he happened to live in an urban area that had an 'isolation hospital' with an available bed." Hard-pressed family members did their best to make the patient comfortable under the guidance of the family physician, with perhaps an occasional assist from his nurse. But most children were forced to remain in this condition, their bodies wasting for weeks and months before a place could be found in an orthopedic hospital or convalescent home.

In order to qualify for a share of the $2,850,000 annual grant-in-aid budget that Congress provided to implement the crippled children's program, states had to submit plans that included specific descriptions of how they would carry out the enumeration, screening, diagnosis, hospitalization, and aftercare services of crippled children. They also had to submit their facilities to inspections.

The Children's Bureau, which supervised the federal grants-in-aid program, empaneled a committee of independent professionals to advise on technical issues, and APA sent Mildred Elson. A charter member and the first president of the Wisconsin Chapter from 1932 to 1936, Elson worked persuasively to make APA's own standards of professional training and conduct the bureau's standards as well. This had a pass-along effect on virtually every state, assuring that henceforth physical therapists working for state and local agencies would have to meet APA and AMA prerequisites in regard to education and practical experience.

Almost overnight, hundreds of physical therapists who had found it as difficult as everyone else to work full time during the Great Depression were in a position to pick and choose among positions. (The *Review*, ever the conscience of the organization, reminded members in a November-December 1936 editorial that, while

*Sarah "Sally" U. Colby, active in the Southern California Chapter, led the Association from 1934 to 1936.*

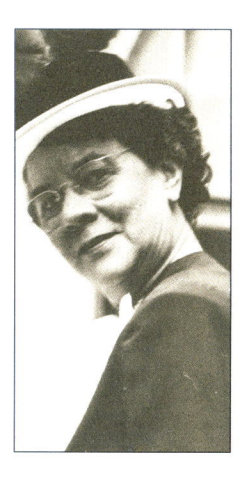

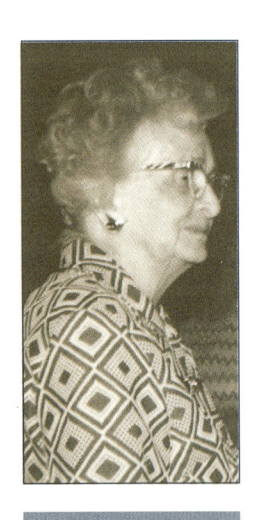

*Constance Greene brought the presidency back to Boston. Greene, pictured here in later years, directed the education program for physical therapists at Bouvé-Boston and led the American Physiotherapy Association from 1936 to 1938.*

improved employment opportunities were welcome, what was more important was the "opportunity to assist in the development of a finer plan for the welfare of the crippled child," a cause for which they had fought unwaveringly since the founding.)

Physical therapists were needed to work in diagnostic clinics, in treatment programs at outpatient centers, in convalescent homes, in orthopedic hospitals, in schools for crippled children, and as instructors of others in supportive and restorative activities. Field work in rural homes was perhaps the most difficult, for the physical therapist had to use all her skills, human and practical, to assist families who were often ill-informed, frightened, and without hope. Going on house-to-house rounds, they carried out muscle tests, taught parents the next crucial steps in muscle reeducation, adapted equipment in the home for the bedridden patient's comfort, and even improvised temporary frames, splints, and braces until proper ones could be fitted at a hospital. One of the leaders in this service was Jessie Stevenson, who was on the supervisory staff of the Visiting Nurse Association of Chicago. Stevenson's knowledge and ability in training others to do polio aftercare were recognized by the NFIP soon after it was established, and she was given one of its first research grants.

Because the great majority of physical therapists delivering polio aftercare worked on their own, without the benefit of regular training and retraining to upgrade technique as more was learned, educational materials were of critical importance. Once again, the Social Security Act became a key factor in seeing that such materials were disseminated. Influential contributions in this category were a monograph and a five-reel film produced by Henry and Florence Kendall under the sponsorship of the United States Public Health Service's Title VI outreach program. USPHS Bulletin #242, *Care During the Recovery Period in Paralytic Polio*, sold for 20 cents and became the standard against which all other systems of examination and aftercare were judged. USPHS funds also helped distribute the Kendalls' five-reel movie on polio aftercare, made in association with the Maryland League for Crippled Children and finished in 1936.

By 1939, when R. C. Hood, M.D., appeared before the Eighteenth Annual Conference of APA in Denver, he was able to report that every one of the 48 states now had a functioning program that in some way addressed the crippled children population, which he estimated at 165,000 youngsters. While many health professionals were involved in the delivery of remedial care, physical therapists were especially in demand because chronic conditions, by definition, required ongoing care. In the most recent year, Hood said, physical therapists had given some 350,000 treatments under Title V's crippled children's program.

Hood concluded his talk to the conference with comments on important work yet to be done. He noted that three groups of children continued to be underserved for lack of understanding. One group was the youngsters with spastic paralysis, by which he meant a heterogeneous group

*Healing The Generations*

of disorders of movement and posture often termed "cerebral palsy." Although cerebral palsy had been recognized as a distinct condition for many years, it had only recently been subjected to study. Hood observed that with the right combination of specialized care, in which the physical therapist was the pivotal person, remarkable gains were possible.

The second and largest group, constituting perhaps three out of four crippled children, according to Hood, comprised young orthopedic patients. Once their crippling deformities were pronounced unamenable to surgery, they were unlikely to be sent to "aftercare," when in fact muscle reeducation directed by the trained physical therapist could rehabilitate them substantially. (Working to reeducate the public and improve the care of these youngsters was the newly organized National Easter Seal Society, which raised $47,000 in its first sale of "penny seals" in 1934.)

The third group, said Hood, comprised the polio patients who were still too often mishandled because anxious parents allowed "irregular practitioners" to overtreat muscles in the acute phase of the disease. Hood urged his audience to develop the kind of research information — what we now know as "outcomes research" — to make every state agency see how critical "intelligent" physical therapy care was to each of these patient groups.

### TYING UP THE LOOSE ENDS

Not surprisingly, the growing recognition of physical therapy's place in health care brought additional challenges to APA and its leadership. Near the top of everyone's agenda was finding some way to lighten the volunteer workload of members of the Executive Committee, whose contributions in unreimbursed time were running an average of 44 hours per month. In 1933, Edith Munro's Constitutional Revisions Committee proposed a management reorganization, the highlight of which was the hiring of a paid executive secretary to handle APA's routine business. The costs, Munro said, would be met by a "temporary" increase in dues, to $8.00. After some fiscal soul searching, the membership agreed, and in 1934 the reorganization became a formal part of APA's fourth Constitution and Bylaws.

Another pressing need, the leadership felt, was having a permanent address to call its own. Even the hiring of an executive secretary had not fixed APA geographically, for the position simply followed the president. The address problem was finally solved in 1938, when the *Review* ceased its migratory career and came to rest in Chicago, replete with a desk, a phone listing, and a part-time editorial assistant to look after things. Ida May Hazenhyer, editor-in-chief at the time,

*In 1934, the Executive Committee met to go over Association business. Shown here, left to right, are Sue Roen, treasurer; Margaret Campbell Winters, Board of Directors and past president; Jefferson Brown, secretary; Sally Colby, president; Catherine Worthingham, vice-president; and Lucille Grunewald, vice-president.*

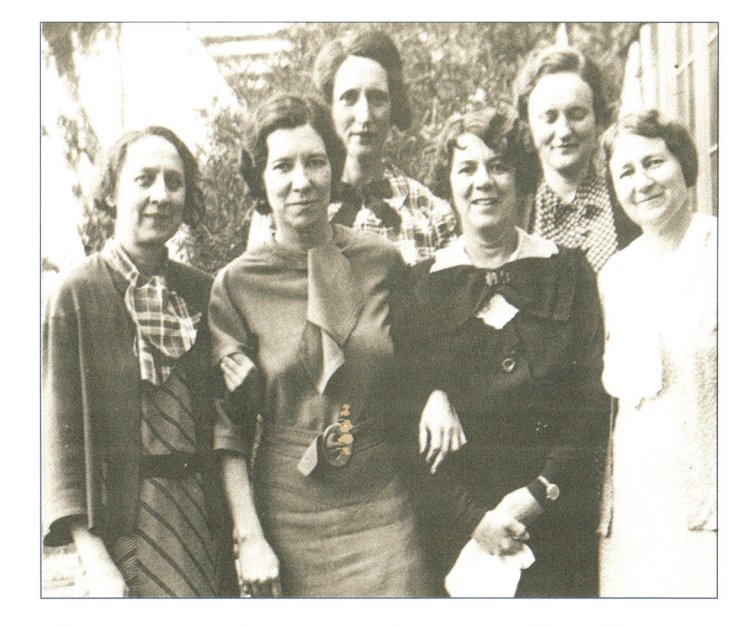

recalled, "This was a day to talk about. . . . Now the entire Association felt that it had 'headquarters' even though the business of the Executive Committee was not transacted there. Members travelling to or through Chicago stopped for visits." The office also became a central location for storing the Association's records, which up to that time had been scattered from Boston basements to San Francisco attics. Still eluding Hazenhyer and her harried colleagues, however, was a reduced workload and the chance to "sit on a cushioned chair, with feet on the desk while directing the work. . . . The midnight candles continued to burn."

One issue that kept APA leaders working late was concern about a professional credentialing process. In the 1920s APA had approached the American College of Physical Therapy, the organization of physicians specializing in the use of therapeutic modalities, for help. But the college's solution — a job bank of sorts — had missed the mark and was soon abandoned. APA approached the physicians again in the early 1930s, and in 1935 a seemingly satisfactory resolution was reached.

With APA's good friend John Coulter as its guiding force, the American Registry of Physical Therapy Technicians was created to examine and certify the competency of physical therapists. Sponsored and controlled by the American Congress of Physical Medicine, the ARPTT took as its standard the minimum educational requirements on which APA and the AMA had previously agreed. Anyone joining APA after June 1935, regardless of prior education or experience, had to pass a written examination in order to use the term "registered" as part of her or his professional title. As a courtesy, all APA members currently enrolled in APA were also deemed "registered." The council held its first examination in September 1935 and some months later sent out impressive-looking certificates to 31 successful applicants. The ARPTT, later recast as the American Registry of Physical Therapists, would continue to serve as an outside accreditation agency until 1976.

If having an outside registry was a sign of approaching professional maturity, so too was the introduction of APA's first "Code of Ethics and Discipline" in 1935. The Code not only expanded upon the primacy of the physician's diagnosis and prescription in carrying out physical therapy treatments, but also prohibited the procurement of patients through advertising as well as the criticism of doctors or colleagues in the presence of patients. Not included in the formal Code, but driven home forcibly in occasional *Review* editorials and articles, were other "ethical" and "moral" issues, such as how to behave around patients. Here, in an article by Christopher McLoughlin, a Fellow in Physical Medicine at the Mayo Clinic, are some gems of advice to the physical therapist: "Never consider an invalid 'a case.' Each sick person is an individual. . . . Always make a point of knowing the name of the patient. . . . Sense when the patient is inclined to be taciturn and do not bore or annoy him with small talk. . . . Do not inflict your personal problems on the patient; they often add to his worries and confusion. . . . Personal cleanliness is an intrinsic requirement for the physical therapy technician. Absolute freedom from bodily odor and a clean and neat appearance are essential. . . . Extreme 'hair-do's' with many curls are as much to be frowned on as uncombed or disarranged hair. . . . The uniform always should be neat, clean and modest. It should fit well enough to insure neatness and yet loosely enough so that there is not too much accent on physical contours. Stockings should not be rolled in such a way that the roll shows below the hem of the uniform. . . . Deep or startling shades of nail polish should not be used. . . . Hands stained from nicotine are unsightly. No jewelry should be worn."

### TRANSCENDING THE MATERIALISTIC

With so much accomplished professionally and the nation's economic picture improving, it was reasonable to suppose that APA's members were finding their own fortunes on the rise. To find out for sure, the Association undertook a survey in 1938, only to discover that despite their advanced education and their responsibilities, members still commanded a median salary of only $1,650, putting them on a par with schoolteachers. According to an article appearing in the May-June 1939 issue of the *Review*, the standard fee paid a physical therapist in the state of Washington was $2 per treatment in the hospital clinic setting.

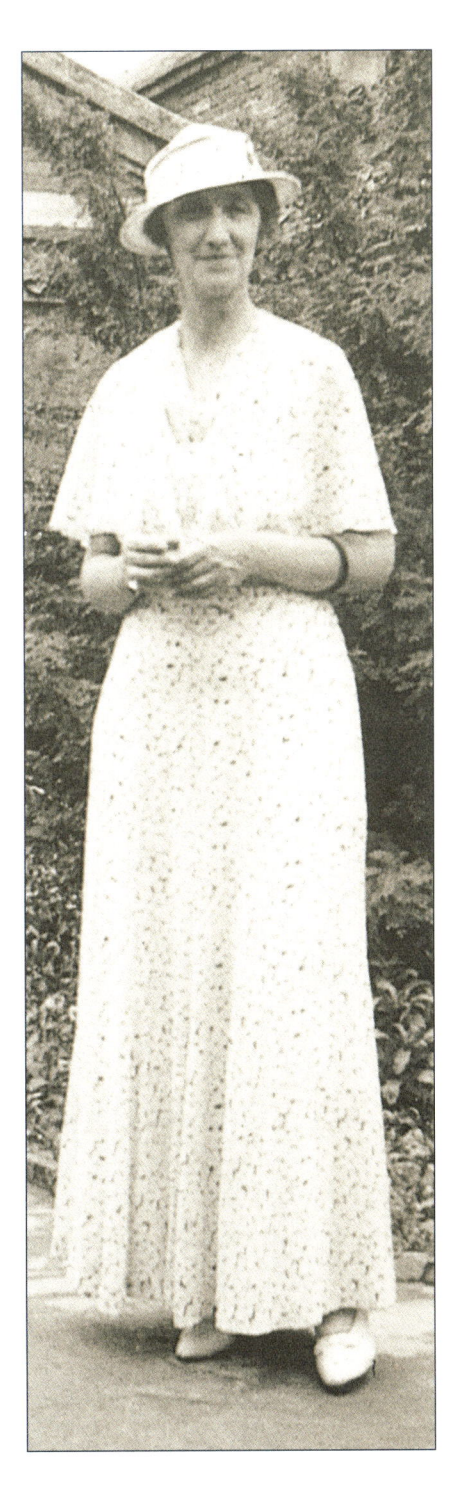

The survey also found that of the 916 members enrolled in 1938, roughly half were employed in hospitals, where the provision of room and board was considered a strong attraction. Ida May Hazenhyer, commenting on the findings in a *Physiotherapy Review* editorial, concluded sadly, "One who anticipates following physical therapy as a vocation does need a vision which can transcend the materialistic."

Mollie McMillan would certainly have agreed. The year before, she had embarked on a challenging assignment at the Peking Union Medical College to train Chinese physiotherapists. Now, as she read Hazenhyer's words in the latest issue of the *Review*, she could hear the occasional sound of enemy gunfire in the distance.

*Mary McMillan poses in the courtyard of Peking Union Medical College for her 1939 Christmas photo. McMillan's letters to APA friends back home inspired others to join the effort to teach, promote, and practice physical therapy abroad.*

CHAPTER 4

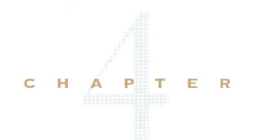

# The World War II Years
# 1939 – 1946

*The start of World War II found Emma Vogel directing the Walter Reed General Hospital education program for physical therapists. Vogel was soon redeployed to direct War Emergency Training Courses at 10 army hospitals.*

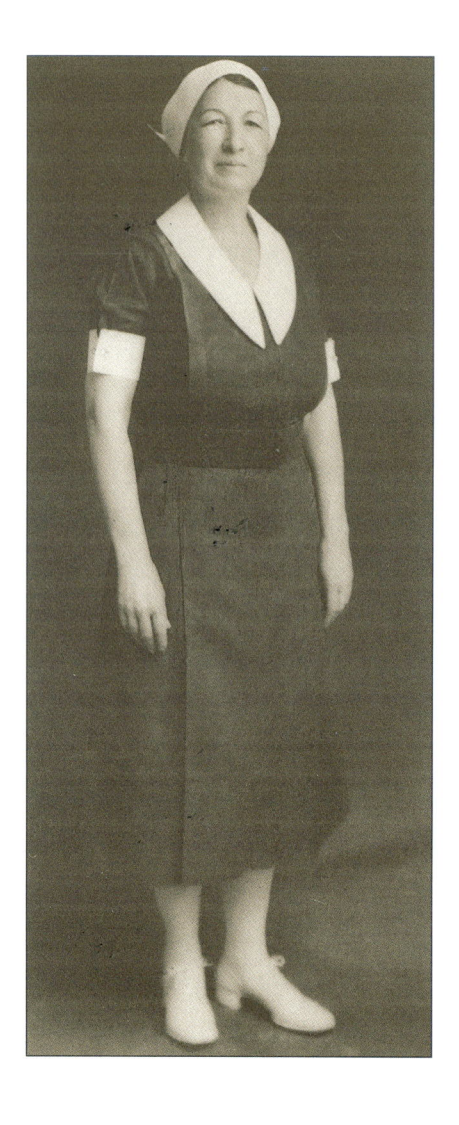

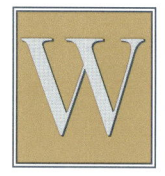

Within days of Germany's invasion of Poland and the outbreak of open warfare in Europe in September 1939, President Roosevelt declared a national state of emergency. The United States began preparations for its own defense. Included in the planning was the medical care of United States military forces.

As in World War I, the responsibility for putting military hospitals and their staffs at the ready fell on the Army Surgeon General's Office. The task was no less formidable than it had been a quarter century earlier. Depression-era cutbacks and a mind-set that was both isolationist and anti-military had left the United States defense establishment with a force of civilian support personnel scarcely more adequate than that which existed in 1918. There remained in army hospitals just 36 of the reconstruction aides who had received their education in the Walter Reed General Hospital training program between the wars. And all of these women were paid out of funds allocated by the Civilian Conservation Corps, a bookkeeping nicety instituted during the lean years when the Veterans Bureau subsidies were withdrawn. Equipment and hospital facilities were also generally outdated and inadequate.

Perhaps the only bright spot in this bleak Medical Corps picture where physical therapy was concerned was the continuing presence of the civilian director and charter member of APA, Emma Vogel. Now 50 years old, Vogel had been with the army, if not of it, since she trained under McMillan at Reed College in 1918.

104  *Healing The Generations*

A dedicated teacher and natural leader, "Emmy Lou" had succeeded McMillan at Walter Reed General Hospital, where she inaugurated the first peacetime program in the United States devoted solely to physical therapy. Although teaching had come to be her principal vocation in the years between the wars, Vogel had never stopped working to resolve what she regarded as an inefficient, misguided, and even dangerous government policy in regard to its discriminatory treatment of women physical therapists. She recognized, as did many other members of APA, the government's failure to give PTs working for the army their due. This was a key reason for the chronic shortage of personnel serving in military hospitals. Should war break out and casualties begin to mount, the army would find itself severely shorthanded once again.

During a period of several years, Vogel had tried, with the full support of her fellow professionals in APA, to persuade those in authority to alter the policy and give women a reserve connection with the peacetime army. Some Medical Corps officers had come to see the virtue of her arguments and had carried the message to the Surgeon General's Office and to the secretary of war, but to little avail. Throughout the 1930s, salaries remained at rock bottom, job security at a minimum, and morale low.

The first sign that something might change regarding status came from Congress in the late winter of 1939. Military Affairs Committee Chairmen Senator Morris Sheppard of Texas and Representative Andrew Jackson May of Kentucky, both with some personal knowledge of the frustrations suffered by civilian staffers at WRGH, introduced identical bills conferring military status on women working within the Medical Corps. But before the bills left committee, Secretary of War Harry Woodring let Congress know that such a change was simply too expensive to be practical. Woodring also said that even in the event of war, physical therapists would certainly not be sent overseas this time, so there was no administrative need to change their current status. The bill died. Unswayed by Woodring's argument, Sheppard and May tried again in 1940 and in 1941, but with similarly discouraging results.

At about this time, the Surgeon General's Office asked John Coulter to make an estimate of the number of "physical therapy technicians" the army would need in case of open warfare. Coulter, following his usual penchant for thoroughness, took his time, contacting a number of authorities in the field and analyzing his data carefully. Basing his calculations on the presumption that the United States would have field armies in the European theater of war only, a presumption that was soon proved wrong, he concluded that the army would need to organize 300 general hospitals of 1,000 beds each (this in distinction to battlefield hospitals, in which PTs were not expected to serve). Following then-current staffing formulas of seven physical therapists to 1,000

*Making its way through the legislative process for the second time, Andrew May's H.R. 8542 fared no better in 1940 than it had in 1939. Not until 1942, with the nation facing wartime emergency, did resistance weaken, at which time women PTs were accorded military status.*

*When Helen Kaiser stepped into the presidency in 1938, there were 956 active members. Associated with the Ohio Chapter, Kaiser is the only president to date to represent that state.*

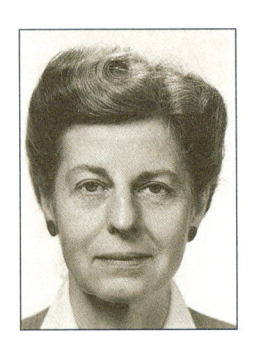

beds, the army would have 2,100 PT positions to fill.

Coulter then went on to survey the United States civilian sector. It was already having trouble finding personnel to treat current case loads, a result of the huge increase in polio patients, the recently inaugurated crippled children's program, and the growing acceptance of physical therapy as a critical part of health care generally. Ideally, said Coulter, civilian hospitals should retain 1,584 physical therapists; crippled children's schools, 1,682; and field service programs for the Children's Bureau, 710. By Coulter's calculations, then, the nation had a total need of slightly more than 6,000 physical therapists.

The gap between "need" and current reality was staggering. More or less coincident with Coulter's study for the Surgeon General, APA had surveyed its own membership in 1940. Of its 1,077 members, 493 were in civilian hospitals and clinics, 154 in schools, 94 in physicians' offices, 87 in private practice, 79 in facilities devoted to crippled children, 66 with the Visiting Nurse Associations and United States Public Health Service, 9 with industrial organizations, and just 37 with the military. Rounding out the survey were 58 "unidentifieds" plus perhaps another 250 PTs who were not members but whose qualifications were sufficient to gain them recognition by the Registry. In a separate survey, APA found that approved schools were currently graduating 135 students per year. To Coulter's way of thinking, this shortfall constituted nothing less than a national emergency in the profession.

Writing to the *Review*, Coulter declared, "The time is now at hand for every member of the American Physiotherapy Association to . . . make the necessary sacrifice. . . . Your country and your profession needs your active cooperation." He urged those readers who were physically qualified for service to volunteer immediately, and those who could not, to give their time and effort to recruiting eligible college graduates who could. He also proposed that approved schools begin offering emergency "abbreviated" courses of six months' duration to candidates with either two years of college, including physics and biology, or a degree from a nursing school or physical education school. And he suggested that "assistants," working under the direction of trained personnel, be brought into civilian hospitals and other large facilities to relieve some of the trained physical therapists for military service. It was a daring suggestion, considering APA's long history of working to raise educational standards. But no one could doubt that the shortage, so long predicted, was truly serious now.

APA, which had initially balked at giving any cooperation to the army in light of its discriminatory policies, now decided to put professional pride aside in recognition of the national emergency. It urged members to respond to a survey being conducted by the American Red Cross for the Surgeon General's Office sounding out a willingness to volunteer immediately in the event of war. However, the Association also urged that members who taught physical therapy at accredited colleges and universities hold themselves apart from the call-up. And just in case anyone needed to have the point driven home more forcefully, the *Review* published an honor roll of therapists whose continuing service as teachers they considered vital. The list of names totaled 54, only two of whom were men. (The list gives us some idea of the relative size of teaching programs in those years: Bouvé-Boston had a staff of three physical therapists; Children's Hospital, Los Angeles, nine; D. T. Watson, Leetsdale, Pennsylvania, four; Children's Hospital, Boston, four; Mayo, Rochester, Minnesota, three; Hospital for Special Surgery, New York, four; Northwestern, Chicago, eight; Sargent College, Boston, five; Stanford University, five; University of Minnesota, six; and University of Wisconsin, three.

### Back In Uniform

In the summer of 1941, six months before the bombing of Pearl Harbor, Emma Vogel initiated the first War Emergency Training Course of World War II at Walter Reed General Hospital. The course consisted of six months of concentrated "didactic" instruction to be followed by six months of supervised practice at a military hospital. Ten students were enrolled in that first session, including Fran Tappan, Jane Carlin, and Dorothy Hewitt, who would become influential educators in the field of physical therapy as well as lifelong friends. Because it was obvious that a program capable of turning out far larger numbers of prepared physical therapists was needed, similar courses were started by Vogel protégés at Fort Sam Houston Hospital, San Antonio, Texas; the Army and Navy General Hospital, Hot Springs, Arkansas; O'Reilly General Hospital, Springfield, Missouri; and Fitzsimons General Hospital, Denver. Later, still more courses were added at Bushnell General Hospital, Salt Lake City; Ashford General Hospital (the Greenbriar Hotel), White Sulphur Springs, West Virginia; Percy Jones General Hospital, Battle Creek, Michigan; Lawson General Hospital, Atlanta; and Fort Huachuca Station Hospital, Arizona. This last was a segregated education course for black physical therapists who were subsequently posted to the 944-bed station hospital or to one of the smaller black hospitals overseas. The official records of the Huachuca hospital and education course were lost in a fire after the post closed, but the names of three staff physiotherapists, Katherine Alexander, Maude Davis, and Carmen Patton, are known.

As further inducement to potential volunteers, these courses and others at Stanford University, the University of Wisconsin, and the D. T. Watson School of Physiatrics were offered at government expense. And in an appeal to patriotism and adventure, a blitz of posters, magazine articles, movie shorts, and pamphlets were generated by APA, the National Foundation for Infantile Paralysis, the American Red Cross, and a host of other service organizations. APA, for example, ran a story headlined "Attractions for a Physical Therapy Aide in the Army," in which the writer gushed, "Life in an army camp is interesting and thrilling. Even in this time of war there is sufficient social activity. Enjoyable evenings at the club or recreation halls afford excellent means of relaxing after a hard day's work." For anyone who loved the outdoors, army life was said to be punctuated by tennis, riding, and recreational swimming.

The reality of being a physical therapist in an army hospital was

*Graduates of the June-December 1942 War Emergency Training Course at the University of Pennsylvania line up for their group portrait. In the back row, left to right, are Ann Harmon, Fern Green, Routh Dixon, and Leila Holly Green; in the foreground, left to right, are Ann Gaither, Alice Earhart, and Mary Alderman Hall.*

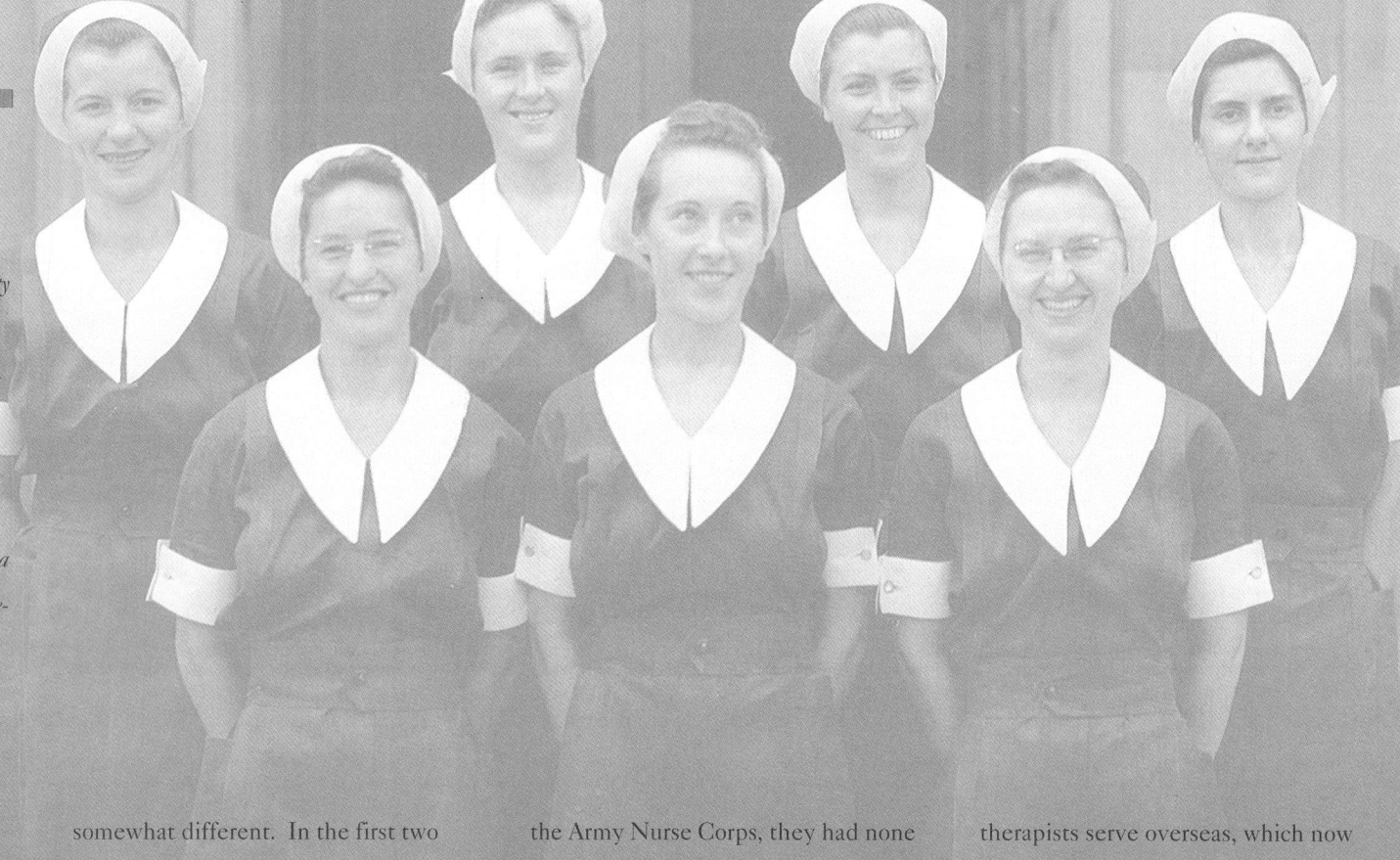

somewhat different. In the first two years of war mobilization, the army increased its hospital facilities in the United States from 45 to 66, precious few of which had tennis courts or much else to amuse physical therapists, whose work sessions were often long and arduous. The problems inherent in the PTs' neither-fish-nor-fowl status were dramatized by the circumstances they found. Although physical therapists were required to conform to the same social rules as members of the Army Nurse Corps, they had none of the benefits. Often the physical therapists had to find housing off-base, and with gas rationing in effect, just getting to work could be a serious problem. Their salary of $160 per month barely covered board, room, and uniforms; certainly it afforded no room for emergencies or the purchase of sports gear. Hospitalization and dental care, as well as transportation to the first assignment, had to be paid out of pocket. Should volunteer physical therapists serve overseas, which now seemed inevitable, they would not be entitled to the provisions of war-risk insurance. If disabled in the line of duty and returned to the United States, they were essentially on their own, just as they had been in World War I.

As for work duties, the volunteer was likely to find herself the only physical therapist on base, responsible for assembling equipment and, more than likely, educating a group of enlisted men as to what they were there to do. Nonetheless, by early 1942 perhaps 150 APA members had volunteered.

Ex-Reconstruction Aide Mary Lee Castleman was one of the first to sign up, and she brought a wealth of experience to the assignment. A graduate of the Harvard Emergency Course with Robert Lovett and Janet Merrill, a veteran of army and Public Health Service hospitals and a successful private practitioner, Castleman dropped everything to go to the army hospital at Pine Camp, New York.

Writing to fellow APA members in the *Review*, she explained: "After Pearl Harbor I felt a total urge to get into the army again. . . . It was not too easy to persuade the Surgeon General's Office that I was still young enough for the strenuous job ahead of me, but they agreed to try it out when they found I really had Civil Service Status and would get rid of my business, also my home, and that I was ready to go way off for the duration."

Castleman loaded her dogs and all the furniture she might need to set up a physical therapy unit into her old Ford, and set out for adventure. She found a remarkably smooth-running operation, thanks to the work of her predecessor, APA member Maude Baum, who was preparing to ship out for Europe. With seven assistants and another five corpsmen in training, the new director got busy with the treatment of 100 to 150 patients a day. While the work was varied enough to be interesting, Castleman reported that the largest share of complaints among the new enlistees arose from foot problems brought on by hours of marching daily. "We had six duplicates made of the corrective foot board," Castleman reported, "and we really go to town using them. The patients like them much better than the marble exercises, and they are much more comprehensive. The foot boards, massage plinths, and corrective exercise equipment are all made in the hospital carpenter shop."

In her spare time, Castleman often treated physicians and nurses, seeing in the repair of their aching muscles an opportunity to demonstrate the value of physical therapy. "So we pioneer on, even in this new army. We are very busy and happy. Who could ask for more?"

Much younger and greener was Mary Flickinger, but her joy in finding herself at a 65,000-man Army Air Corps base in north Texas was much the same: "I had just received my certificate in physical therapy from Northwestern University in February 1942, and the army was my first job. I arrived at Sheppard Field to discover the Physical Therapy Department consisted of one whole ward of the station hospital. There were seven treatment tables, one Hubbard tank, one leg and arm whirlpool, six heat lamps, and an ultraviolet lamp. That was the extent of my equipment. Six enlisted men were assigned to physical therapy and the only treatment they administered was to turn a heat lamp on a patient for twenty minutes. There was no physical therapist, so no one received exercises. About eighty patients a day were going through the department. Most of them were victims of the obstacle course, and many had post operative knee conditions. There I was, fresh out of school, with

*The World War II Years 1939 - 1946*   109

*Catherine Worthingham, noted Stanford University educator, became the Association's two-term president during World War II. She would later become a major figure at the National Foundation for Infantile Paralysis, from which position she was instrumental in advancing the physical therapy profession.*

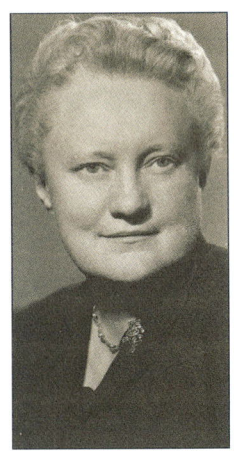

no experience, and having to cope.... Had I been older and more experienced, I probably would have been defeated by the enormity of the job."

Flickinger put in a desperate request for an assistant, and on the last day of August an "assistant" did materialize. To her embarrassment and delight, it was the 44-year-old Signe Brunnström. Despite the former's senior rank and the latter's superior experience, the two quickly worked out a modus vivendi, whipping their department into shape and becoming fast friends in the bargain.

### MILITARY FOOTING – FINALLY

Emma Vogel, who had been called in periodically as an advisor to the Surgeon General's Office on issues concerning the education and assignment of physical therapists, was appointed part-time director of the army's physical therapy program immediately after the Japanese attack on Pearl Harbor. For six months she attempted to juggle her difficult duties as program coordinator while managing the day-to-day affairs of running Walter Reed General Hospital's physical therapist education program and delivering care to patients. But it soon became apparent that no one could properly manage personnel appointments and standardize programs at dozens of hospitals scattered around the country without ever leaving Washington.

In August the SGO asked Vogel to leave WRGH and to work full-time at running the department and its satellite centers. Meanwhile, the army had begun to rethink its position on the civilian status of PTs in light of the fact that numbers of them were needed in war zone hospitals. At the secretary of war's request, Congress passed Public Law 828 on December 22, 1942, offering qualified women physical therapists and dietitians the same rights, privileges, and benefits as members of the Army Nurse Corps. Now they were recognized as members of the Army Medical Department but not precisely of the army itself. Applicants were offered the rank of second lieutenant at a base pay of $150 a month, plus quarters and subsistence allowances of $66 per month, for the duration of the war plus six months. Those who volunteered for overseas duty were to receive an additional 10 percent of salary per month.

Following this changeover, Vogel became director of the Army Physical Therapy Branch and the first woman to receive the rank of major. By the curious administrative terms of the time, Major Vogel held a "relative" rank in the Medical Department, which made her eligible only for the lower pay and allowances due a captain. Following right behind Vogel were six WRGH physical therapy graduates, including Lieutenant Colonel Agnes Snyder who, as Vogel's principal assistant, became the second officer commissioned. (Snyder would go on to become president of APTA in 1958.)

One of Vogel's first acts was to campaign for an upgrade in the job title of physical therapists. The term "reconstruction aide" had been officially discontinued in 1926. Since that time, PTs associated with army hospitals had been known as "physiotherapy aides," which seemed to equate them with "nurses' aides," a class of medical worker whose training was substantially less than that of nurses. That year, 1943, Congress rectified the inequities inherent in Public Law 828 with new legislation authored by Representative Frances Bolton of Ohio. Public Law 78-350, popularly known as the Bolton Bill and passed on June 22, 1944, finally insured full commissioned status to "physical therapists," nurses, and dietitians, marking another milestone reached in the advance of the profession and of women.

It must be added here that male physical therapists remained outside the loop, administratively. Despite protestations by APA, neither P.L. 828 nor P.L. 78-350 contained provisions covering the professional status of male physical therapists. Those men who did serve during World War II — and the precise numbers are unrecorded — entered service at the noncommissioned rank of army sergeant or navy pharmacist. (Robert Teckemeyer and Sam Feitelberg, both of whom would go on to become APTA Board members, served, respectively, as a navy pharmacist's mate at Mare Island Hospital, Vallejo, California, and as an army SP3 at Fort Sam Houston in San Antonio. Feitelberg also performed "PT duties" at WRGH from January 1955 to September 1956.) Also excluded from military status were women occupational therapists; because their work never took them overseas, it was concluded that they did not need the protection associated with a military commission.

Within three months of passage of the Bolton Bill, 279 of the 354 fully trained and qualified women physical therapists serving the army had accepted military status. A handful of others, including Signe Brunnström, had enlisted in the WAVES (Women Appointed for Voluntary Emergency Service). The navy, it should be noted, in presenting Brunnström with her lieutenant's papers, used the only existing form they had for commissioned officers. Her certificate of commission refers to the good lady throughout as "he" and "him."

The evolution in status of physical therapists during a relatively short time was mirrored in the progressive modification of uniforms. In the beginning, PTs attached to the army were ordered to wear the same ankle-length dark blue cotton hospital uniform that had been authorized back in the time of the reconstruction aides. When one APA member heard that, she dashed off a note to the *Review*. "Surely that rumor is a mistake," she sputtered. "Surely, in this streamlined age of progress, it can't be that Aides are going about in those same house-maid uniforms which used to stick forward below the waist line no matter how the P.T. (Poor Thing) tried to hold it in. . . ."

*With ready-made uniforms in short supply in wartime,* the Review *helpfully provided members with simple patterns and sewing instructions.*

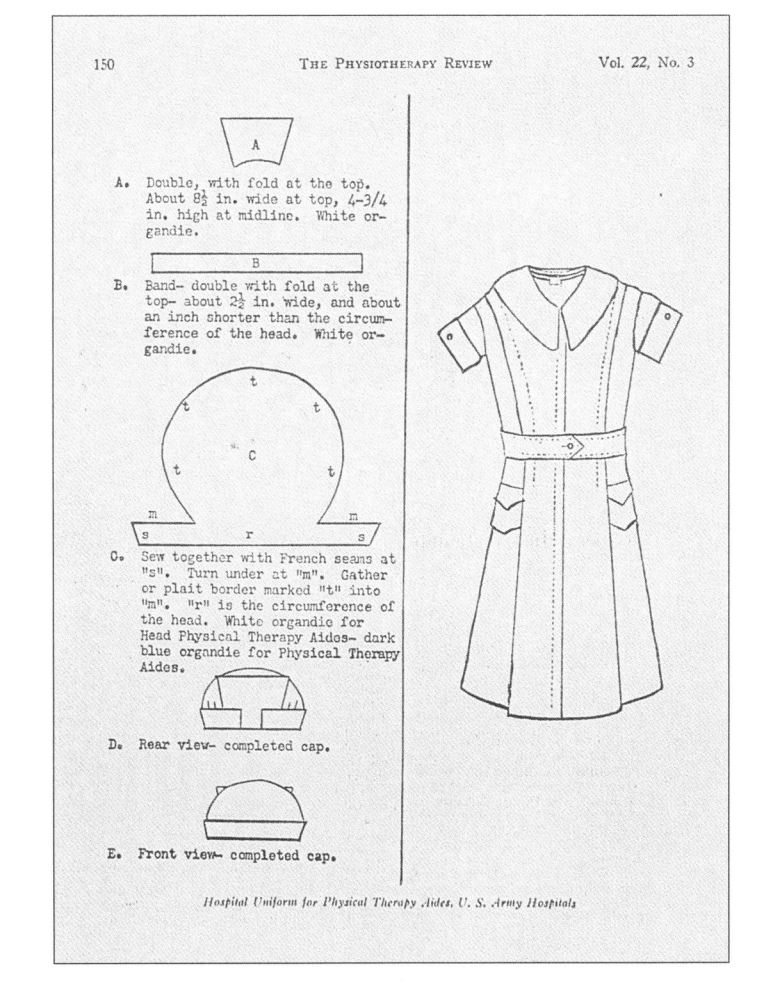

*Navy physical therapists were much envied for their trim uniforms. Here, Ensign Betty Edwards snaps to attention for a photographer at the Navy Hospital, Mare Island, Vallejo, California.*

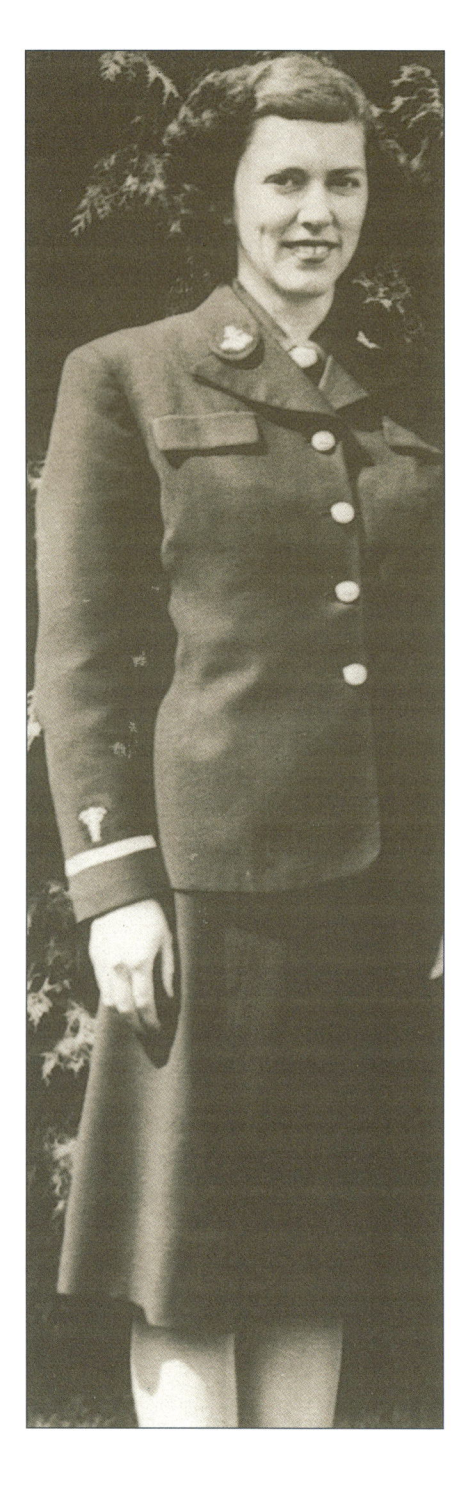

Those uniforms were the jokes of those days, even. And today, when soldiers and sailors and marines are so sleek in revised uniforms, and the WAACs and WAVES in their tailored lines — please, dear Editor, write to me and tell me that the rumors are unfounded. Why should the Aides be singled out in such deplorable manner? Are they not as good as any femme serving her Uncle Sam?"

The former reconstruction aide had a point. The "femmes" in the nursing corps were positively glamorous in their trim-fitting uniforms, which had been chosen by means of a contest among New York fashion designers. And the OTs were dealt an equally smart-looking white dress after Lieutenant Colonel William Porter, chief of the Neuropsychiatric Service at WRGH, complained to his superior that the OTs' old uniform was detrimental to their work. Porter wrote, "A. It is clumsy, unflattering to the female form and suggests that its origin is contemporaneous with Florence Nightingale. B. It is a laundry nightmare. C. Its color is depressing alike to normal and psychotic persons."

Meanwhile, the *Review* published a sketch of the dreary one-length-fits-all dress that was to be the PTs' lot, together with its specifications. It was to be "a one-piece, straight line uniform, with one knife pleat one inch wide down each side of front and back, stitched to a few inches below the waist line. No buttons. Large patch pockets. Detachable collar and cuffs of white pique." A cap of pleated dark blue organdy and white headband finished off the costume. Initially no "United States" insignia nor unit sleeve patch was permitted, so the only means of identifying the wearer as a citizen of the United States was a flimsy paper ID meant to be carried in the pocket.

The *Review* editor commented with evident lack of enthusiasm, "We feel that although it may seem a trivial matter, the appearance of an individual is important not only to her own morale but also that of the patient. We all feel better when well dressed and a uniform that is too long according to current styles and fashioned in such a design that physical therapy aides are mistaken for ward helpers is not conducive to good morale."

112    *Healing The Generations*

Unflattering design was not the only problem with the uniforms. The designated cloth was in chronic short supply, so the first physical therapists to volunteer for overseas duty often had no alternative but to go in civilian clothes, which looked distinctly peculiar, not to say unsoldierly, when worn with pistol belts, canteens, musette bags, helmets, and life belts. One physical therapist sent to England in the summer of 1942 described how her unit coped: "We were encouraged by our commanding officer to buy something — anything that even vaguely resembled a uniform. So we supplied ourselves with dark tailored suits, topcoats, and overseas caps. With this 'uniform' we wore the pin of the American Physiotherapy Association." Shortly after arriving overseas, the unit was issued the uniform of the Army Nurse Corps, but told to snip off the brass military buttons and replace them with plain dark ones. No sooner was this done than new orders and new specifications came down; off came the plain buttons and back on went the brass ones. Finally, in the spring of 1943, they were issued white duty dresses and an olive drab or beige suit or dress as street uniform. Military insignia and a caduceus bearing the letters "P.T." were also authorized and eventually supplied.

### CREATING A DEPARTMENT

Vogel had the examples of Marguerite Sanderson and Mary McMillan as professional inspirations, but in organizing the Physical Therapy Department of the Army Medical Corps, she really had few administrative precedents on which to rely. Nonetheless, her work proceeded with remarkable efficiency and few major glitches, an accomplishment later recognized in her being accorded the army's Legion of Merit for "outstanding accomplishment and unselfish devotion to duty."

Between March 31, 1943, when the first group of women physical therapists received their military commissions, and V-J Day, September 2, 1945, the department grew to 1,688, of whom approximately 1,000 either received their entire professional training or completed apprenticeships in courses organized by Vogel and offered at one of the United States Army emergency training programs. (The vast majority of these students applied for membership in APA as soon as they graduated, accounting in large part for the Association's 87 percent growth during the next four years, to a record total enrollment of 3,841.) Although the majority were in their twenties, more than 100 of those commissioned were over the age of 40, and four were veterans of the World War I reconstruction aide program — joining Vogel and Castleman in this distinguished company were Lieutenants Lelia Zernow and Ethel Dreyer.

Given the shortage of personnel, dispersing physical therapists to the various hospitals in the United States and overseas was, to say the least, an exercise in "doing the mostest with the leastest." Therapist-to-patient ratios were determined on the basis of the kinds of cases presented, and in no instance were there ever enough physical therapists to achieve desirable ratios. Within the Zone of the Interior, which included stateside hospitals, physical therapy departments typically offered one of two principal classes of care, and PTs were trained and de-

*Jessie L. Stevenson of New York succeeded Worthingham as president in 1944 as the Association approached its 25th anniversary and the war was nearing its end.*

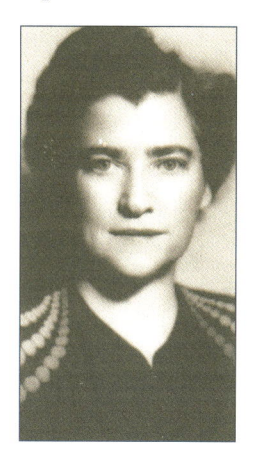

ployed accordingly. Station hospitals, for example, treated the usual assortment of stress injuries associated with intensive education and conditioning of raw recruits being readied for combat. U.S.-based general and specialized hospitals, on the other hand, were specifically responsible for treating and rehabilitating severe and long-term casualties returning from battle theaters. Hospitals in the so-called "Communications Zone" behind the lines were also divided into station and general hospitals, but the areas of responsibility tended to be less clearly divided, with crossovers occurring frequently as the circumstances of engagement changed.

At general hospitals and specialized treatment centers in the United States, the regulation ratio of physical therapists to patients was 1:250, with amputation, neurosurgical, and arthritis wards receiving additional personnel on the rare occasion that someone could be spared from other duties. Station and regional hospitals were staffed at the same basic levels. Convalescent hospitals, which received large numbers of severely injured patients in the last year of the war, demanded and received somewhat greater complements of physical therapists to patients.

If these levels were not daunting enough, overseas hospitals were even more underserved in terms of sheer numbers, with a single physical therapist staffing the average 750-bed hospital and two PTs assigned at hospitals of a thousand beds. While the quality of the care delivered remained excellent, procedures often had to be kept to the barest essentials, and much of the routine work was carried out by enlisted men who received on-the-job training from the physical therapist. In times of particularly heavy case loads, as following the D-Day invasion, treatments had to be limited to instructing patients in exercises they could perform on their own during their evacuation home. Chiefly these procedures were meant to prevent deformities and maintain muscle tone and strength until such time as the patients were back in the United States and under extended care. Initial planning had also called for two physical therapists aboard hospital ships, but the first voyage of the *U.S.H.S. Acadia* proved that plan to be impractical; crowded conditions and a rough crossing made treatments too difficult to justify the shipboard deployment of physical therapists when their services could be used so much more effectively elsewhere.

With staffs as small as they were, there was minimal need for command structure within a hospital physical therapy unit. Theoretically the hospital's chief of the surgical service, who in most cases was an orthopedic surgeon, was charged with directing individual patient treatment. In actual practice, however, the responsibility often fell upon the senior physical therapist, whose duties were broad indeed. She not only supervised a team of PTs and trained and supervised the enlisted men assigned to assist the department, but she examined and evaluated the condition of each patient, scheduled treatments, maintained records, set policy, and acted as the eyes and ears of the surgical chief, doing weekly rounds with him.

Hospitals located in the Zone of the Interior followed a shared set of guidelines, which made the role of the physical therapist in one location generally like that in another. By contrast, each overseas physical therapy department ran itself more or less according to its own rules and reported only to local hospital headquarters. This "seat-of-the-pants" method of management was not one that Vogel or her subordinates thought advisable, and over and over again she argued for the appointment of theater coordinators to standardize procedures. But it was not until she made a tour of inspection of the European and Mediterranean theaters in March 1945 and was subsequently able to present convincing evidence to support her requests that the SGO relented. She then appointed as supervisors Captains Jean Beatty, Lois Ransom, and Felie Clark. By all accounts, the value of this supervision was well demonstrated by improvements in both care and department morale.

As time went on, many of the stateside hospitals came to specialize in particular disabilities — amputations, peripheral nerve injuries, spinal cord injuries — as a means of increasing efficiency. While specialization sometimes meant that wounded soldiers received rehabilitation far from home, it also meant that scores of medical teams were given the unusual opportunity to see how well current techniques worked on large numbers with similar conditions and to make constant improvements in technique. In this, physical therapists were major participants.

Vogel, summarizing the work after the war, cited several particularly challenging programs of which physical therapists could be proud. In the category of major amputations, she said, there were 15,000 patients, including 80 percent lower-extremity cases, for which the physical therapist was given primary responsibility following surgery. As developed at Walter Reed General Hospital, one of the largest amputation centers, continuous physical therapy treatment stretched from wound healing and stump preparation through prosthesis fitting, to gait analysis and education in satisfactory ambulation. In the treatment of extremity wounds with peripheral nerve involvement, a noteworthy program was developed at Percy Jones General Hospital, in Battle Creek, Michigan, using the prototype of a device that would come to be known as the Golseth-Fizzell Constant Current Stimulator, or EDX. When its value in testing for neurological dysfunction was established, the EDX became a useful tool for physical therapists.

In the treatment of orthopedic patients, Captain Thomas DeLorme, a physician on the staff of Gardiner General Hospital, Chicago, experimented with heavy resistance exercise coupled with low numbers of repetitions and came up with the forerunner of progressive resistance exercise programs. His technique was almost immediately incorporated into the work of physical therapy clinics throughout the army.

Spinal cord injuries, Vogel declared, also underwent a major evolution in treatment. Patients for whom total immobility had been the presumed outcome a decade earlier were now taken through an arduous convalescence of progressive exercises that led, in 70 percent of cases, to ambulation with braces and crutches. And thoracic injuries, which in World War I had sentenced most who incurred them to a life as a "chest cripple," with

*Bella Abramowitz Fisher took her education at Walter Reed General Hospital with her to the 27th Station Hospital on New Caledonia during World War II. Pictured, above, demonstrating exercise with boxing gloves and, opposite, with a patient (continued opposite)*

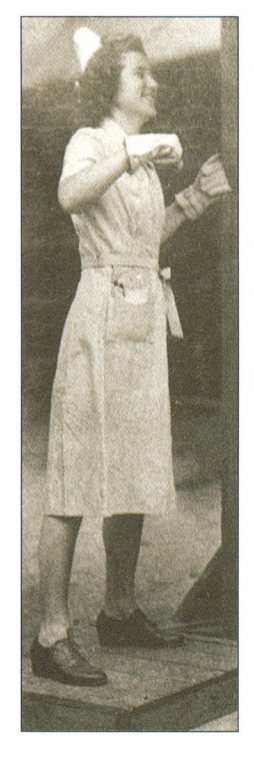

marked scoliosis, weakness, and deformity, now resulted in substantial recoveries through posture instruction, breathing exercises, and general reconditioning.

### PHYSICAL THERAPISTS OVERSEAS

Before the U.S. declared war, there were only four physical therapists serving overseas with the Medical Department of the Army. Three were civilians on duty in Hawaii, including Barbara White, who wrote to the *Review* afterward to describe what happened when the Japanese struck Pearl Harbor on December 7, 1941. "I was on duty that day — went on duty at seven — and just happened to be at the Emergency when the first victims were brought in with the report that one of our own bombs had gone off accidentally. I went about my business on the wards trying to convince myself and the patients that we were having a fancy alert. But we weren't to kid ourselves or anyone else very long — the radio was too specific — which was a good thing, as it kept people from tearing out to see what was going on.

The nurses did a land-office business in Luminal (phenobarbital). It wasn't long before the ambulances started coming in — from then on I worked at the Emergency entrance — and I saw things I never expected to live long enough to see." White concluded her long letter with what she called the "main item." "We in 'far off Hawaii' are much pleased to be a Chapter of APA. We were getting under way nicely, but darkness, distances and gas rationing stopped our evening meetings. We'll be going again before long in the afternoons!" (The Hawaii Chapter had joined just months before the attack.)

The fourth overseas civilian, Brunetta Kuehlthau, was assigned to Sternberg General Hospital in Manila, the Philippines. Shortly before the Japanese invaded Manila in January 1942, Kuehlthau was part of a hospital team evacuated to Corregidor and later to Bataan. On April 8, following the United States surrender there, she was captured and returned to Manila for internment at Santo Tomás, where Mary McMillan, captured en route back to the United States, also was being held. Kuehlthau, dubbed one of the "Angels of Bataan," was awarded a commission in absentia. She survived imprisonment, her spirit kept alive, she would later say, by the sense of achievement she felt in keeping the prison camp's makeshift physical therapy clinic going.

Within a year, the number of overseas PTs expanded to 44 in the so-called "Communications Zone" behind the lines. Although the complement of physical therapists would never reach the desired level, a massive effort to sign up additional women brought the numbers of personnel serving overseas by late 1945 to a grand total of 644, with the largest group in the European theater. Metta Baxter, who served in Italy, was a POW and would return with the Legion of Merit for heroism; Helen Filbert and Bella Abramowitz Fisher each received a Bronze Star "for meritorious achievement" — Filbert for serving the wounded in the steamy jungles of the Netherlands East Indies, and Fisher for her service on New Caledonia and at the war front on Okinawa.

Whenever possible, the army sent fully formed units made up of volunteers from a single civilian hospital. Because the physical therapists were initially in such short supply, many of these units departed understaffed. Nurses, nationals living in the area, convalescent patients, and, in at least one facility, cooperative prisoners of war were put to work as the emergency might require. Once a physical therapist was on the scene, she was assigned a complement of enlisted personnel who, after a period of education, were able to carry out many routine procedures. In these ways, "a few heads and many hands" were able to accomplish small miracles of service.

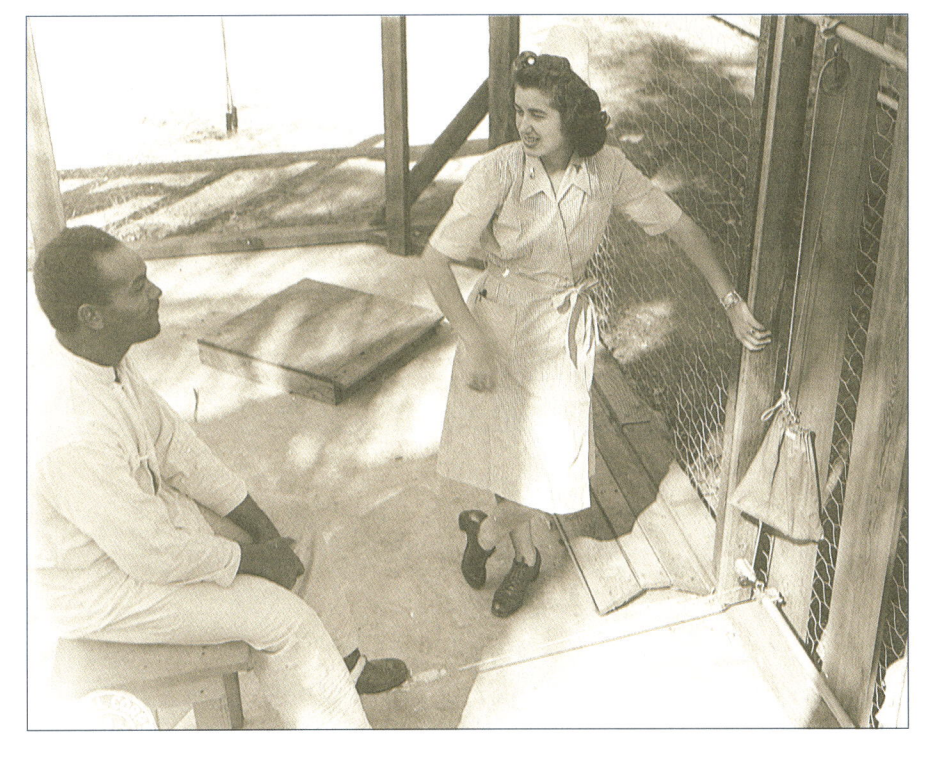

Scattered from Ireland and the European Continent to North Africa, Australia and New Zealand, India, Burma, China, and the islands of the South Pacific, the overseas departments read like a Cook's tour of the globe. Although usually safely removed from the fighting, a few were all too close to danger. Surely the most infamous of these were the two facilities at which Brunetta Kuehlthau found herself in the spring of 1942: the crowded, stifling "tunnel hospital" under Malinta Hill on Corregidor and Hospital #2 in Bataan, which in the days before the surrender handled as many as 1,000 patients in open tents. The Manila hospital in which Fran Tappan served following MacArthur's return was also in the combat zone initially. Tappan treated wounded soldiers within earshot of the nerve-shattering sound of exploding shells for nearly a month before the last of the enemy were driven out of Manila's suburbs. From that time on, she lived with a degree of hearing loss.

Clinics were as varied in space and completeness as the hospitals to which they were attached. Some were installed in buildings originally designed as hospitals and looked not unlike their civilian counterparts stateside. Nearly as good were the hospitals installed in army-issue prefabricated Quonset™ and Nissen huts. Such facilities were likely to have a collection of standard equipment as set forth in a formal procurement list worked up by the AMA's Council on Physical Therapy before the war, including portable bakers, infrared and

*in the outdoor gymnasium she constructed "based on my memory of the various equipment at Walter Reed," she later earned a Bronze Star for her diligent and caring treatment of marines at the front on Okinawa.*

*The World War II Years 1939 - 1946*   117

mercury arc lamps, whirlpool baths, and portable sinusoidal machines. Even in these relatively complete set-ups, however, diathermy machines were rare. Not only did their radio waves tend to interfere with critical military radio reception and transmission, but the government had forbidden the manufacture of these machines early in the war out of fear that some would fall into the hands of enemy agents and be converted to shortwave radios. Also absent were any kind of U.S.-manufactured therapeutic exercise apparatuses, which the Quartermaster Department regarded as low priority among its shipment requirements.

Other departments, generally farther from central supply points but sometimes thrown up amidst the ruins in the days following a major battle, might be set up in makeshift tents, thatched huts, churches, or schoolhouses. On Saipan, where PT and First Lieutenant Barbara Robertson served following the island's capture in late 1944, a small unfurnished tent was all she was given to work with. "I insisted that a floor was essential. . . . Finally, although we were told there was absolutely no lumber available, the powers-that-be consented to let us use lumber salvaged from boxes in which beds had been crated. . . . As there was nothing suitable for a foundation, the floor was just put down, cuddling the contours of Mother Earth. Consequently, we have a rollicking, rolling floor with quite a decided slope, which makes you wonder what has happened to your equilibrium." Robertson also found the temperature within the tent insufferable, given the combination of a hot, humid climate, a black, sun-absorbing top, and the heat treatment lamps inside. She made a false ceiling by hanging white bed sheets overhead on wires, a solution that not only cooled the place down slightly but earned the clinic the name of "the Palace."

In this insubstantial building, which swayed alarmingly in the lightest breeze, there was no way to keep even the semblance of cleanliness. "The floor had either a covering of dust which had blown in, or one of mud which had been tracked in. Large slimy snails, which crawled in at night leaving grayish white trails in every conceivable place, were a constant source of annoyance." She also reported that rats frequently scurried underfoot.

As concerned exercise equipment, it seemed that every physical therapist was on her own, and many devised original and ingenious devices, often with the help of enlisted assistants in their department. Scavenging from trash heaps and junk piles, they made everything from stationary bicycles and rowing machines to wrist rollers and resistance weights. Metta Baxter, who served with the 21st General Hospital in Italy, constructed measuring devices and an exercise bicycle from odds and ends lying about the supply depot, and with the help of a couple of plumbers, she turned the bottom of a kitchen steam table into two whirlpool baths.

Posture mirrors were very hard to come by almost everywhere, but some PTs found workable substitutes. One fashioned a single looking glass out of dozens of smaller mirrors taped together. Another procured a length of shiny sheet metal, fastened it to an easel, and was able to tip the "mirror" down for gait instruction and up for muscle reeducation in a case of facial palsy. In still other locations, physical therapists and department personnel made exercise wands from tree branches and mop handles, sitz baths from used oil drums, paraffin treatments from melted wax candles, and sponge rubber hand exercisers from the foam rubber salvaged from wrecked airplane cockpits. Even relatively sophisticated modalities were devised. In one instance an old-fashioned clothes iron became the instrument for heat-treating certain back injuries; a chair, a set of wheels and tracks, and a couple of pulleys salvaged from a sunken ship became the materials for a quadriceps resistance exerciser.

Whether to maintain general body tone, improve morale, or substitute for labor-intensive massage and heat treatments, many military physical therapy departments adopted a program of general exercise for hospitalized patients in all stages of recovery. The program, which appears to have been introduced in 1942 by APA member Edna Blumenthal (later a first lieutenant) at the 5th General Hospital, Northern Ireland, was later incorporated as a principal element in the army's total rehabilitation program. Participants were classified by the chief surgeon into classes A (full military calisthenics, no restrictions) through E (bed patient, very mild general exercise) and put through a half-hour of group exercises five days a week. Where appropriate, many were also enrolled in group remedial work for shoulder, hand, foot, trunk, and one or both legs.

Workdays in the clinics were typically 9 to 10 hours long, with another hour or two devoted to record keeping and muscle testing at night. Climatic conditions were sometimes so different from home as to require the physical therapists to change standard practices. In the North African theater and in hospitals in India, heat was a constant problem that had to be taken into account when designing treatments so as to avoid excessive fluid and electrolyte loss on the part of patients and overworked PTs as well. At the 31st Station Hospital on New Caledonia, a tent facility, one PT wrote, "We had been taught never to remove our hands from a patient during massage, but the author of that idea must never have worked in a mosquito-ridden swamp land. We learned to massage with one hand and swat with the other."

### War's Unique Challenges

For most physical therapists, whether in the Communications Zone or the Zone of the Interior, war service introduced injuries previously unknown or rarely seen. Certainly civilian life had not fully prepared them for the frequency with which they met amputations, although anyone having passed through either Vogel's Walter Reed General Hospital course or one of the War Emergency Training Courses that it spawned would have received a heavy dose of instruction. (Amputations were a specialty of Vogel's on which she wrote and lectured often.) Severe burns resulting from the explosion of shells and combustibles; cold injuries due to periods of severe exposure to the elements; penetrating and lacerating wounds of soft tissues, often compounded by fractures and peripheral nerve damage injuries, traceable to grenades and gunfire; and combat-related brain and spinal cord injuries were also among the all-too-common injuries sustained in the fighting. Each case was likely to require urgent and prolonged attention, first in evacuation hospitals overseas and later in rehabilitation centers back in the United States.

To ensure that every department clinic was privy to state-of-the-art therapeutic measures, Vogel's Physical Therapy Branch produced and circulated a number of instructional aids. Captain (later Major) Mary Lawrence was technical advisor for a dozen or more films that proved to be so useful that civilian agencies borrowed them. One of these, *Toward Independence*, a narrative concerning the successful rehabilitation of a patient with paraplegia, was subsequently awarded an Oscar by the Academy of Motion Picture Arts and Sciences as the best documentary of the year in 1949. Vogel, who had begun publishing papers as far back as 1941, also contributed several bulletins on specialized physical therapy treatments.

### ON THE HOME FRONT

While the circumstances of war naturally captured the individual attention of every member of APA, the Association continued to grow as an organization, quietly and purposefully, under the leadership of Catherine Worthingham. A member of the faculty of Stanford University and the first physical therapist to hold a doctoral degree (in anatomy), Worthingham served an unprecedented five years as APA president, from 1940 through 1944, at the request of the Executive Committee, which felt that the war years were no time to install new, inexperienced officers. Most of her Board, also residing in California, continued on for a second term. During this era, incidentally, the Association actually had a small second-floor office over a store in Palo Alto. Though New York is conventionally said to have been the first location of a national office, Californians can claim with some merit that their "digs" were really first. A part-time secretary occupied the space, and Worthingham used it to conduct regular Association business, though the *Review* remained in Chicago.

The annual meetings held during the war years became more professional, taking on the aspect of continuing education programs. The first of these was held at Stanford in 1941. The Association's agenda was worked in around four days of coursework that ran from 8:00 a.m. to 5:00 p.m. Offered by panels of experts, the sessions were designed to give members an opportunity to delve more deeply into clinical practice issues than had been possible at previous conferences. And for the first time, a special four-week post-conference graduate course was offered to members able to extend their stay. The idea was obviously a good one, for 37 members signed up, gaining credits in advanced kinesiology, therapeutic gymnastics, skeletal muscle and motor activity in health and diseases, and "the psychology of the invalid and handicapped." Subsequent meetings did not quite live up to these high standards, but not for lack of good intentions. The Office of Defense Transportation curtailed civilian travel during the war, causing APA to cancel its 1943 and 1945 conferences altogether and limiting the size of the others.

The governance structure of APA also changed substantially to accommodate increased responsibilities, growth of membership, and a more national outlook. When the practice of voting on the business of the Association through chapter delegates became too unwieldy in 1944, the APA membership voted for a constitutional change that provided for a separate "legislative" branch, henceforth known as the House of Delegates (HOD), a term and structure probably inspired by that of the American Medical Association. Thenceforth, all legislative powers, including the power to amend or repeal the Bylaws of the Association, were vested in the HOD, whose delegates were duly elected by the separate chapters. The House was also deemed an advisory body for the Executive Committee and a coordinating agency between the Executive Committee and the general membership.

Along with building up the structures within the organization, APA also found in the war emergency an urgent need to coordinate with other professional groups, particularly those engaged in the work of rehabilitation. The Relations Committee, which had been formed in 1940, had begun this process by appointing APA members as advisors to a number of medical commissions and federal health agencies. This positive experience led, in turn, to the passage of a resolution at the 1942 Annual Conference at College Camp, Lake Geneva, Wisconsin, inviting representatives from all agencies interested in the welfare of the injured and disabled to form a so-called Allied Council.

The council's first formal meeting in August 1942 was a notable success on many levels. First, it showed APA's readiness to take on a leadership role outside its own membership; second, it brought together 39 organizations representing nearly 1,400,000 constituents all told. Among those joining APA as council participants were the American Association for Health, Physical Education, and Recreation; National Society for Crippled Children; U.S. Department of Labor; Joint Orthopedic Nursing Advisory Service; National League for Nursing Education; American Occupational Therapy Association; Council on Medical Education and Hospitals of the AMA; American Public Health Association; National Foundation for Infantile Paralysis; and American Congress of Physical Therapy. From this initial effort was born the National Council on Rehabilitation.

Paralleling APA's efforts to reach out to other organizations in the United States were efforts to forge ties with physical therapists in other countries. Mollie McMillan's work in China had set the example, and other APA members had followed, with Katherine Lorrilliere and Helen Kaiser going to Greece to carry out relief missions, particularly among the children; Alice Lou Plastridge heading to Belgium to assist in a wartime outbreak of polio; and the organization of physical therapy services in a Rockefeller-funded hospital in Venezuela.

The experience of Army Medical Corps PT veterans had further enriched the Association's "world point of view," as Jessie Stevenson termed it in her 1946 President's Report. Members had worked shoulder to shoulder in overseas hospitals with their English,

*Past president Helen Kaiser took her physical therapy skills to war-torn Greece in 1946. Here, she visits the Children's Rehabilitation Center in Athens.*

Australian, and Canadian counterparts in physical therapy, consciously sharing their knowledge with one another. Others had seen, in the most heart-wrenching detail, the need for more and better services in war-ravaged countries in Asia, Eastern Europe, and North Africa. Mollie McMillan, who attended the first post-war Annual Conference in Blue Ridge, North Carolina, that same year, confirmed this view in her stirring speech "Physical Therapy from the Embryo on Three Continents," in which she spoke with particular fondness of her work in Asia and of her concern for the health and safety of her former colleagues in China. In a spontaneous burst of affection and shared commitment, McMillan's audience, knowing of her life-saving project to send vitamins and medical supplies to Peking, took up a collection that they presented to her.

APA's Executive Committee consequently took it upon itself to open talks with other national associations concerning reciprocal exchanges of research and educational and technical materials, which would become the first exploratory steps toward world confederation.

The war years also brought the election of the first male member of APA to a national leadership position: in 1942 Paul Campbell, a physical therapist who was active in the Pennsylvania Chapter, was elected to the Board of Directors and two years later was elected national treasurer — a post he held until 1948.

APA's first "sections," as its special interest groups are known, were mentioned in 1941 and were included in the scheduling of the 1942 Annual Conference program. One was a section designed to focus on the problems and issues surrounding Crippled Children's Schools; the other was concerned with Physical Therapy Schools. Only the latter survived to become a permanent fixture, initially as the "Schools Section" and later as "Education," making it the oldest continuous special interest group in the Association and the only one not established under the aegis of the House of Delegates.

### The Politics Of Polio

Of all practice issues, none remained more pressing — or political — than that of polio care. In the two decades preceding World War II, the search to find better methods of managing patients with acute and chronic poliomyelitis had been the principal engine driving the advancement of physical therapy. And even during the war, despite the terrible toll of wartime wounded and the demands their rehabilitation placed upon so many in physical therapy, the disease continued to be a central concern of the health professions. Polio incidence, which had been rising gradually, suddenly began to take on alarming proportions in the 1940s. Not only were the very young falling prey in greater numbers, but unprecedented numbers of adults were also becoming infected, many, but not all of them, veterans of war campaigns in southern Europe, North Africa, and the Pacific. The public, which was now intimately aware of the annual outbreak of polio thanks to extensive radio and newspaper coverage, watched with alarm as each summer season brought another record-breaking set of polio statistics.

The health care community's response was threefold. First, public and private funds were poured into expanded research aimed at developing a polio vaccine for what was now known as an intestinal infection. Second, additional monies and minds were focused on expanding knowledge of the clinical course of polio, and consequently on finding better methods of aftercare. And third, specially trained medical personnel were organized into "shock teams," which were dispatched to areas of severe outbreaks to assist local doctors and hospitals. In all of these efforts, APA and its staff were deeply involved.

In the matter of aftercare techniques, the road to consensus was rocky indeed. Where there had been essentially one basic approach, tracing back through Legg and Merrill to Lovett and Wright, there were now two. At the heart of the controversy was a middle-aged Australian nurse known as "Sister" Elizabeth Kenny, who had a remarkable talent for self-promotion, a charismatic personality, and some convictions about the nature of polio that left her more soft-spoken adversaries at a loss for words. Sister Kenny's arrival in the United States in 1940 and her assault on traditional polio aftercare polarized the medical community for nearly a decade. Kenny's crusade also gave ample demonstration that the science of physical therapy needed a stronger foundation, that too much was still done on the basis of anecdotal experience without the research to prove its worth.

Contrary to the traditional therapy of bed rest and immobilization of weakened limbs during the acute phase of polio, Kenny believed in aggressive physical therapy from the outset. Strongly opposed to splinting or bracing of any sort, she treated patients with round-the-clock hot "fomentations," or hot, wet packs applied to afflicted areas. Once or twice a day, she also instituted passive exercise and massage.

In another departure from orthodox theories, Kenny claimed that in all cases of paralysis, the loss of muscle function was due to reversible "muscular spasm" in the hamstring muscles and not to the permanent destruction of the motor neurons controlling the affected, flaccid muscles. According to the Kenny scenario, the painful spasm had to be dealt with quickly before it led to "incoordination," by which she meant the involuntary substitution of one muscle for another. In like manner, Kenny claimed that the spasm was also likely to evoke "mental alienation," which was the inability of the patient "to produce a voluntary, purposeful movement in a muscle in spite of the fact that the nerve paths to that muscle are intact." It was the responsibility of the physical therapist, she said, to keep the paralyzed patient mentally in touch with physically alienated muscles, lest he or she permanently forget how to use them. Kenny claimed that in the vast majority of paralytic cases, the long-term disability experienced by so many patients was attributable to the immobilization of muscles and not to "true" paralysis. Orthodox practitioners, she declared with undisguised contempt, were thus "treating a disease that didn't exist." By implication, these same practitioners were responsible for any resulting paralysis and weakness.

Kenny's techniques, about which she spoke with messianic certainty, had been developed during years of working in the sparsely settled Australian outback, where polio had erupted with surprising frequency during the 1930s. Knowing virtually nothing about the disease when she first encountered it, the bush nurse had simply improvised methods of easing pain with materials available in the homes of her impoverished patients. These treatments centered on the repeated application of hot, moist towels and torn flannel blankets to inflamed muscles, coupled with daily massage and a generous dose of reassurance to the anxious family. Patients did experience some relief from Kenny's therapy, and when word of her favorable results spread, she attracted the notice of the wider British medical community. In the late 1930s, Sister Kenny was invited to England to demonstrate her method before a committee of medical experts. The British observed her at work, queried her theories at length, and finding her explanations at variance with current science, pronounced the "Kenny System" without merit. But Kenny was nothing if not persistent, and she took her message of hope to the public, which was eager for any new approach to the intractable disease.

In consequence, when the 54-year-old Kenny came knocking on doors at the U.S. medical establishment in 1940, her reputation had preceded her. She was received cordially if cautiously by representatives of the AMA and ultimately given a six-month demonstration grant from the National Foundation for Infantile Paralysis. Arrangements were made for Kenny to carry out her work at the Minneapolis (now Hennepin) General Hospital and the University of Minnesota Medical School. Given a 22-bed ward at the city hospital and another 17 beds at the university, she was "loaned" a staff of some 20 physical therapists who were to carry out her techniques.

In January 1941, when the six-month period was nearing its end, the NFIP sent observers to Minneapolis to see what progress the Australian visitor had made. Included were Mildred Elson and Gertrude Beard of Northwestern University, Alice Lou Plastridge of the Warm Springs Foundation, and Henry and Florence Kendall of the Baltimore Children's Hospital School. All were people whom Kenny considered the pillars of orthodoxy, diametrically opposed to her methods, and she met them in a spirit of combativeness and impatience.

Plastridge, in her report to the NFIP, has left us with a vivid recollection of the woman: "Sister Kenny has a most unusual personality. She is a tall, heavily built person with an almost majestic bearing. She is a white-haired Irish woman with dominance, belligerence, intolerance and stubbornness predominating — hard and defiant." Plastridge added that the observer team was frequently confounded by Kenny's Australian terminology, so that they were often unsure as to what symptoms and physiological events she was talking about. However, they had been warned by their Minneapolis hosts not to raise questions or objections nor to expect any free discussions or comparisons as Kenny was notoriously quick to take offense and might even terminate the meeting prematurely if challenged.

Plastridge found the entire proceedings difficult to follow and sometimes illogical. Kenny's sketchy documentation made it impossible to differentiate cases of "abortive" or nonparalytic polio from paralyses that had actually been reversed as the specific result of her controversial treatments. At the same time, Plastridge found merit in the hot packs, which were applied every half hour for a period of 12 to 24 hours during the painful acute stage, though she thought them too labor-intensive for chronically understaffed clinical settings. Plastridge also noted that the patients did appear to experience relief more quickly than was frequently the case in the sort of immobilization practiced at Warm Springs. And she declared that whether or not Kenny's theories of "mental alienation" were correct, the personal attention intrinsic to her system and her insistence upon the mental as well as physical cooperation of her patients surely had a positive effect on outcomes. She marveled that Kenny was able to train children as young as six to know their own musculature, to locate the precise points where actions took place, and to carry out certain simple "muscle reeducation" exercises on cue.

The Warm Springs observer concluded her report by saying that only scientific investigation could ultimately prove what parts of Kenny's "system" were valid and worthy of adoption by American physical thera-

*"Sister" Elizabeth Kenny demonstrates her controversial methods of polio treatment to a group of physical therapy students. Though the NFIP funded her efforts, hoping to find a miracle cure, eventually Sister Kenny's method was abandoned.*

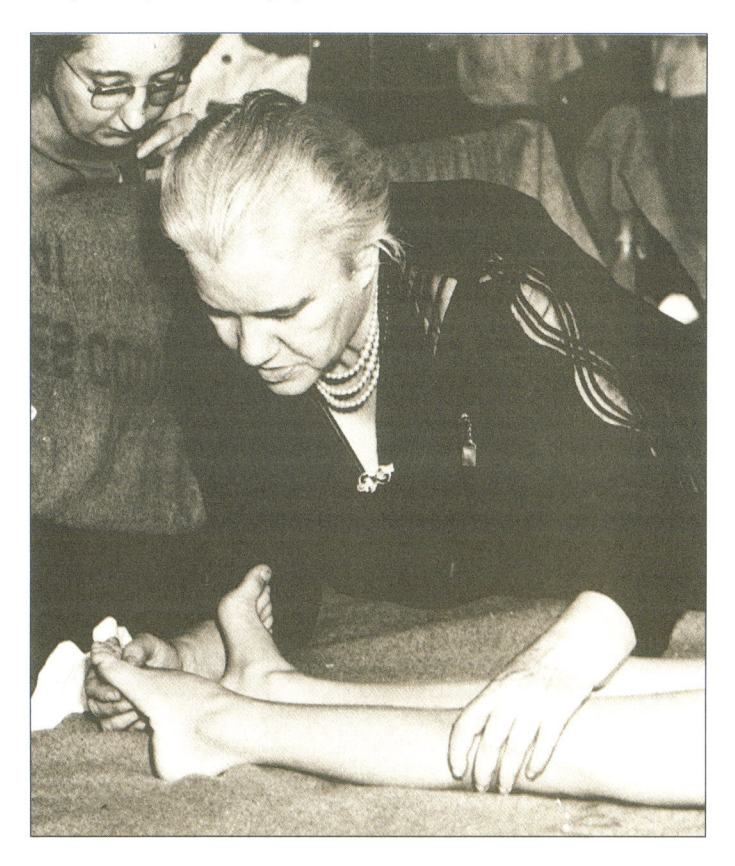

*The World War II Years 1939 - 1946*  125

pists, but "she is getting such unusually good results that it does not seem possible that they could all be a matter of chance." "One thing is certain," she added generously, "her controversial theories have given a tremendous stimulation to further research in this field, and made many of us take serious stock of ourselves, and the type of physical therapy we are doing. . . . That in itself is a forward step."

The Kendalls, who came to Minneapolis knowing they were specific targets of Kenny's crusade, also prepared a report for the NFIP. As Florence Kendall described the meeting, she started with a peace offering, telling Kenny that she hoped that discussion would prove that many of Kenny's so-called "twelve points of difference" would turn out to be not so different after all, but rather misunderstandings of each other's terminology. Kenny retorted that no such accommodation was possible, that her system was diametrically opposed to that of the Kendalls, and that she had no intention of "proving" to them how or why she was right. Such proof, she claimed, was self-evident in her published papers.

Taking another tack, the Kendalls asked to see Kenny working with some of her patients; Kenny said she did not wish to do so. Even more frustrating to the observers, Kenny would not allow any form of manual muscle testing on the grounds that it would exaggerate "incoordination" and thereby slow patients' recovery. The Kendalls concluded in their report to the NFIP that Kenny's system held many implied risks to the patient. Though the Kendalls also thought her hot pack treatments could be employed more widely during the acute phase, they declared her wrong in her abandonment of splints and casts, which in their opinion were still the best way to support and protect affeced muscles from overstretching. Regarding Kenny's assertion that polio was primarily a disease of muscle tissue, the Kendalls declared that the Australian nurse was simply wrong as a matter of scientific fact. All evidence indicated that the primary lesions were located in the nerve tissue. And as for Kenny's claims to cures — "55 percent well in 36 days" — they found such numbers meaningless, because

there were still no accurate ways to measure or compare polio treatment outcomes.

To address this problem, the Kendalls recommended what would seem obvious today but was novel in 1941: "a thorough statistical study . . . which should include not only the number of cases that are restored to normal function by the end of the first 6 weeks after onset, but a careful study of the eventual degree of recovery among those cases which are still weak or paralyzed." They also urged that, for purposes of comparison, all patients undergo detailed and accurate muscle tests, both to establish a record of neuromuscular status at the outset of treatment and to track progress. Until such time as these kinds of rigorous studies were made, the Kendalls suggested, any group recommending wholesale adoption of the Sister Kenny System was working in the dark, at best.

The Kendalls, for their part, were mobilized by the Kenny challenge to defend their own "common sense" approach to polio treatment with more rigorous documentation. The results of these efforts, which reflected modifications of their earlier USPHS Bulletin #242, were eventually published in a wide-ranging article titled "Orthopedic and Physical Therapy Objectives in Poliomyelitis Treatment" in a 1947 issue of the *Review*.

Meanwhile, the controversy over Sister Kenny's methods simmered on with various factions trading shots. Several influential physicians, including John Pohl, director of the Infantile Paralysis Clinic at the Minneapolis General Hospital, Frank Krusen of the Mayo Clinic, and Miland Knapp, director of the physical therapy program at the University of Minnesota Hospital, not only defended Kenny but wrote articles on her behalf, winning her a wider backing among other members of the medical profession. At the 1942 annual meeting of the AMA, where Kenny was invited to give demonstrations four times a day, she reportedly took her message to a total of 3,500 doctors and nurses. Many physical therapists who were looking for a way to improve their own less-than-satisfying record with polio rehabilitation applied to take her specialized education in Minneapolis.

When the Committee on Research for the Prevention and Treatment of Infantile Paralysis endorsed Kenny's work at a scientific meeting sponsored by the NFIP later in the year, Kenny's triumph was virtually assured. The APA Executive Committee, which discussed the various viewpoints at length, decided that it too saw major benefits in Kenny's system and made their Australian guest an honorary member by bestowing upon her their Gold Key Award. The *Review* editors, for their part, gave her article the lead position in one of their 1942 issues.

The demand for training in the Kenny method soon overwhelmed the existing facilities, and the city of Minneapolis gave Kenny a building in which to set up a separate Sister Kenny Institute. (With generous private support, it became the Sister Kenny Foundation in 1943.) When even the combined resources of the three hospitals were still insufficient to take the patients and physical therapists applying, the NFIP created six "satellite centers" around the country where the expanded work was carried on. In 1943, for example, Boston Children's Hospital sent Dorothy Frederickson for nine weeks' instruction under Sister Kenny. Frederickson returned to take over the polio isolation ward. Janet Merrill, Frederickson's supervisor, describes the buzz of activity that followed: "Under her direction 12 to 15 physical therapy students carried out the packing schedule in the morning (as the nursing staff continued it the rest of the day). Groups of three rushed the boiling hot cloths from the central sterilizer to tubs near the patients, ran them through hand wringers, and applied as many as 20 to a child, wrapping them in outside covers to maintain the heat. At one time, 28 children were receiving hot packs every two hours, . . . and it was done the hard way, for electric wringers could not be obtained for our direct current in this time of shortages." Had the Kenny treatment proved as effective as Kenny claimed, all the rushing and packing undoubtedly would have been worth it, but a year later, after observing results firsthand and struggling with a severe shortage of physical therapy students, Merrill concluded that "restoration of properly

*Kenny's treatments, detailed in the pamphlet below, included the application of "hot packs" to the patient's legs at half-hour intervals when the disease was in its acute stage. Though this technique provided some comfort, no effect on paralysis was observed.*

controlled muscle function and flexibility seemed . . . better accomplished by other methods." Boston Children's Hospital returned to the older ways.

Remarkably, it was nearly four years before anyone in the medical profession took the time to analyze systematically what was and was not occurring with the Kenny System. When this was finally done by John Pohl of the Minneapolis General Hospital and comparisons were made with orthodox treatments, what had been claimed regarding the superior outcomes of Sister Kenny's methods was cast into question again. Of the 364 patients in Kenny's care, it was revealed that 6 percent died and another 16 percent were extensively paralyzed, a far cry from newspaper reports that claimed a success rate as high as 90 percent. Maurice Visscher and Jay Myers, two of Kenny's adversaries at the University of Minnesota, declared in a guest editorial in the August 1945 issue of the English journal *Lancet* that, while such numbers were not worse than those found at the general run of traditional treatment centers, they fell below the performance levels of some of the specialized hospitals where "orthodoxy" was practiced at its best. The writers concluded that it was difficult to see how anyone could continue to support such "pseudomedical theorizing" in light of "the enormous mass of neuropathological and neurophysiological evidence" to the contrary. Visscher and Myers reminded their readers once again that rational therapeutic practice should be based upon better and more objective research rather than "international publicity . . . salesmanship, and wishful thinking. . . . Science is the search for truth. . . . Fidelity to sound science is not a glamorous pursuit, nor a financially lucrative one, but it does enhance one's self-respect, and in the long run brings the respect of the world."

Meanwhile, the NFIP, finding it had "a tiger by the tail," plotted how and when to let go of Kenny safely, but in 1945 she raised the level of discourse to a point at which the foundation had no other choice. During a series of Congressional hearings into the treatment controversies, Kenny spoke of "petty annoyances by sniping medical groups" and accused her critics of willfully engineering "disappointments and humiliations." At the same time, she applied to the NFIP for $840,000 in grant monies. Without further discussion, the NFIP replied curtly, "Your request is refused." The Kenny Foundation, claiming to be glad to regain its independence, promptly found other private sources of income. Ultimate resolution of conflicts between the Kenny System and orthodox polio treatment would not occur until the next decade.

### PATRONS AND ALLIES

APA had never lacked for ambitions, but a precarious financial state in the early years made many a worthwhile plan difficult if not impossible to execute. One program particularly dear to APA's Executive Committee was to find creative ways to attract more qualified candidates into the profession. The *Review* regularly reminded members to recruit promising young people to the profession, and with this in mind, it twice published "Physical Therapy as a Vocation," a thoughtful article by former editor Ida May Hazenhyer on the moral and financial rewards to be found in joining this young profession. Clearly the hope was that members reading the piece would pass it along to someone perched on the brink of choosing his or her life's work. But the Executive Committee also recognized that the high cost of tuition — averaging $500 per year in 1947 — was scaring away numbers of potential candidates. Young women in particular were being excluded from contention because they were far less likely to receive family financial assistance for advanced schooling than were their male peers in those years.

APA approached several organizations to ask for scholarship funding. The first and consistently largest source of grants and loans turned out to be the National Foundation for Infantile Paralysis, which was fighting another war within the United States in these years — the expanding polio crisis in the civilian population. The NFIP opened APA's scholarship drive in 1942 with an initial grant of $10,000 and gave increasingly larger amounts thereafter. Other substantial scholarships came from the Rosenberg Foundation of California, the Pi Beta Phi sorority, and the W. K. Kellogg Foundation.

In 1945, the NFIP set aside an additional $1,267,600 for the expansion of physical therapy on several fronts; funding allocations included scholarships to assist nearly 90 candidates in their undergraduate studies, a dozen exchange fellowships with Canadian physical therapists, still other fellowships to provide additional instructors in approved schools of physical therapy, and monies to underwrite various surveys and slide and film programs for distribution to schools and APA chapters. The very first candidate to receive a scholarship under this new grant was physical education instructor Marjorie Ionta, twin sister of First Lieutenant Margaret Ionta, a physical therapist with the Army Air Corps. Marjorie Ionta would go on to attend the Harvard Medical School Course for Physical Therapy, graduating in 1946, and to carve a distinguished place for herself in the history of physical therapy.

As it turned out, the scholarship program became the instrument for bringing the NFIP and APA closer together on many other matters of mutual interest. This "marriage" was made possible by the wise matchmaking of three distinguished members with deep interests in polio care. The first was Catherine Worthingham, who, as president of APA, led the Association through two terms of vigorous growth in the early 1940s. In December 1944, Worthingham left Stanford to move to New York as the NFIP Medical Department's Director of Professional Education. The second was Jessie Stevenson, who had come to New York City to be headquartered at the office of the National Organization for Public Health Nursing while completing a book on polio care. Stevenson succeeded Worthingham as APA president, from which position she continued to work closely with her friends at NFIP. The third was

Mildred Elson, one of the founding members of the Wisconsin Chapter and for eight years editor of the Chicago-based *Physiotherapy Review*. Elson has the distinction of being APA's first salaried executive director, a post she assumed in late 1944.

In that year, the NFIP earmarked a grant of $5,000 to help the American Physiotherapy Association open its first full-fledged national office at 1790 Broadway, near Columbus Circle, in New York City. The office was a mere 350 square feet in size and furnished with little more than a couple of secondhand desks, plus a stack of cartons filled with files. But to the membership, it seemed a momentous achievement, symbolic of the Association's arrival at a level from which it could exercise a truly national outlook. Having an executive director to maintain chapter relations meant that the officers and Executive Committee could be relieved of much detail work. This not only freed them to devote their energies to policy issues, but it meant that fewer face-to-face meetings were needed, and this in turn allowed the Nominating Committee to draw up slates of candidates who could be chosen entirely on the basis of talent rather than on geographical convenience. In 1945, in a change that was radical but surprisingly nondisruptive, members of an Executive Committee drawn from as far afield as California, Tennessee, Maryland, and Ohio were able to complete their duties through just two formal meetings, keeping in touch on the general business of the Association through bulletins composed and sent from the national office staff.

Writing of that period, Elson recalls, "The spirit was as it always has been . . . that of confidence and optimism. We never realized how small we really were and no one scared us. . . . One great factor in our strength was the oneness of purpose of the membership, the elected officers, and headquarters staff. Ours was a profession not just to develop but to *save* — and we (I mean everyone) did just that." Elson's first effort at "saving" APA was directed at elevating physical therapists in government service from subprofessional to professional classification within the Civil Service rating system. Surviving countless meetings with Washington officialdom, she orchestrated a letter-writing campaign by some of the medical profession's most respected individuals and finally won the sought-after recognition for members. Shortly after Elson moved in, the *Review*'s business office was transferred to New York as well, and the editorial office, under the direction of Louise Reinecke, followed later.

Still another NFIP grant was made at APA's request to underwrite the hiring of an education secretary — Barbara White (formerly of Hawaii). White's central task was to give more active counseling to schools regarding curriculum planning, but her mandate also included giving counsel and guidance to research groups as to the areas of physical therapy practice that were in most urgent need of scientific study.

### The "Rehabilitation Movement"

Long before the war was over, Bernard Baruch, son of the great nineteenth-century physician/hydrotherapist Simon Baruch and himself an ardent supporter of physical therapy, became convinced that too little was being done to ensure the rehabilitation of the war wounded. The army's surgeon general had declared the Medical Corps legally responsible only for the "reconditioning" of below-par personnel to make them fit for military service; "rehabilitation," which involved helping the permanently disabled soldier adapt physically in ways that made possible his future economic usefulness, was something the SGO preferred to turn over to the Veterans Administration as soon as practicable. But the VA was neither ready nor eager just yet to take on the massive task, and the dedicated physicians and physical therapists within the Medical Corps were reluctant to cede responsibility that they thought was rightfully theirs.

Into this breach stepped the pro-rehabilitation faction of the corps, including Howard Rusk, director of the Army Air Corps Reconditioning and Recreation Program. Rusk in particular gained Baruch's ear, and the financier in turn persuaded Roosevelt to expand the army's mandate at least until the war's end.

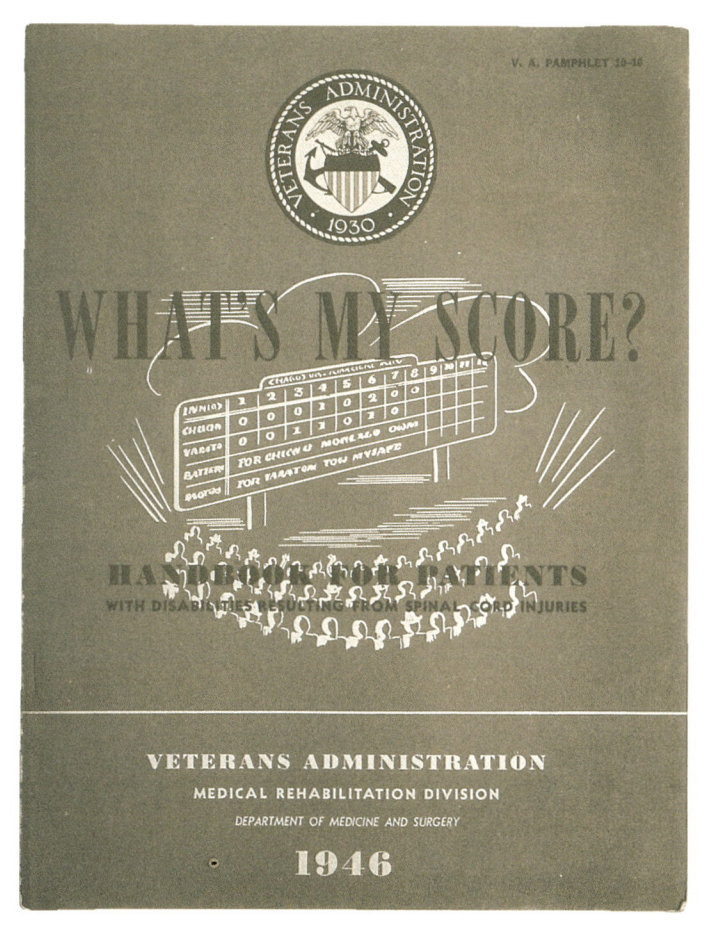

Much had to be done, however, to make the promise of rehabilitation a reality. To speed the process, Baruch funded a committee, comprising more than 40 specialists in medicine and the basic sciences, to consider what avenues of research and clinical development were most needed. When it was found that the greatest effect could be rendered through expanding medical school courses, Baruch parcelled out gifts totaling $1,100,000 to the medical schools at 10 universities across the country to be used for the teaching of physical medicine, which was generally understood to encompass reconditioning and rehabilitation through "scientific" diagnosis and treatment. Another $100,000 was earmarked for fellowships and residencies for promising medical school graduates who would make physical medicine their specialty.

Baruch's patronage of physical medicine not only played a major part in redirecting the specialty's focus toward rehabilitation, but it also was to have tremendous repercussions for the growth of physical therapy in the

*The morale of patients was often valued as equally important to their recovery as the physical treatments. This handbook for patients with disabilities related to spinal cord injuries was designed to encourage and assist individuals in tracking their own rehabilitation progress.*

*Ida May Hazenhyer's four-part history marked the Association's 25th anniversary. The first part appeared in this, the January-February 1946* Review.

rehabilitation sphere. Through the Baruch Committee and its physician director, Frank Krusen, model programs were funded at such prestigious institutions as Columbia University and New York University. NYU was thus able to open the pioneering Institute of Rehabilitation Medicine in 1947 where, under the leadership of Howard Rusk, senior director, and George Deaver, medical director of the physical therapy teaching program, a distinguished physical therapy faculty was assembled, including Beth Addoms, Mary Eleanor Brown, and Signe Brunnström.

In a related development in the so-called rehabilitation movement, a "crash" program was launched to develop better-performing artificial limbs and orthoses. Funded at first by the army and later by the Veterans Administration, the research was carried out variously by staff at the National Academy of Sciences, the U.S. Army Prosthetic Research Laboratory, and selected medical and engineering schools. Particularly productive were projects established at the University of California, Berkeley, on lower-extremity design; at UCLA, on upper-extremity prostheses; and at the Institute for Rehabilitation Medicine at NYU, on the quadrilateral suction socket. Even some high-tech industrial companies, such as Northrop Aviation, whose designers had a wealth of wartime experience in using state-of-the-art lightweight metals and plastics, made contributions to the search. Among the notable developments to come out of this war-related research were the voluntary-closing hand, a finely engineered metal mechanical hand covered by a flesh-colored rubber glove, from the Army Prosthetic Research Laboratory (APRL); Northrop's alternating-lock elbow unit, operated from the harness for transhumeral amputations; and an imperfect but promising electrically powered arm conceived with the help of IBM.

Many physical therapists became intimately involved as hands-on clinical investigators in developing the underlying biomechanical studies of tissue and locomotion, but none made a larger contribution than Signe Brunnström. Both as physical therapy officer at Mare Island, the navy's West Coast center for the rehabilitation of people with amputations, and later through her teaching, lecturing and writing, Brunnström set a high standard for the treatment of patients with amputations.

### THE NAME THING – AGAIN

The expanding environment in which "physical therapy physicians" were now operating led this specialty medical field in 1944 to reconsider the sensitive matter of what to call itself. After having contested for nearly two decades with the physiotherapists (alias physical therapy technicians) their proprietary right to the term "physical therapy," the physicians were not sure they had chosen the right name after all. Following much soul-searching and two years of debate about the relative merits of "physiatrician," "physicologist," and "physiatrist," the Council on Physical Medicine declared itself in favor of the last designation. Submitted to the parent AMA for approval, the new name was formally recognized in 1946. It was not that the physicians had had a change of heart; it was simply a reflection of the new reality: their use of physical agents was no longer limited to practicing "therapy" but encompassed a wide range of diagnostics as well, for which they felt the old name was too restrictive.

To no one's surprise, members of APA saw nothing but good in this change of course. In an editorial in the September 1946 issue of the *Review*, editor Louise Reinecke declared, "As the field of physical medicine expands, so will the professions which are an integral part of it. Physical therapists must be informed concerning new developments and be aware of the trends in treatment. Our growth depends upon the intelligent practice of physical medicine and it is our responsibility to be interested in its future."

Physical medicine's evolutionary change also presented an opportunity to right what members regarded as an old wrong. Before the dust had begun to settle on the name discarded by the medical men, the House of Delegates polled the APA's 44 chapters via bulletins regarding changing the organization's name to the American Physical Therapy Association, or APTA. By an overwhelming majority, the chapters voted to proceed, and at the annual meeting in 1947, the deed was completed through an amendment of the Bylaws. The timing was significant, for it came as the Association embarked on its second quarter-century of life. Tidying up one more of its rough edges, the reenergized organization showed once again its extraordinary capacity for change and growth.

*The APTA pendant below belonged to Lucy Blair, who served as a lieutenant with the WAVES before joining the Association's staff. Blair, a well-loved member for whom an Association award is named, was stationed at navy hospitals in California, Oregon, and New York during World War II.*

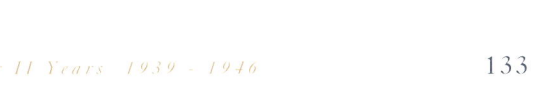

*The World War II Years 1939 - 1946*

## Physical Therapy's Ambassador To Asia

For a decade after World War I, Mollie McMillan prospered in Boston. In addition to her voluntary work as founder and first president of APA, she was co-director of ten successive sessions of the famous Course 442 at Harvard and carried on as principal physiotherapist in the office of Dr. Elliott Brackett. She also managed to travel widely overseas, usually for the purpose of observing other methods of physical therapy. In 1927 she took a three-month-long sabbatical at Rollier's Clinic in Switzerland to study the "sun cure." Then in 1932, when the China Medical Board of the Rockefeller Foundation advertised for a new chief physiotherapist for the Peking Union Medical College, she applied, stating in her application "[I] have always been interested in seeing how other people in different parts of the world live." The board briefly wondered among themselves whether McMillan was too old for the strenuous undertaking — she was 52 at the time — but her exceptional reputation and experience ultimately overcame their concerns. They appointed her to a four-year term, at a handsome salary of $3,000 per annum.

McMillan and the 360-bed Peking Union Hospital turned out to be a perfect match, and she remained there far beyond her original contract. "It isn't exactly easy to start work in a country where one knows nothing about the people or their language," McMillan later told attendees at APA's twenty-fifth anniversary Annual Conference in Blue Ridge, North Carolina. "I think the thing that perhaps helped me in my early days in Peking was these lines — 'To get adjusted to the world is, after all, the better plan — it won't adjust itself to you, for it was here before you came.'" She taught scores of young Chinese in the science and techniques of physical therapy, oversaw day-to-day care of patients, and lectured doctors on the rationale of Western physical therapy. In her spare time, she immersed herself in the life of her host country, traveling off into the hinterlands aboard donkey carts and decrepit trains to climb mountains and visit historic sites. Within less than a year she had progressed so far in her language studies that she could run her department in Chinese when necessary. As she had so many times before, she earned herself a great circle of devoted friends and admirers.

Indeed, when the clouds of war began to form in Asia, and the U.S. State Department advised Americans in China to come home, McMillan wanted to remain where she was needed. Late in 1941, however, when her employers ordered the evacuation of all foreign personnel, McMillan had no choice but to depart with them. Arriving in Manila where she was to transfer to another vessel early in December, she was caught by the Japanese bombing of Pearl Harbor and the U.S. entry into war in Asia.

As usual, Mollie volunteered to help, this time in caring for the huge numbers of bombing casualties being brought into the U.S. Army's Sternberg

Hospital. For three weeks the 61-year-old physical therapist lived and worked at the hospital under the most difficult of conditions, all the while expecting Japanese invasion. "We were obliged to spend Christmas Eve and Christmas morning in a trench, helmet and gas mask in place, . . . the sickening dread of immediate danger to one's self and to one's friends close by," she recalled.

Finally, early on the evening of January 2, with the Japanese invasion of the city imminent and the hospital having been hurriedly evacuated, McMillan martialled two companions and a large hotel delivery truck to collect the great quantities of precious medical supplies left behind. "Three women looted drugs and medical supplies . . . by flashlight, not knowing at what moment the Japanese might come and find us." Working feverishly for more than an hour, their pockets bulging with thermometers, pressure cuffs, and specula, their necks strung with as many stethoscopes as they could carry, the lady marauders managed to fill the truck, deliver the contents to the Red Cross, and return through the back gate of the hotel by midnight.

Before dawn the next morning, McMillan's hotel was seized and she and the other occupants were arrested. Ordered into the street and bravely singing "Where Do We Go From Here" as they went, they were herded along with 3,200 other foreign civilians into the walled grounds of Manila's ancient Santo Tomás University. Living conditions in the prison were, by any measure, extremely difficult. Malaria and dysentery were rife, warm clothing and blankets rare, and food so scarce that the majority of prisoners lost 30 pounds or more during the first year. Living accommodations were also primitive.

Mollie made her bed in an inverted wooden filing cabinet to avoid sleeping on the ground, and she shared four toilets and three showers with 469 other women. But with her indomitable spirit, she still managed to set up a physical therapy clinic for the prisoners, performing miracles with her clever hands, hot water, a few pails and towels. As one admirer would later recall, "Aching backs and arthritis from sleeping on cold cement, pulled muscles, painful feet, infected bedbug bites and rashes — all manner of aches and pains were brought in. And every day people went away feeling better." It was, McMillan said, her duty and her joy: "A physical therapist must never let her patients go without hope. . . . Hope helps to chase away fears."

After nearly nine months at Santo Tomás, McMillan was transferred. She traveled 10 days and nights in the hold of a Japanese cattle boat, with only space enough to lie down, no drinking water, and a rancid gruel of rice and fish heads as sole sustenance. Incarcerated at Chaipei prison near Shanghai, she fell seriously ill but survived to be part of a prisoner exchange completed on October 19, 1943, in the Indian Ocean. McMillan sailed home aboard the Swedish "*S.S. Gripsholm*."

Mildred Elson later recalled the moving speech a recuperating McMillan gave to the 1944 Annual Conference in New York: "Still pain-racked from the effects of beriberi and peripheral neuritis . . . with a voice not quite strong . . . her unquenchable spirit, deep religious faith with its accompanying inner strengths shone through her every word."

## CHAPTER 5

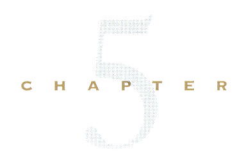

## "Progress Is A Relay Race"
## 1946 – 1959

*Susan Roen of the Southern California Chapter was elected president in 1946, a period of rapid growth for the Association. During Roen's tenure membership grew from 3,146 to 3,731.*

President Jessie Stevenson, in her annual address to the membership in 1946, reviewed the many advances that had taken place within the profession and the Association during the war years. Membership had more than doubled, the organization's financial solidity had improved substantially, a permanent national office and an executive secretary had been put in place, a new association name had been adopted, and many changes had been made within the Constitution and Bylaws to assure greater national unity. With peace at hand, she said, the time was ripe for everyone to slow down a little, get some perspective on where they were, and consider what further steps the organization needed to take to reach maximum effectiveness.

As the Executive Committee saw it, several issues commanded early attention. With regard to the level of therapeutic care, developments in polio and neuromuscular rehabilitation were at the forefront, requiring everyone's commitment. Some organizational matters, particularly the relationship between the national office and the chapters, needed additional refining. And in the matter of professional growth, educational enhancement and improved credentialing were essentials. Indeed, in the era dawning, the two seemed indivisible.

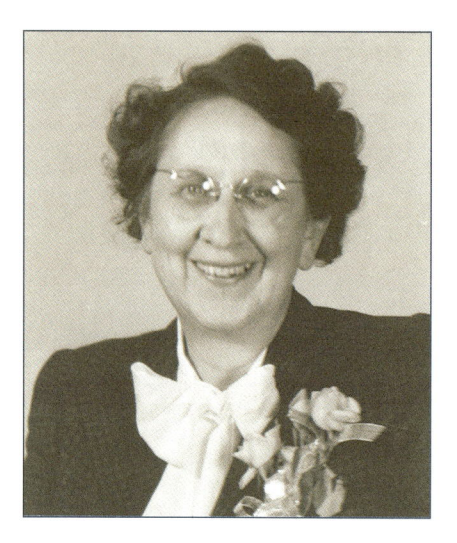

### RAISING THE GRADE ON EDUCATION

The first and most effective area in which APTA could exert its growing influence was in the educational arena. With war's end, all of the army schools and two civilian schools had been discontinued. That left just 21 approved schools producing 480 graduates annually. With an estimated 15,000 or more physical therapists needed in practice by 1960 — roughly five times the actual numbers — and with the net gain in PTs annually (after allowing for attrition due to retirements, deaths, and other causes) at just 200, the gap between supply and demand was on the way to becoming a chasm. As Mildred Elson, executive secretary of APTA, reminded everyone repeatedly, it was inevitable that the health care system would have to hire less-skilled practitioners if the situation didn't change. Something needed to be done about raising the number of physical therapy students quickly.

APTA consequently stepped up the campaign to get more universities and medical schools involved in teaching physical therapy and to expand the opportunities for graduate-level education. In this effort, the national office had the strong support of the fledgling Schools Section (forerunner of the Section for Education) which, beginning in 1946, met at least once a year to make recommendations regarding admissions, curricula, education, and administration of physical therapy schools. Within the section those members who served as program directors at accredited schools also established the Council of Physical Therapy School Directors. By 1947, the numbers of approved schools had increased only modestly, but many curricula had lengthened from nine months to twelve. Four schools now offered post-baccalaureate certificate programs; these were the Medical College of Virginia, Northwestern University Medical School, Stanford University, and the University of Wisconsin Medical School.

Three years later the record was still better: there were 31 accredited schools, 19 of them offering four-year, integrated bachelor's degree programs and eight offering post-baccalaureate certification.

One of these was the School of Allied Medical Professions (SAMP), which was established by the University of Pennsylvania in 1950. Probably the first "allied health" school in the nation, SAMP started with two departments: one evolved from a 30-year-old program initiated at the Philadelphia School of Occupational Therapy; the other, from a post-baccalaureate certificate program in physical therapy that traced its roots all the way back to 1915 and the Philadelphia Chirurgical Hospital, which was itself a forerunner of the Graduate Hospital of the University of Pennsylvania. The Occupational Therapy and Physical Therapy Departments were joined in 1952 by a Department of Medical Technology offering an undergraduate degree program. Among the physical therapists staffing the school were Dorothy Baethke and Jane Carlin.

*On April 16, 1947, President Truman, posing here with Major Emma Vogel, far right, and other senior officers, signed Public Law 80-36, establishing the Women's Medical Specialist Corps in the Regular Army. The AMSC's medallion, left, reflects this founding date and the name change that occurred when male PTs were accepted in 1955.*

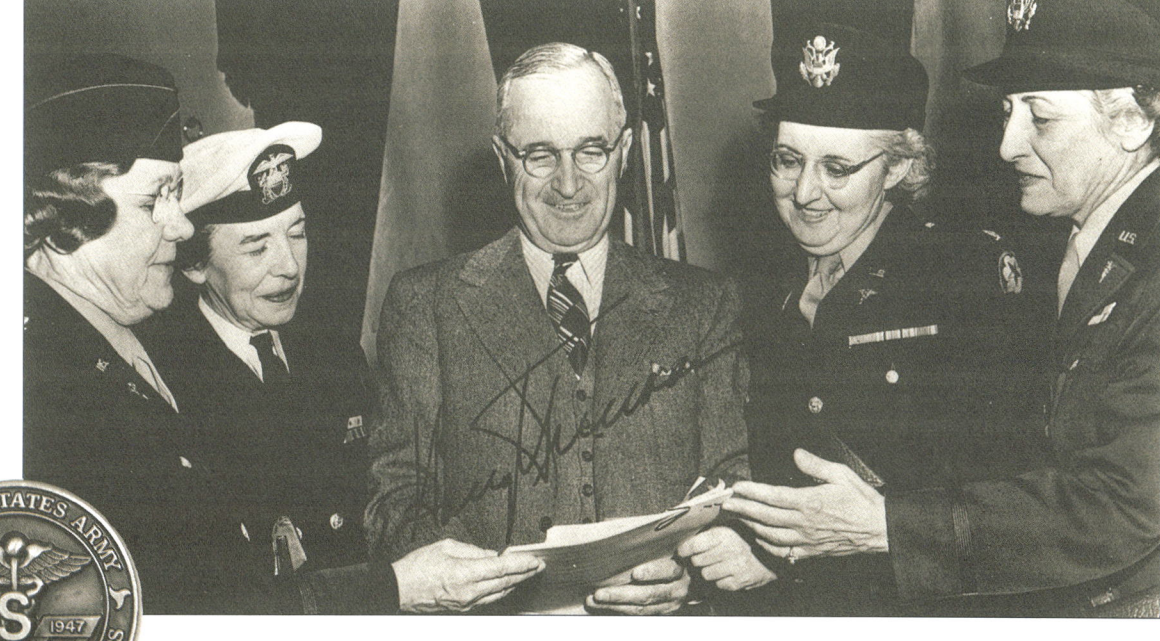

"Progress Is A Relay Race" 1946–1959   137

*Physical therapy, occupational therapy, and dietetics are traditionally joined in partnership in the military services. Shown here is a commemorative coin used by the Army Medical Specialist Corps from 1952 to 1992.*

Meanwhile, as part of APTA's continuing effort to enhance educational offerings, the Association invited the technical directors of approved schools of physical therapy to a three-day conference in French Lick Springs, Indiana, in 1950 to discuss common concerns. The leadership was gratified to have 26 schools send representatives. Among the issues covered were vocational guidance, the lack of adequate laboratory and practice space at many schools, the chronic shortage of staff instructors, the difficulties of integrating physical therapy programs within established university programs, the need for internships as an extension of education, and what was generally perceived as a terribly outdated set of minimum curriculum standards which schools were using as their guide in designing course work.

The standards were those set by the AMA's Council on Medical Education, which had been responsible for accrediting "Acceptable Physical Therapy Schools." Their evaluations, in turn, were based on a set of "Essentials" that, except for minor changes in 1943 and 1949, was essentially identical with that issued by the AMA Council in 1936. Helen Hislop, in the first of what would become scores of articles she would publish in the *Review*, argued in her 1953 "Survey of Physiology Teaching Programs in Schools of Physical Therapy" that 78 percent of schools were offering inadequate education in this most critical subject. Many other subjects were also getting short shrift.

Concerns about the adequacy of the "Essentials" were made greater still by information that 18 medical colleges and universities were clamoring to establish their own programs. Though Margaret Moore, then APTA's staff educational consultant, confirmed that many more schools were needed, she also thought that poorly planned and executed programs would be worse than none. "Quantity should never take the place of quality in our work," she wrote in the September 1951 *Review*. The new Council of Physical Therapy School Directors, in concert with APTA's Department of Education, decided to come up with a new set of recommendations for entry-level education.

Managed by Moore with the help of many volunteers, the Curriculum Revisions Committee labored for several years before coming up with a set of recommendations that were adopted by the AMA in 1956. They included a four-year baccalaureate degree with major work in physical therapy, though they also allowed for the continuation of a certificate course for individuals who sought physical therapy education only after completing college work in some other major.

One source of the dissatisfaction about curricula derived from the fact that physical therapists had limited direct input into the accreditation process. Another was the result of an evolutionary change in the process by which prospective physical therapists entered the profession. Once students typically had taken their physical therapy training only after earning their baccalaureate in other fields, such as physical education, nursing, or the biological sciences, with the clinical skills taught later in special courses attached to a hospital. By contrast, students preparing to become physical therapists were now likely to earn their physical therapy degrees in a university setting, with less opportunity for clinical exposure and very little preparation for the teaching part of their profession.

Notable in the revisions was a 35 percent increase in total numbers of class hours, with much of the increase concentrated in physiology, tests and measurements, and clinical practice. These content additions were a clear reflection of the changing role of the physical therapist. No longer was it sufficient for the practitioner to be educated in basic anatomy and kinesiology and to have mastered a series of basic procedures; now it was also necessary to understand the rationale for every application, which often lay in neurological principles.

At the same time, the national office pleaded with the chapters to organize membership drives, to send speakers into the high schools, and to look for opportunities to explain to their communities what physical therapy was all about and why its professionals found their work so gratifying. In the words of Lois Ransom, APTA president in 1948, "We have sold our profession as a service. We must now sell it as a career."

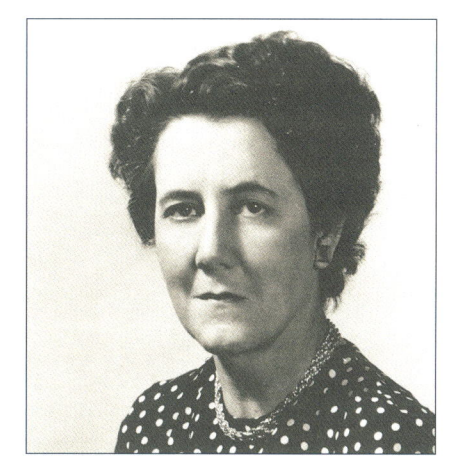

Through all of APTA's labors on behalf of education, the National Foundation for Infantile Paralysis played a unique role as stalwart friend and financier. When APTA began its effort to strengthen physical therapy schools, the NFIP offered to subsidize the position of education secretary, a position first filled by Barbara White, followed in 1949 by Jane Carlin and in 1950 by Margaret Moore, who carried the revised title of educational consultant. When more and better-prepared students were sought, the NFIP provided funds for the writing and printing of recruiting materials. When, early in 1953, the Executive Committee authorized the most extensive recruitment program ever launched, with a goal of 1,000 new students by the fall, the NFIP paid for more than 40,000 mailings, a recruitment film, filmstrips, and a poster contest whose winning submission by staffers at the National Society for Crippled Children and Adults was distributed in the form of 50,000 posters.

When the shortage of instructors proved a sticking point to the continued growth of physical therapy schools, the NFIP underwrote teaching fellowships — 49 of them by late 1955 — and provided direct assistance to 13 struggling schools in the purchase of needed instructional equipment. When APTA declared that the schools of physical therapy would benefit from a curriculum update, the NFIP provided the Association with a grant to cover most of the costs.

*Lois Ransom of Washington, D.C., left, was elected APTA president at the 1948 Conference in Chicago. A notable innovation at this year's meeting: for the first time, members were invited to present research papers. The brochure, below, published in that year, helped publicize the growing professionalism and popularity of physical therapy as a career.*

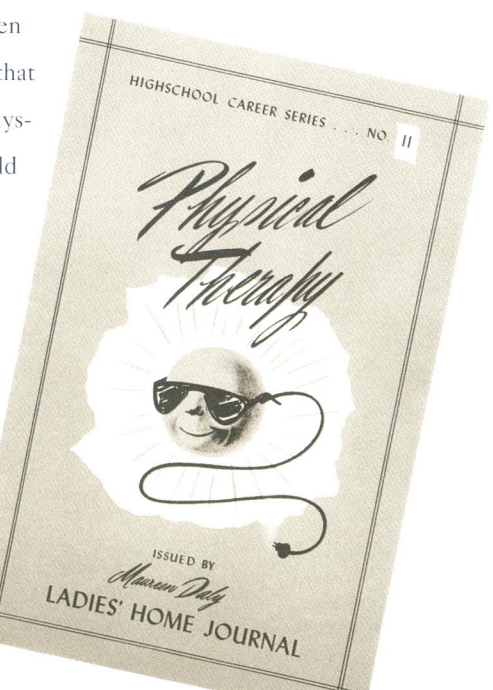

"Progress Is A Relay Race" 1946 – 1959     139

Indirectly, the NFIP also financed a study undertaken for APTA by the New York University Testing and Advisement Center. The center was asked to design a scientific evaluation program that would assist school admissions directors in predicting applicants' suitability — both intellectual and vocational — for the work. (With admission spaces so limited, the Association hoped to reduce the number of students who, for lack of sustained commitment or academic ability, ultimately failed to enter the profession.) And in its greatest gift of all, the NFIP provided academic scholarships and funding for travel abroad. By the end of 1955, more than 2,700 physical therapists, or one third of the nation's total, had shared in the nearly $4 million that the "March of Dimes" had authorized for educational financial aid. It was certainly no coincidence that the increase in student enrollment and the level of education sought grew in proportion to the grants-in-aid available. As for the travelships, numbers of practicing physical therapists were given the opportunity to observe and report on work of colleagues overseas, visiting hospitals, rehabilitation centers, and long-term residential facilities. By 1955, nearly 81 percent of current physical therapy students were in degree programs. In all of these cooperative ventures, Catherine Worthingham, a former APTA president and current director of professional education for the NFIP, was always the wise counselor and friend to APTA.

### Credentialing

Coincident with upgrading the educational base of physical therapy, APTA began a campaign to firm up its legal position within individual states. In the war's aftermath had come many new challenges to the physical therapists' turf. Chiropractors probably represented the largest single competing group, but "corrective" or "exercise" therapists presented a more acute risk. Most corrective therapists (CTs) were men with degrees in physical education. They worked principally in VA hospitals, where their physical strength equipped them for the heavy work of exercising patients with paraplegia. But as VA hospitals were not required to abide by the AMA's professional codes, prescribing physicians had a tendency to treat CTs as interchangeable with PTs in many other therapeutic tasks for which they were not trained. It was just a matter of time, the APTA leadership reasoned, before corrective therapists would also be allowed to treat civilians and children in the general run of hospitals. Another area in which new and stronger regulations were needed was in the realm of services increasingly performed outside the usual hospital and clinical settings; many "irregulars" were finding it particularly easy in the home-care milieu to call themselves "physical therapists" and go unchallenged.

Registration through the AMA-controlled American Registry of Physical Therapists had provided a weak form of protection to the extent that it conferred a formal title and certified that individuals so registered met or exceeded the AMA's standards of minimum professional competence. Physicians and hospital administrators seeking physical therapy staff knew that, at the very least, a candidate on the Registry had successfully completed an approved physical therapy curriculum. But such private certification came at a price that increasingly caused strains within APTA. With no physical therapists sitting on the Registry board initially, physicians wrote and administered tests that APTA viewed as poor measures of professional competence in physical therapy. In 1946, for example, of the 671 applicants examined, only 10 failed. Charles Magistro, who passed the Registry exam in May 1950, recalls that the test was the physical therapist's equivalent of "reciting the Baltimore Catechism, a test of rote memorization skills only."

But if the title "Registered" was relatively easy to secure, it could also be taken away by the Registry board on grounds that APTA felt were inappropriate, even self-serving, as in the case of physical therapists disciplined for maintaining a private office "independent of medical supervision and direction." Another problem with the Registry was that it offered registered physical therapists no legal protection. Municipal, state, and federally operated hospitals, along with other services, were free to staff their facilities with non-registered, non-certified physical therapists when convenient. By 1949, Catherine Worthingham, Jessie Stevenson, and Mildred Elson concluded that the Registry was, at best, "a temporary device," and, indeed, history would prove them right. Meanwhile, in a reversal of APTA's earlier wariness concerning state licensure, they called for the enactment of state practice acts as soon as possible.

In contrast to the Registry, state practice acts not only regulated the use of relevant occupational titles but also controlled the right to practice the profession in the name of protecting the public from unskilled impostors. Such powers typically emanated from a designated state licensing board or agency, usually the State Board of Medical Examiners, which already regulated physicians, surgeons, and the nursing profession. The licensing board set up formal criteria for each profession (education, experience, ethical requirements) in consultation with the professional leadership in the state and administered a licensing test, again relying on the guidance of professionals in the field. Persons passing the test were judged to be capable of performing their profession in the public interest and were licensed to practice within a set of published rules and regulations. Those who did not pass were denied a license and thus prohibited by law from practicing within the state or using the title "physical therapist." Licensed professionals who failed to abide by state regulations were subject to discipline, including the loss of license.

Although state licensure could and did evolve through a variety of mechanisms, it was generally left up to interests within each state to initiate the process through application to the governor or legislature. Licensing in Pennsylvania and New York had developed through such a process decades earlier. Pennsylvania had its first licensing mechanism in 1913, New York in 1926. Now Mildred Elson challenged APTA chapters in the other states to get the ball rolling in their separate jurisdictions. Offering advice and counsel was APTA's Standing Committee on Public Laws, formed in 1947 under the able leadership of Floy Pinkerton, director of Columbia

*Mildred Elson served as the first executive director of APTA from 1944 to 1956 and the first president of the World Confederation for Physical Therapy from 1951 to 1955. She also served the profession as editor-in-chief of the* Review *from 1936 to 1944 and as a consultant on physical therapy to the U.S. Army and Veterans' Bureau.*

University's School of Physical Therapy. It was to take "prodigious work." By 1950 Connecticut, Maryland, and Washington had joined Pennsylvania and New York in having Physical Therapy Practice Acts; by 1953 the number had grown to 15 plus the territory of Hawaii; by 1959, related legislation had been approved by 30 additional states. The stringency of the regulations varied considerably at first, with some mandatory, some "permissive," but gradually all states moved toward the stiffer standards.

Meanwhile, APTA decided to take the initiative in developing an objective test to evaluate individual competency. The reasons were twofold. First, such a test would give states another option to the cost and burden of developing and grading their own tests, a boon that might spur them to tighten regulations sooner. Second, it would provide a nationwide standard of competency which existed separate from the diversity of state licensing practices; thus, a physical therapist could readily move from one state to another and enjoy reciprocal licensure in most states, without having to be examined anew each time. In 1953 the Association approached Dr. Lillian Long, director of the Professional Examination Service of the American Public Health Association, for technical assistance in developing a suitable examination. The Association then assembled its own examination committee, including Elizabeth Addoms of New York University, Lucille Daniels of Stanford, and Mary Elizabeth (Mary Lib) Kolb of the D. T. Watson School of Physiatrics, to lay out the overall objectives of the test, and they, in turn, recruited another 200 or so members to write and review them. The result, completed in 1954, was a seven-hour-long multiple-choice examination with 310 questions spread over the basic sciences, clinical sciences, and theory and procedures. The roughly $12,000 cost of preparing the initial test was borne entirely by APTA. This cost, plus additional expenses for regular revisions, was gradually recovered through the $10 per capita fee charged for each test administered. Florida was the first state to avail itself of the APTA-PES exam, and 11 others had followed suit by 1958, with many more to come.

Coincident with APTA's efforts to improve its credentialing process, the Joint Commission on Accreditation of Hospitals (JCAH) was formed in 1951 by five major associations in the field of medicine and hospitals. Although the JCAH's recommendations did not carry the force of law, the standards it proposed did serve to encourage the raising of standards in institutional staffing and health care.

### FOREIGN RELATIONS

APTA had long been working to strengthen its relations with other groups on the world stage, and the postwar era provided a particularly favorable climate for pursuing that goal. In the most visible example, Mildred Elson became a guiding force in forming the World Confederation for Physical Therapy. Not only did she attend the very first discussions in London in 1948, but when the 11 founder-members — Australia, Canada, Denmark, Finland, Great Britain, New Zealand, Norway, South Africa,

Sweden, the United States, and West Germany—held their inaugural session in Copenhagen in 1951, she was elected first president of the organization. She went on to preside over the first international congress held in London in 1953 and the second congress, which was hosted by APTA in New York in June 1956. That Elson and the others had anticipated a real need is demonstrated by the attendance records: at the New York meeting, more than 2,000 physical therapists representing 34 countries were in attendance!

Continuing in the noble tradition of Mary McMillan, individual APTA members also reached out to the international community as consultants, clinical workers, and teachers. Edith Buchwald Lawton is but one of many notable examples of teachers whose teachings reached far beyond U.S. shores. While director of postgraduate education at New York University–Institute of Physical Medicine and Rehabilitation, Lawton taught state-of-the-art rehabilitation techniques to some 150 professional physical therapists from 40 foreign countries. Other APTA members served Fulbright Teaching Fellowships in Rome, Milan, and Greece; held polio demonstrations at international congresses; accepted lengthy Red Cross assignments in Morocco; served with the International Refugee Organization and UNESCO; and carried out shorter training missions in such far-off places as Belgium, Cuba, Egypt, Haiti, Italy, Saudi Arabia, Czechoslovakia, Thailand, and Japan. An "epidemic unit" from Boston Children's Hospital was rushed into occupied Berlin in 1947 to assist in the polio emergency.

The written works of APTA members, chiefly in the form of clinical training guides, were increasingly translated and published abroad, too, a clear sign that American professionals were growing in stature and accomplishment. Especially appreciated were works on polio, cerebral palsy, and retraining for people with amputations.

### THE PHYSICAL THERAPY FUND

Over the years there had been many articles in the *Review*, both encouraging and scolding, on the subject of physical therapists providing better scientific data on their work, one of the hallmarks of a true profession. Several articles came from physiatrists who had strong ties to the Association: Dr. Nina Covalt's "The Challenge of Physical Therapy" (1947); Dr. Harry

---

*The first international congress of the World Confederation for Physical Therapy in London, 1953, was made possible by the increased cooperation and visibility of physical therapists in the European theater in World War II. Aware of the professional benefits of collaboration, thousands of PTs from all over the world attended to show their support for the Confederation.*

*Marguerite Irvine of Seattle, Washington, became APTA president in 1949, the year that saw the* Physical Therapy Review *mature into a monthly.*

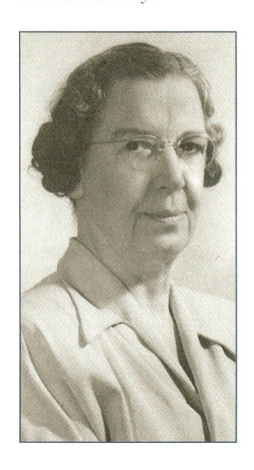

M. Hines's "What Research Means to a Profession" (1951); and Dr. Frances Hellebrandt's "The Communication of Ideas as a Professional Responsibility" (1951). All made outstanding cases for research in physical therapy. Similar themes were explored by physical therapists Sara Jane Houtz in "The Challenge of the Scientific Method" (1951) and Jane Carlin in her *Review* editorials on "record keeping" (1957) and "documentation" (1958), among others.

A few members obliged with worthy contributions to the research literature. Among the more impressive works were Margaret Moore's three-part "Goniometric Measurements" (1949) and Marian Williams's comprehensive "Manual Muscle Testing, Development and Current Use" (1956), both of which appeared in the *Review*. But as a general rule, physical therapists were too busy practicing their profession to find the needed time and funds to undertake and record well-documented studies.

Research grants from outside organizations, both private and public, had offered encouragement to a few would-be researchers, but there was a growing conviction among APTA's leadership that the Association should, in effect, put its money where its mouth was and do something on its own. In 1955, Jane Carlin and Mildred Elson brought before the House of Delegates the idea of establishing an internal fund to foster scientific, literary, and educational projects in physical therapy. After lengthy discussions the House of Delegates gave the proposal an enthusiastic go-ahead, and in 1957 the Physical Therapy Fund was established. To ensure that the fund remained independent of the Association and tax-exempt, it was incorporated as a separate entity under the laws of the state of New York, with APTA as sponsoring agent. The fund's first board of trustees consisted of Jane Carlin, Lucy Blair, and Mary Haskell, all executives in the national office. Members of APTA were invited to make voluntary donations large and small as an investment in the future of their profession.

The fund's first gift was a 1957 bequest from the family of Ruth Whittemore, a former staff polio consultant at APTA's national office and lifetime member who had died earlier that year after 19 years as a member. Over the next decade, the fund would disburse nearly $80,000 in research awards and educational grants. The initial grant of $1,500 went to Robert Kruse and the Northern Midwest Section of the Council of Physical Therapy School Directors in 1958 to assist in their study of the frequency of use of various modalities, procedures, and treatment techniques in clinical situations. Unfortunately, the fund experienced chronic problems in maintaining a purse adequate to the research ambitions of APTA's leaders, and in the late 1970s it would be reorganized as the broader-based Foundation for Physical Therapy, described in the next chapter.

### FEDERAL INVOLVEMENTS

The postwar era was a period of tremendous change and expansion in federal health programs, the most important of which was the revolution in the scope of activities of the U.S. Public Health Service and the spending to go with it. One has only to compare the $65.6 million in annual PHS appropriations in 1945 with the nearly $1.9 billion appropriated for the year 1965 to recognize that unprecedented changes were involved. While all phases of the PHS expanded, the largest growth was in research, training, and the development of medical facilities. It is also evident that within each of these categories a gradual shift was taking place from the earlier preoccupation with communicable diseases to a new concentration on serving chronic diseases and disabilities. Also changing was the PHS's mechanism for getting things done. Building on the positive experiences of the 1935 Title VI of the Social Security Act, which had authorized the Surgeon General to grant $8 million a year to strengthen state public health programs, the postwar PHS was permitted to carry out much of its expansion in pass-throughs to the states.

Certainly the most visible example of the expansion in pass-throughs was manifested in the Hill-Burton Act, which was introduced in 1946 and enlarged repeatedly thereafter. Known officially as Public Law 79-725, the Hospital Survey and Construction Act, the far-reaching program was sponsored by Senators Lister Hill of Alabama and Harold Burton of Ohio as an antidote to the sorry state of postwar hospitals. The Great Depression and World War II had brought to a virtual standstill the construction and modernization of public and private hospitals, and the legacy was a shortage of modern medical facilities in virtually every part of the country. In its initial form the bill authorized $75 million a year in federal grants to assist states and local communities in constructing general hospitals and public health centers. In more than 400 towns and cities that previously lacked any hospital facilities, new hospitals were built; in 165 other locations in which existing facilities were very old-fashioned, major upgrades were undertaken; scores of established hospitals, including major teaching hospitals, were also helped to modernize and expand. In subsequent amendments, the figure for hospital construction was enlarged to $150 million and an additional $60 million annually was set aside for specialized health service facilities such as rehabilitation centers and chronic disease treatment facilities. During the next three decades, Hill-Burton and the Public Health Service spurred new building programs in every state in the nation. Initially, the monies went to the most basic sorts of construction — patient wards, operating rooms, diagnostic facilities — but as the need for other kinds of services was recognized, substantial sums were funneled in their direction as well. In all, some $3.7 billion in federal grants were matched with $9.1 billion in state funds.

Other key social legislation affecting public health and physical therapy included Congress's approval of U.S. participation in the new World Health Organization in 1948; the restructuring of the National Institute of Health into the ambitious, multidivisional National Institutes of Health (NIH) in 1948; the creation of the new Department of Health, Education and Welfare, of which the PHS became a part, in 1953; the passage of various health amendments authorizing educational grants to physical therapists and other "allied health" professionals;

*With the establishment of the Women's Medical Specialist Corps, the status of physical therapy in the army was secured. Better equipment, such as this whirlpool bath, right, complete with an aerator and a temperature gauge, was provided for physical therapy units. However, the shortage of actual PTs to staff these units that (continued opposite)*

and a series of laws designed to innovate the nation's vocational rehabilitation services.

In this last category, the transformation was carried out by the Veterans Administration for World War II veterans with service-connected disabilities and by the civilian Office of Vocational Rehabilitation (OVR) for members of the general population with disabilities. The VA, which ultimately employed 625 physical therapists in its ambitious program to rehabilitate the war wounded, showed the nation what could be done to restore those with severe disabilities to meaningful lives and careers. The civilian OVR program, which was able to benefit from the VA's example, was built upon foundations in the Social Security Act of 1935 but went far beyond the original goals of "training around" existing disabilities. Under the 1943 Barden-LaFollette Act and the 1954 Vocational Rehabilitation Amendments, thousands of civilians with disabilities were given their first opportunity to get better.

Not only were state rehabilitation facilities enlarged substantially at very low costs to the states, but for the first time, cities and counties could apply for federal funds to build and staff rehabilitation centers, and educational institutions and private nonprofit agencies engaged in rehabilitation research could also receive financial help for their programs. For example, in 1956 APTA was given $10,000 to manage a week-long institute on the "Correlation of Physiology with Therapeutic Exercise" at the University of Oklahoma. With this sum, the Association was able to introduce representatives of 35 physical therapy schools to the latest rehabilitative techniques of Edna Blumenthal, Signe Brunnström, Florence Kendall, Laura Smith, and other leaders in the field. Two years later, the OVR granted APTA $40,000 to produce and distribute the Association's first public relations film, "The Return." The film was made at the New York Rehabilitation Hospital in West Haverstraw and focused on the role of physical therapists in rehabilitating traumatically injured

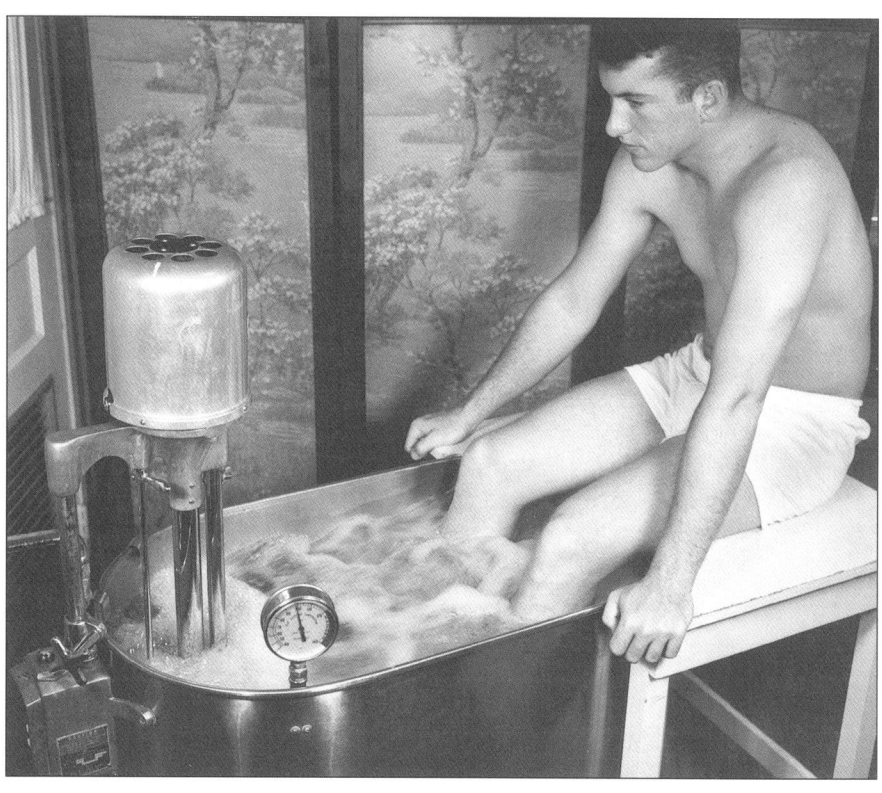

146  *Healing The Generations*

patients. It was distributed for showing in each of the states and was recognized as the "Outstanding" educational film of 1959 by *Scholastic* Magazine.

Coincident with the sweeping revisions of 1954, President Dwight Eisenhower challenged the nation to more than triple the current figure of 60,000 persons being rehabilitated annually to reach all of the estimated 200,000 newly disabled each year. The actual growth in rehabilitative services was, however, considerably slower than hoped for, in part because state rehabilitative services were slow to reorganize administratively and in part because there simply were not enough people trained in the rehabilitation field to carry out the work. (A principal bottleneck in staffing was at the "head" of the rehabilitation team, where physiatrists remained a relatively underpopulated medical specialty. Between 1953, when physiatry redescribed the field as Physical Medicine and Rehabilitation, or PM&R, and 1960, the number of board-certified physiatrists had risen to just 394.) Still, if the growth failed to live up to optimistic projections, it was moving in the right direction: by 1960 nearly $80 million in combined federal and state funds were being spent annually to rehabilitate 88,000 Americans, an increase of roughly 45 percent in less than six years. At the same time, another $13,574,000 was going to research, demonstration programs, education, and traineeships in the rehabilitation field. In every facet of this growth, physical therapists were heavily involved.

One name that particularly stands out in the early years of rehabilitation is that of Mary Eleanor Brown. Brown came to the profession of physical therapy by way of dance, which she studied briefly with Martha Graham, and exercise training, which included work with Bess Mensendieck and the Mensendieck System of Functional Exercises. But it was only after meeting Signe Brunnström and being persuaded to take up physical therapy at New York University that she found her true calling. Studying nights for her physical therapy certificate, which she obtained in 1945, Brown worked days as research assistant to the noted rehabilitation specialist George Deaver at the Institute for Crippled and Disabled (ICD) and taught several courses at the NYU Physical Therapy Program, where Deaver was curriculum director. She went on to hold directorial positions at a number of rehabilitation facilities, including the New York State Rehabilitation Hospital at West Haverstraw. Along the way, Brown carried out pioneer studies in "activities of daily living" (ADLs), a phrase she is often credited with having coined.

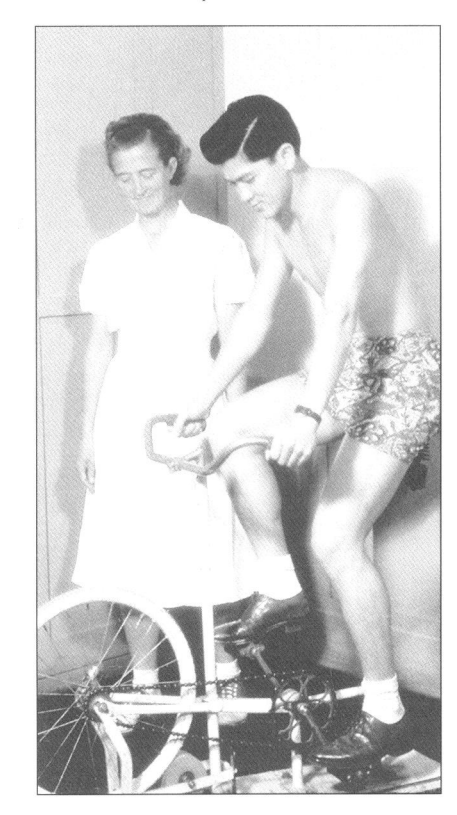

*had plagued the army in World Wars I and II was evidenced in the Korean War as well. With less than half the staff it needed, the WMSC instituted a brief training course to teach enlisted men how to administer the more basic treatments and to supervise therapeutic exercise such as performed on the exercise bike pictured, left.*

*Mary Clyde Singleton, below, professor of physical therapy and anatomy at the University of North Carolina, presided over APTA from 1950 to 1952. Shown at right is Col. Emma Vogel, first chief of the Women's Medical Specialist Corps, shortly before her retirement in 1951.*

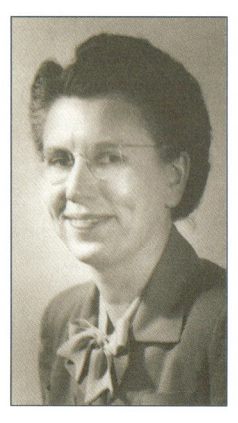

Geneva Johnson, herself a specialist in rehabilitation physical therapy, recalls her former teacher fondly: "Mary Eleanor brought a joyous sense of wonder to the practice of physical therapy. She had amazing self-discipline, curiosity, attention to detail, with the result that she was always discovering something. For example, she'd come around at lunch time and get all of the new graduates to act out particular ADLs while she ran her stopwatch and made notes. She was also unflappable when it came to taking her disabled patients places. Long before there were any public accommodations for the handicapped, she'd take a group into the city on a train and spend the day with them building their confidence and physical capabilities. She was a natural-born teacher, and very possibly physical therapy's first clinical researcher."

### The Korean War

The ongoing effort to achieve full military recognition for women physical therapists serving in the armed services ended successfully when in March 1947 the 80th Congress passed a law establishing the Women's Medical Specialist Corps (WMSC) within the regular army. Major Emma Vogel was made chief officer of the peacetime corps, which included Dietitian, Occupational Therapy, and Physical Therapy Sections, and was promoted to the rank of colonel. Those women remaining in uniform following World War II received peacetime commissions, and those who chose to return to civilian life but made themselves available for involuntary mobilization in emergencies retained reserve commissions. Men with the same credentials and education, on the other hand, were frozen out, because the WMSC was, by definition, a women's corps.

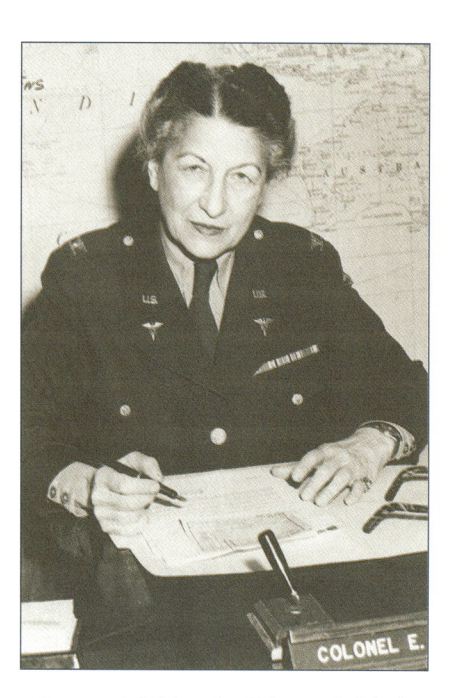

Vogel's all-women command had scarcely adjusted to its new status when the United States became embroiled in another war, this time in Korea, in June 1950. As with every other part of the army, five years of demobilization and postwar austerity measures had left the corps far below fighting trim, with 340 officers, only 135 of them physical therapists. Another 39 physical therapists had transferred over to the air force when that service had been given a separate identity in 1949 and were now under the command of Colonel Miriam Perry, another physical therapist.

Involuntary call-ups brought in a small number of physical therapists, as did patriotic appeals for qualified volunteers in the *Review* and the earnest support of Mildred Elson, who was appointed as civilian consultant to the WMSC. But neither Vogel nor Colonel Nell Wickliffe, who succeeded as chief upon Vogel's retirement in November 1951, were able to muster more than half of the projected need.

148　　*Healing The Generations*

Similar problems existed in the smaller Air Force Medical Service. The entire complement of commissioned physical therapists never exceeded 255, and this to care for an army that, when fully mobilized, amounted to 1.5 million men.

Combat in Korea, especially in the early months, was fierce, and casualties were heavy. Along with the wounds inflicted by gunfire and bombs, there were large numbers of men sidelined with polio, encephalitis, tuberculosis, fungal infections, and severe frostbite. More than 4,000 cold-injury patients were treated by physical therapists in one command hospital in the first brutal winter. Not surprisingly, the Far East command hospitals — some in South Korea, others on hospital ships off the coast, in Japan, and stateside — were chronically struggling with shortages of trained personnel to handle case loads. To ease the situation, staff physical therapists instituted informal "on-the-job" training for enlisted men assigned to the clinics. When the stopgap program proved to be surprisingly effective, U.S. Army headquarters formalized 12-week training courses, and through this approach, the crisis was met and mastered. Several members of the WMSC were recognized for exceptional service during the war, including Major Ethel Theilmann, with the Legion of Merit; and Captain Mary Torp and Major Elizabeth Jones, with Bronze Star Medals.

Throughout the Korean conflict, the disparity in military status that existed between men and women physical therapists proved a particular sticking point. In a curious reversal of the discriminatory policies that women had fought against for so long, the male physical therapist could expect no more than the rank, privileges, salary, and benefits accorded any other enlisted man. The arrangements were such to discourage, not to say anger, the most dedicated individuals, and it was bound to have a bearing on the corps' difficulties in meeting wartime staffing goals.

Reporting in the September 1950 issue of the *Review*, Executive Director Elson reassured members that her office was acutely aware of the inequities and was working hard to do something about it. Male commissions had, in fact, been a hot topic of debate in the House of Delegates for some time, and the recent conflict only served to intensify matters. Finally, in 1955, Representative Frances Bolton succeeded in pushing through Public Law 84-294. Henceforth, qualified male physical therapists were admitted at the same second lieutenant rank as women, the Women's Medical Specialist Corps was retitled the Army Medical Specialist Corps, and a new, more inclusive insignia was issued. The first enlisted men to receive the hard-won commissions were Sheldon Saffren and Philip A. Canton, both members of APTA, who were sworn in late in 1955. Virginia Metcalf, AMSC staffer at Brooke General Hospital, Fort Sam Houston, San Antonio, Texas, at the time, recalls that "there was much fear and apprehension among the women PTs, who had worked so long and hard to attain recognition in the army, that the men would come to dominate the corps. But as it turned out, the change went remarkably smoothly."

A major factor in making the smooth transition was the cooperative

*Col. Harriet Lee was APTA's 16th president, leading the organization from 1952 to 1954. Lee went on to serve as chief of the WMSC from 1954 to 1958.*

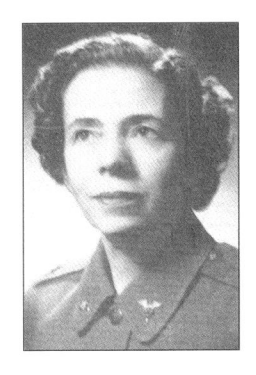

leadership at the top of the corps and APTA, which continued to work for common goals of excellence and professionalism. Indeed, there was so much overlapping between the two organizations during the 1950s that it was sometimes difficult to see them as having separate identities. In 1952, even before the Korean War had ended, Colonel Harriet S. Lee, chief of the Physical Therapy Section of the corps, was elected president of APTA. Lee held the presidency until 1954, when simultaneously she was promoted to succeed Colonel Wickliffe as Women's Medical Specialist Corps chief and returned to APTA's Board of Directors. Lieutenant Colonel Agnes P. Snyder, a Physical Therapy Section chief in the AMSC, served as speaker of APTA's House of Delegates from 1956 to 1958, at which time she took over the president's gavel, serving in the top APTA post from 1958 to 1961. Lieutenant Colonel Beatrice Whitcomb, on the faculty of the Medical Field Service School at Brooke, was selected an associate editor of the *Physical Therapy Review* from 1952 to 1956 and from 1960 to 1962. Lieutenant Colonel Barbara Robertson Friz, Physical Therapy Section chief from 1958 to 1962, served as chairman of the *Review* editorial board during most of those years.

### FAMILY BUSINESS

If the face of military physical therapy was changing, APTA had already undergone something of an internal transformation on the gender front. By 1955, large numbers of World War II male veterans, aided by the GI Bill, were graduating from civilian physical therapy schools. Where men had represented single-digit percentages of physical therapists graduating before the war, they now made up as much as a third to half of some classes. Lucy Ryan Anderson's 1946 class at the Graduate Hospital, University of Pennsylvania, had six men and 13 women. Five years later, Vilma Evans's class had near parity between the sexes: 18 women and 14 men, Eugene Michels among them. The 1951 class at the University of Connecticut had five men and one woman. (It was, incidentally, the inaugural class at UConn, with Fran Tappan making her debut as assistant dean and program director.) At New York University, the 43-member class of 1950 counted an unprecedented 34 men! Among them were Jack Hofkosh, Jay Schleichkorn, and Justin Alexander. The result was that by 1953 men constituted as much as 20 percent of the APTA membership rolls; the annual attrition rate, which had hovered around 10 percent due to women leaving to marry and raise children, had consequently dropped to 7 percent.

The increased male presence was also beginning to be reflected in the Association's leadership. By the late 1950s an average of four men were serving on the national board at any given time, with comparable representation occurring in many of the chapters. Among the first men to reach the top rung of chapter leadership were Arthur Brown of New Jersey, Anthony DeRosa of New York, and Robert Teckemeyer of California.

Other minorities were not faring as well. Though membership records were not kept by racial or ethnic category, it appears that the numbers of African-Americans and Black-Americans, Hispanics/Latinos, Native Americans, and Asian-Americans entering the profession and the Association in these years remained disproportionately low. The reasons were many, but surely at the top of the list were lack of exposure to physical therapy as a career and the absence of physical therapy educational opportunities in the South — there was not a single accredited physical therapy school in the South open to African-Americans and Black-Americans before 1963.

With the exception of the special WMSC class at Ft. Huachuca, Arizona, in 1943, the only African-American or Black-American physical therapists practicing during the war years are believed to have been Mary Ellen Spurlock Alexander in Cincinnati and Marge Franklin, who taught an introductory course in physical therapy to physical education students at Alabama's Tuskegee Institute. Franklin, in turn, became the mentor of Elizabeth Campbell and Helen Brown Mayes, both of whom left the South after graduation to take their advanced training in California. (The neighboring Tuskegee Air Force Base also had a physical therapy unit operated by an African-American enlistee who received on-the-job training.) About the same time, Thelma Brown Pendleton became the first African-American to graduate from Northwestern in 1947; Thelma Petty Williams was graduated from the University of California in 1947; Betty Mansfield graduated from NYU in 1947; Theodore Corbitt, mentored by Mary Ellen Alexander, completed the NYU course in 1948; and Vilma Evans came out of the University of Pennsylvania in 1951. Still others, like Beverly Brown and Joycelyn Elders, who would go on to become a pediatrician and, in 1993, U.S. Surgeon General, received their education through the AMSC Medical Field Service School at Fort Sam Houston.

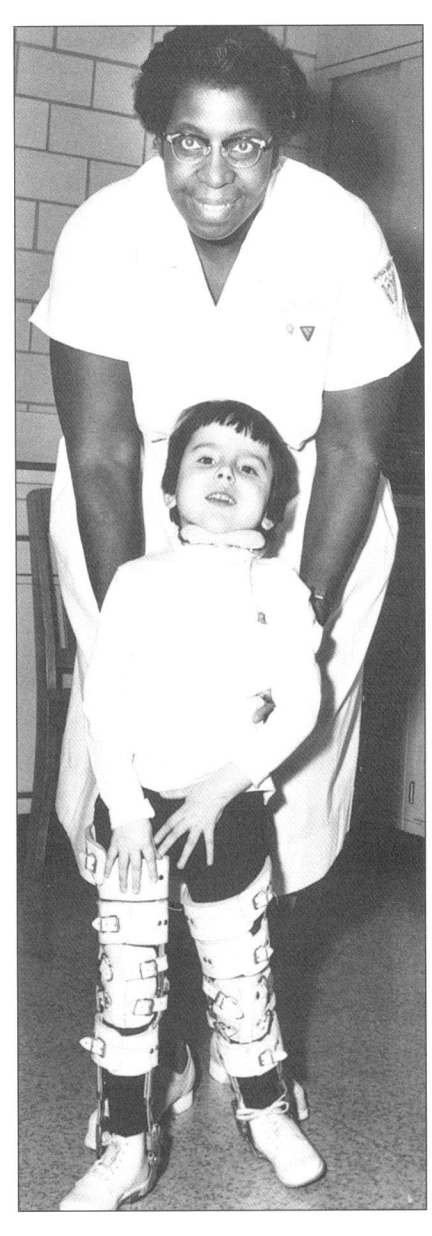

Thelma Petty Williams recalls that Basil O'Connor of the NFIP took a special interest in finding bright young African-American women to enter the physical therapy profession. Vilma Evans and Arretta Smith were two who were recipients of the March of Dimes (NFIP) Scholarship in 1950. Williams also remembers that the membership of APTA was generally welcoming to minority members, although problems arose when the Association chose Dallas as its Annual Conference site in 1953.

*Vilma Evans, one of the hundreds of physical therapists who got their start in polio work, is shown in a treatment room at St. Elizabeth's Hospital, Danville, Illinois, shortly after she became director of the physical therapy facility there.*

Attending her first Annual Conference, Vilma Evans travelled aboard a segregated train from Illinois to Dallas. When she arrived at the Baker Hotel, which was the official meeting location, she was told that there was no record of a room reservation and that the rooms were already full. Evans soon learned that her predicament was shared by five other African-Americans: Evelyn Prince of Columbia University and Louis Ballard, Erle Williams, Wilmotine Jackson, and Garfield Crawford — fellow graduates of the University of Pennsylvania. All had to secure lodgings in "the colored section" of Dallas and taxi to the meetings each day.

Meals were another problem. On the day of the big APTA awards luncheon, Evans and two other minority attendees were initially kept from entering the banquet hall. After much negotiating, the three were given a table in the rear of the dining room near the kitchen door. To circumvent the meal problem the rest of the time, Clara Arrington ordered "room service" lunches for everyone each day in her hotel room, and in this way the attendees managed to eat between morning and afternoon sessions.

During these enforced get-togethers, the "Texas Six," as they came to call themselves, decided to take their protest to the House of Delegates. After some discussion, the House resolved that none of its members should ever be put in such a blatantly discriminatory environment again as a result of attending the Annual Conference. Though little could be done to erase the painful memories of the Dallas meeting, plans to hold the 1954 Conference in Florida were promptly changed, and the next meeting was rescheduled for Los Angeles.

The profession and APTA were growing up in other ways, too. Two important constitutional revisions were undertaken. Notable in 1948 were the tightening of membership qualifications and the creation of a new student membership class; the dropping of junior or provisional members; a series of bylaws dealing with component chapters and charters; the first insertions of text concerning the creation, purpose, and governance of sections; and new articles to clarify the powers and duties of the House of Delegates and the Executive Committee. Eight standing committees, up from three in 1937, were also identified. Further constitutional fine-tuning came in 1954, when the criterion for establishing a section was specified as "group interest by at least 50 members," an effort to prevent an explosion of fractional subgroups; and the nine-person Executive Committee (five officers and four directors) was replaced with an equal-sized Board of Directors.

The period also brought new growth to the *Review*, which went from a bimonthly to a monthly in 1949, roughly doubling its annual number of pages (from 320 in 1948 to 584 in 1949), and changed its name from *Physiotherapy Review* to *Physical Therapy Review*. Employment opportunities widened substantially, as reflected in a five-part series on "The Scope of Physical Therapy" appearing about the same time, which focused on physical therapy in the physician's office or clinic, the small general hospital, the children's hospital, state service, and the large hospital. Average PT salaries were reportedly rising steadily, from a base of $2,000 in 1946 to $5,750 in general hospitals in 1959. (The daily charge for hospital care in this same period went up 250 percent to $25! This was balanced to some extent by a decline in average length of stay to 7.8 days.) A new wrinkle appearing in some areas was the physician-owned physical therapy service, in which an entrepreneurial physical therapist might even go into partnership, presumably sharing in the profits. An advertisement appearing in a 1947 issue of *The Archives of Physical Medicine and Rehabilitation* listed such an arrangement at a medical clinic in midwestern Nebraska.

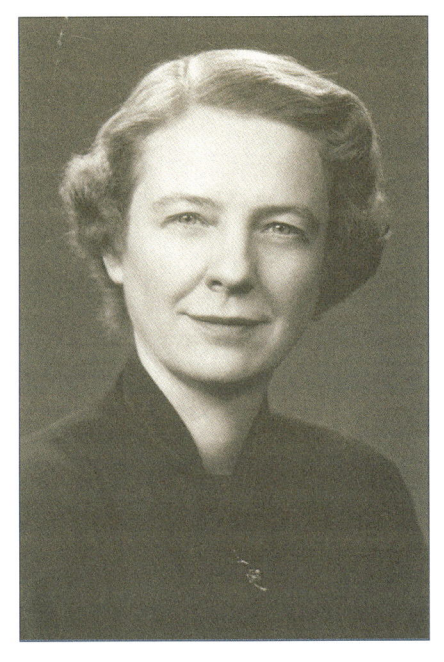

In the same postwar period, the Association's national staff increased from 3 to 21, operating with a budget that went from $16,000 in 1944 to $260,000 in 1957. (Alarmingly, the costs of doing business more than kept pace with income, which was split between dues and grants from the NFIP. In 1953 Margaret Kohli, chairperson of the Finance Committee, announced a year-end budget surplus of $36.36! Kohli asked for a dues increase from $15 to $20, and it was voted in with minimal resistance. In 1958 dues were raised again to $25.)

In a reflection of the dual roles played by many of the national office's administrators in these years, there were frequent changes at the top as individuals felt it was time to return to teaching, to the practice of physical therapy, or to executive positions in allied organizations. In 1956, Mildred Elson resigned after a dozen years as executive director. She was succeeded by Mary Haskell, who held the job until 1958 when she left to return to California and to part-time private practice.

Concurrently, the APTA membership swelled from 3,146 in 1946 to 8,028 in 1959. By 1951 there were just four states or territories without at least one chapter — Alaska, Nevada, North Dakota, and Wyoming; by 1955 all of them had chapter representation. Notable too were the formation in 1955 of the Section on the Self-Employed (later Private Practice), with Robert Dicus the first chairperson, and in 1956 of the Public Health Section (currently Community Home Health), with Clara Arrington its first chairperson.

Members were also becoming more worldly-wise about some of the nuts-and-bolts issues of running a treatment center. An example was the first detailed article on systematizing physical therapy fees, which appeared under the name of Arthur A. Rodriguez in 1955. The fifties brought calls for group health and disability insurance within the membership. The former was introduced by the Association beginning in 1953, and the latter was tabled pending the discovery of an insurer who would offer acceptable group rates. Professional liability insurance was also offered for the first time in 1959.

*A graduate of Bouvé-Boston and a member of APTA since 1929, Mary Haskell was swept up in the search for a cure for polio. She was the first to accept the position of polio coordinator for the Association and served as APTA's second executive director from 1956 to 1958.*

*Mary E. Nesbitt of Boston, Massachusetts, presided over the Association from 1954 to 1956, a time when the nation's victory over polio brought both joy and new concerns to the Association membership.*

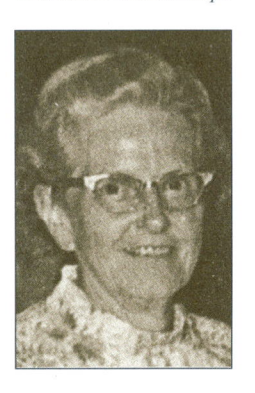

One matter that remained consistent was the national office's role as friendly guide and Dutch uncle, communicated to members through the pages of the *Review*. Scarcely an issue went by that the publication did not urge members to recruit student candidates, to lend a helping hand to new graduates, to protest inequities, to donate blood, to contribute actively in chapter programs and national drives, and to go back to school for more education. One editorial was particularly stern on the matter of treating employers fairly. Members were urged not to get caught up in "bidding wars" among competing hospitals and to give adequate notice before changing jobs. There were even occasional reminders to wear the APTA insignia prominently and to work on personal appearance.

Featured in the June 1953 issue was a commentary by Mildred Heap entitled "Our Looks are Deceiving Us," in which she said that potential recruits were being turned away from physical therapy careers by the sloppy dress of many PTs. "It is one thing to talk to prospective therapists with natural and instinctive enthusiasm, but quite another to show them on the job activities.... Too often, yes, much too often, the therapists' shoes are dirty, run over at the heels, and with shoe strings which might be capable of standing by themselves. At times therapists wear colored shoes with white uniforms. In some institutions the therapists wear street clothes, preferably sweaters, skirts and loafers with a long white coat, although they readily admit that one cannot work effectively in a long white coat. We might take a professional tip from our sister auxiliary groups, particularly like nursing — a profession which has long looked like one."

As the responsibilities of the national office expanded, some would say by leaps and bounds, the physical space it occupied became a nagging problem. Almost since it leased its original two rooms at 1790 Broadway in New York City in 1944, the square footage had been inadequate. Files, publications, reprints, and parts of exhibits were stacked over and under the growing assemblage of desks serving the national office staff. More rooms were added as the *Review*'s business and editorial staffs shifted by stages from Chicago to New York by 1949.

By 1950 still more people had been brought in to work on polio recruitment and emergency placements, and extra space was leased two floors above. The following year, still feeling cramped, the Executive Committee looked at the feasibility of buying shares in a new building to be erected by its landlord, the National Health Council, and went so far as to set aside investment funds for the purpose. But in 1954, when 2,700 square feet of sunny space overlooking 58th Street, Columbus Circle, and Central Park were found on another floor of the same building, plans to move elsewhere were dropped.

Sounding positively euphoric, editor Jane Carlin wrote a brief story in the *Review* about the latest expansion: "The news is a symbol of the growth and status of our profession... an indication of both our achievements and aspirations.... Moving day was March 1, when we came to rub elbows and sometimes bump noses for a week with painters, telephone men, electricians, linoleum layers, and window washers. Did you know that your National Office now totals 21?" With a little space left over to accommodate drop-ins, members were urged to come by and introduce themselves when in town.

The growth in staff was inevitable, of course; the better known the Association, the more responsibilities came its way. One or more staffers were on the road constantly, looking in on chapters, schools, conferences, polio centers, hospitals, and government meetings. In a six-month period in 1951, polio consultants Lucy Blair and Ruth Whittemore were asked to consult in 61 cities, visiting 101 different facilities. Staffers were also having to handle an ever-widening variety of informational services in the office. Elson's replacement, Mary Haskell, reported as routine an unending flow of queries and phone calls from allied professionals, convention bureaus, Association committee heads, and prospective students and their parents wanting information. She was even becoming accustomed to demands from the working press, fielding calls from

"beauty editors of teenage periodicals who consult us . . . on how to give curves to skinny legs and make fat legs alluring or where in New York to find a photogenic physical therapist."

### THE POLIO CONNECTION

The scourge of polio, despite the concerted efforts of the NFIP and legions of researchers and clinical medical people, grew worse in the years after World War II. Although the bruising battle between the Kenny supporters and the medical research establishment had lost much of its steam, fundamental divisions on some particulars remained wide and deep. Henry and Florence Kendall were among those who were determined to regain the ground lost to the well-publicized Kenny System, and their carefully considered report in Volume 27, Number 3, of the *Review*, entitled "Orthopedic and Physical Therapy Objectives in Poliomyelitis Treatment," represented the first stage in that effort.

*Combining an exercise table with adjustable seat and the inherent buoyancy and comfort of water, a physical therapist takes a youngster with polio through a form of progressive resistance exercise. New, more effective treatments for polio were always being sought by the medical community, but old and new treatments alike were given over primarily to the care and practice of physical therapists.*

155

*The Iron Lung, invented by Philip Drinker, M.D., represented the cutting edge of respiratory technology in the 1930s and 1940s. With it, patients who were rendered incapable of breathing on their own were kept alive long enough for therapy and their own resilience to restore them to some degree of independence.*

Among the 1947 article's highlights were discussions of how to tailor specific treatment to the individual patient; the importance of assessing the type of muscle weakness involved before instituting therapy; the critical role of arc-of-motion exercises in treating muscle-stretch paralysis; and the fundamental usefulness of bracing to protect weak muscles, hold joints in alignment, prevent deformity, and facilitate function.

While all the Kendalls' recommendations were probably familiar to fellow practitioners of orthodox polio treatment, the Kendalls also made it clear that no modern physical therapist should be satisfied to carry out treatments to correct "abnormal" conditions without knowing scientifically what constitutes "normal." They then described their own ground-breaking investigations to document normal flexibility in trunk and leg muscles, those parts of the anatomy most frequently afflicted when polio strikes. Based on their measurements of some 4,500 healthy children, ages 5 to 18, in the Baltimore school system and another 500 adults between the ages of 18 and 22, they were able to show statistically, for the first time, that normal flexibility among children is highly variable and that it typically waxes and wanes at various developmental ages.

With this information as their guide, the Kendalls went on to suggest that in testing children with paralytic polio the best way to assess muscle function loss and set appropriate therapeutic goals for recovery was to compare the individual patient's residual strength and flexibility with age-specific norms. Jules Rothstein, editor of the Association's journal (now called *Physical Therapy*) since 1989, has called this early Kendall paper "a remarkable model of clinical reporting for its time. In it the Kendalls defined all the relevant issues, set forth the critical variables, and created the scientific framework in which they and their colleagues could then carry forth needed research. They anticipated the same kind of systematic principles we use today." The research was subsequently incorporated in the Kendalls' *Muscles, Testing and Function*, which upon publication in 1949 became the standard text in its field, going into four U.S. and seven foreign-language editions by 1993.

As for Sister Kenny, she had become something of a folk hero, and whatever the rightness or wrongness of her "system," her fame probably advanced awareness of physical therapy among a public that cared little for the details of scientific controversy. The subject of a popular film with Rosalind Russell in the title role, she was also the focus of countless magazine and newspaper articles. She was showered with honorary degrees and was the recipient of a Special Act of Congress enabling her to enter and leave the United States sans passport or visa — an honor shared only with the Marquis de Lafayette and Winston Churchill. Kenny, however, wanted no part of the fuss anymore. In failing health due to the onset of Parkinson's disease, she was little seen in the United States in the last few years of her life and died back home in Australia of a cerebral hemorrhage in November 1952. The *Review* published a brief but warm tribute, citing "her kindness, reassuring manner, and skillful hands. She will be missed but also remembered for her courage and devotion to the polio patient."

As for medical and physiotherapeutic opinion about how best to treat paralytic polio, a new consensus was gradually forming, one that combined aspects of the Kenny System and orthodox practice in what was a nonsectarian middle ground. Sister Kenny's "hot fomentations," having demonstrated their value in relieving much of the pain associated with the acute stages of polio, were retained by common agreement. And further examination of patients had indicated that muscle shortening was not merely a secondary result of neurological cell damage, but a primary entity in itself and one that benefited from treatment in early stages. So, too, the reduced use of braces and casts combined with daily massage, mild exercise, and gradual reeducation of muscles were all adapted from the Kenny System but with modifications to accommodate what was known scientifically about the need to protect paralyzed muscles from overstretching. (A classic example of this integrated approach is seen in Alice Lou Plastridge's very detailed instruction sheet on "Muscle Reeducation" which she prepared for staff physical therapists at Warm Springs. According to Plastridge, the first level of reeducation — passive motion — was to begin *only* "when any segment can be taken through a small arc of motion without pain, i.e., 20-30 degrees.")

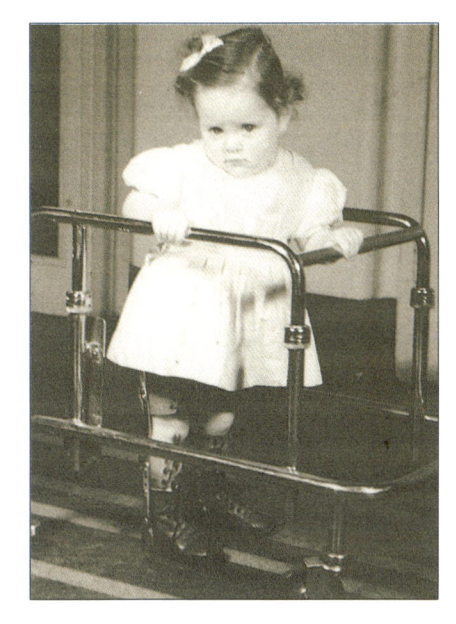

Generally discarded were such faddish practices as using muscle relaxants, like the drug curare, and requiring patients to touch their forehead to their knees to demonstrate flexibility — a Kenny stipulation for discharge. Back in favor, and now supported by more extensive research,

*A rolling walker becomes a critical assistive device in the gait training of this toddler as she recovers from polio. The photo was taken in the early 1950s, when the incidence of infantile paralysis was at its height. In later years the use of splints and braces for treatment of paralysis was lessened in favor of careful passive exercise.*

*Major Mary Ellen Sacksteder, chief of the Physical Therapy Section at the U.S. Army Hospital, Fort Carson, Colorado, teaches a nine-year-old youngster with facial paralysis to self-administer electrical stimulation with the help of a mirror. Physical therapy treatments that could be self-administered allowed the patient minimum inconvenience and the therapist maximum efficiency.*

were such orthodox practices as early bed rest, splinting, and the gradual increase of arc-of-motion exercises in consonance with muscle testing and spontaneous recovery of strength.

### POLIO TEAMS INTO THE BREACH

Meanwhile, new cases of polio were coming along each year, creating ever larger numbers of acute and chronic cases. Up from 10,000 in 1940, 1944 brought 19,270 new cases. In 1946 there were more than 25,000; in 1950, nearly 40,000 (among them, ironically, NFIP Executive Director Basil O'Connor's 30-year-old daughter, Bettyann); and in 1953, more than 57,000. APTA, which had carefully avoided taking sides during the height of the polio treatment debate, worked closely with Catherine Worthingham, NFIP's director of professional education, in recruiting volunteers to help in dealing with the annual epidemics. Initially APTA made annual appeals to members through the *Review*, but responsibility for assigning therapists to particular communities was assumed by the NFIP. In a typical year, as many as 200 physical therapists were thus sent off to assist in the emergency. In 1948, a year when the *Review* declared that the "bottom of the barrel" had been reached in providing physical therapists for emergency work, the NFIP asked APTA to take over full responsibility for recruiting and assigning physical therapists for emergency work. The NFIP gave the Association a grant to support the salary of a polio coordinator.

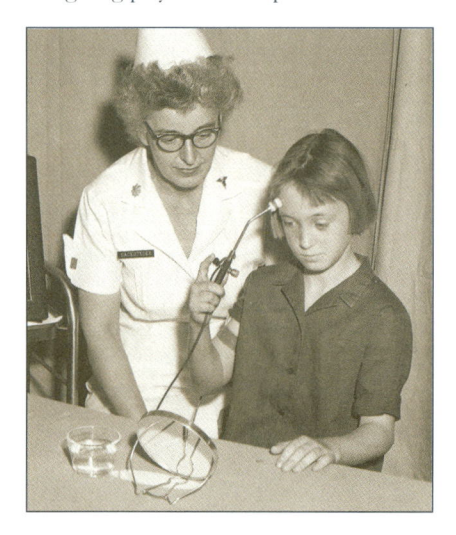

First to take the post was Mary Haskell, a graduate of Bouvé-Boston, a member of APTA since 1929, and current chairman of the Committee on Legislation. At the same time, the NFIP awarded the Association a grant of $31,280 to develop and provide consulting programs in the areas of epidemic and follow-up care planning for hospitals and communities.

Each year, in preparation for the annual explosion of cases of polio, every APTA member was sent a questionnaire regarding her or his availability to assist during the emergency, either part-time or full-time. The information was filed on a geographic basis, ready to be put into action whenever warning signals of an impending crisis went up. Between 1948 and 1960, nearly 1,000 physical therapists participated in the program, among them such new graduates as Vilma Evans, Ruth Sprague, Lenora Grizzell, Ruby Tillman, Carolyn Bowman, Adeline Lewis Berentes, Olivia Parker Cascadden, Margaret Christian, Mildred Griswold Werner, June Kissgen, and Hazel Johnson Fisher.

Emergency service had a curious and disturbing effect on the personal lives of a large number of physical therapists. Lucy Blair, who succeeded Haskell as polio consultant in 1950, filed a report on the matter, stating that she discerned "a pattern of restlessness" among members, a "tendency to follow the epidemics wherever the

National Foundation sent them," like so many medical camp followers. For the benefit of all concerned, she urged that APTA make it a priority to create a more stable framework of qualified physical therapists in permanent positions and to promote a team concept in working with other members of the medical community involved in the care of polio patients. To further this goal, both Haskell and Blair made concerted efforts to place their strongest candidates in well-established centers where they might find long-term employment after the immediate crises had passed. That they succeeded is indicated by comparing the statistics. In 1946, 283 physical therapists were placed in temporary assignments to treat some 25,000 reported cases; in 1952, only 128 emergency physical therapists were needed to swell the ranks of established physical therapy departments treating nearly 58,000 new cases of patients with polio.

At the same time, APTA took on the responsibility of keeping physical therapists current in relation to the changes in the clinical management of polio. With the financial assistance of the NFIP, low-cost workshops and institutes were conducted on a regional basis, and special programs on polio aftercare were regularly included in the programs for the Annual Conference. In 1953, for example, APTA sponsored a gathering of senior physical therapists from five respirator centers around the country for the purpose of improving the care of patients on respirators. One of the attendees, and perhaps the nation's leading authority on respirators at the time, was APTA stalwart Dorothy Graves, who was on the staff of the Los Angeles County Hospital and an instructor at the University of Southern California. Graves prided herself quite appropriately on being able to take apart and reassemble these ornery devices with aplomb. NFIP mobile teaching units, each one organized around a physical therapy school and consisting of a physician, a nurse, and two physical therapists, were tried as well. Traveling from community to community during the polio season, NFIP teams were prepared to demonstrate the latest treatment skills wherever needed. The *Review* also became a forum for articles and news items relating to polio, with the most notable offering being the single-topic, 53-page issue published in July-August 1947.

### THE SHOT HEARD ROUND THE WORLD

The Association and its members also made notable contributions to the development of a polio vaccine. In 1951, prior to the polio season, APTA was asked to help find a physical therapist to go to Provo, Utah, where a team led by William Hammon of the University of Pittsburgh was to run controlled studies of gamma globulin as a preventive agent. Lucy Blair, who was at the time the staff coordinator of recruitment and assignment of physical therapists for the polio emergency, recommended Miriam Jacobs of the D. T. Watson School, and she carried out the detailed muscle tests needed in the evaluation. That Jacobs was chosen was not surprising. The D. T. Watson School, an outgrowth of the Watson Home for Crippled Children located in Leetsdale, outside of Pittsburgh, was a leading center for post-polio work. The following year, as the gamma globulin tests were extended to Houston, Texas, and Sioux City, Iowa, Carmella Gonnella of Texas and Georgianna Harmon of California also participated. In 1953 the PHS asked Blair to recommend still another cadre of 38 therapists to conduct tests on "multiple-case households" scattered across the United States.

To assure the highest degree of uniformity in their procedures, the physical therapists chosen attended a four-day orientation course on Watson's Leetsdale campus during which director Jessie Wright and her staff demonstrated the use of an abridged muscle-grading system and syllabus. Fanning out across the country after the meeting, the physical therapists traveled to 35 states and the District of Columbia to assist in the field trials, in which they performed 2,540 muscle examinations. While the gamma globulin serum ultimately proved unsatisfactory in that it conferred only short-term immunity at a staggeringly high price tag, the favorable results showed definitively that scientists were on the right track.

The nation did not have long to wait. Coincident with Hammon's gamma globulin studies, Jonas Salk was working on another approach in a competing laboratory at Pitt. His preliminary tests, carried out with the assistance of volunteers and staff at the D. T. Watson School, indicated that a killed-virus serum conferred permanent protection against poliomyelitis. Salk was then given the go-ahead to conduct a larger double-blind test, and between March and June 1954, some 1.8 million first-, second-, and third-graders were involved. Of these, 650,000 received the vaccine and the remainder received a placebo. Once again, APTA and Lucy Blair helped, dispatching 63 physical therapists to 44 states. APTA also worked with the Canadian Physiotherapy Association, providing the requisite education to three Canadian physiotherapists who ran the muscle-testing portion of field trials in the Canadian provinces.

On April 12, 1955, the tenth anniversary of Roosevelt's death, the NFIP and Salk held a press conference at the vaccine evaluation center at the University of Michigan. The crowd of invited notables, including Lucy Blair and two other members of APTA's Department of Professional Services, were the first to hear the historic announcement that the Salk vaccine was determined to be safe and highly effective. Immediately, the Food and Drug Administration gave six pharmaceutical houses the green light to produce the vaccine commercially in time for the upcoming polio season, and shortly thereafter mass inoculations began coast to coast.

In the rush, unfortunately, seven lots of improperly inactivated vaccine mistakenly made their way into the program, and within 14 days, reports of children falling sick began to come into the Public Health Service's Communicable Disease Center. The problem was quickly traced to one of the manufacturers, California's Cutter Laboratories, but not before 204 new cases of polio had erupted in California, Idaho, and the city of Chicago; three-fourths of them proved to be paralytic and 11 youngsters died.

It took several weeks to restore the public's confidence, but better control methods were imposed, and before the summer had ended, four million doses were administered without further incident. Since that time, Salk's inactivated virus vaccine has been superseded by Albert Sabin's attenuated live vaccine (1964), and poliomyelitis has largely been eliminated as a threat in the United States, though aftertreatment of a generation of pre-vaccine polio patients continues to be part of physical therapy practice. In recognition of their major contributions, both Salk and Sabin were later elected to honorary membership in the Association.

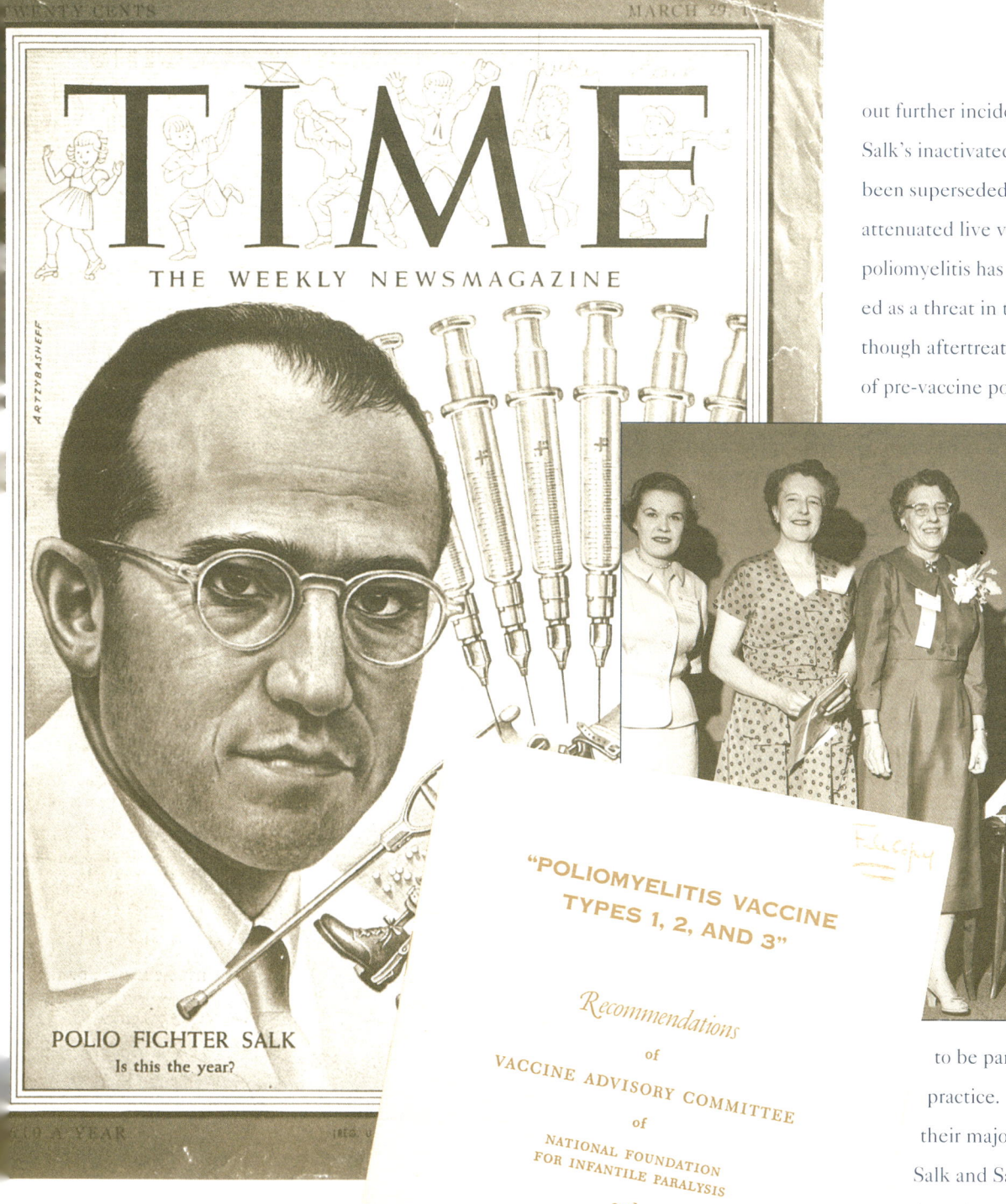

*The Salk vaccine was introduced in spring 1955 to wide acclaim. The following year, Jonas Salk was honored by the World Confederation for Physical Therapy which met in New York. Among the dignitaries shown with Salk in the photo are, left to right, Miriam Jacobs of the D. T. Watson School, WCPT chairperson G. V. M. Griffin of Great Britain, Mildred Elson, and Lucy Blair.*

"Progress Is A Relay Race" 1946–1959      161

*Maggie Knott first gained her reputation as a physical therapist while treating injured mine workers — as many as 200 per day — at the Kaiser Rehabilitation Center in Vallejo, California. Credited with developing many of the principles of proprioceptive neuromuscular facilitation, or PNF, she became a celebrated teacher and author of the classic textbook on the subject.*

### A NEW DAY DAWNING

The prospect of polio finally being conquered naturally brought jubilation among physical therapists, who found the annual toll of illness and disability as painful and perplexing as everyone else. But it also brought some new concerns. Would there be enough ongoing work to occupy the membership, which by 1955 numbered 4,718 active therapists (6,044 total members, including nonpracticing therapists and supporters)? And would the NFIP, or March of Dimes as it was familiarly known, continue to support the Association's many programs and provide scholarships for worthy students?

The funds did gradually diminish, as described in the next chapter, and the Association did go through some difficult adjustments. But as it soon became apparent, whole new categories of patients who could benefit from physical therapy were waiting in the wings. Chief among them were those with neurological disorders — especially stroke and various forms of cerebral palsy — which became the next focus of clinical theory, treatment approaches, and research.

To some extent, the successes of polio aftercare served as a kind of "workshop and showcase" for developing treatment approaches. Certainly the positive results were evidence that seemingly intractable cases of paralysis could be modified with careful, long-term treatment by skilled therapists. And to the extent that polio and the other disorders have a common connection — they are all diseases of the nervous system — it was reasonable for the health care professions at that time to hope that treatments applicable to the former might carry over to the others. However, as soon became apparent, there are also critical differences among these conditions.

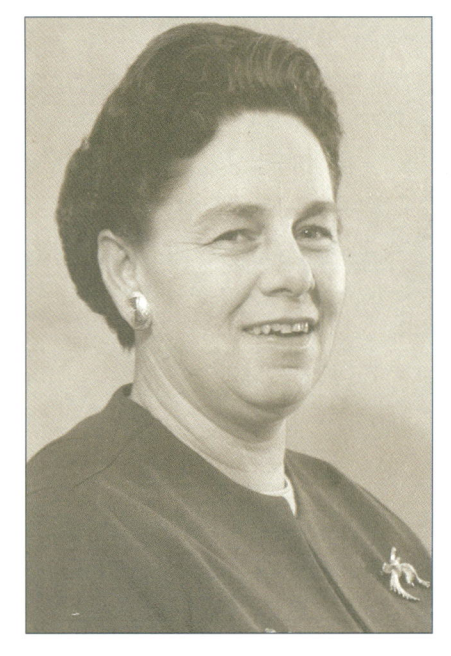

Paralytic polio typically involves lesions in the lower motor neurons, and the resulting damage takes the form of flaccid or extremely weak muscles in the trunk and limbs. Treatment was traditionally based upon "orthopedic" solutions that dealt with the muscles themselves, using manual muscle testing, muscle reeducation, bracing, and surgery to regain some mobility. The other major central nervous system (CNS) disorders, by contrast, are less likely to manifest flaccidity and less likely to respond favorably to such care. These impairments typically arise from damage to higher centers of the central nervous system, such as the cortex, brain stem, or tracts in the spinal cord. The consequences of these lesions often take the form of impaired motor performance that may be exaggerated by spasticity expressed not so much in individual muscles but in altered patterns of movement by groups of muscles. As the deficit is central rather than peripheral, the proponents of neurotherapeutic remedies maintained that remedies must focus on the central nervous system itself.

Due to the tragic circumstances of World War II and the huge numbers of neurologically impaired veterans who survived to need and benefit from rehabilitation, much new information relevant to treating this group of neurological disorders came to light more or less coincident with polio's retreat from center stage. Neurotherapeutics appeared to physical therapists to be an exciting, not to say relatively uncharted, new area of clinical care and research, and many were eager to explore this area in hopes of discovering better treatments for a large class of underserved patients.

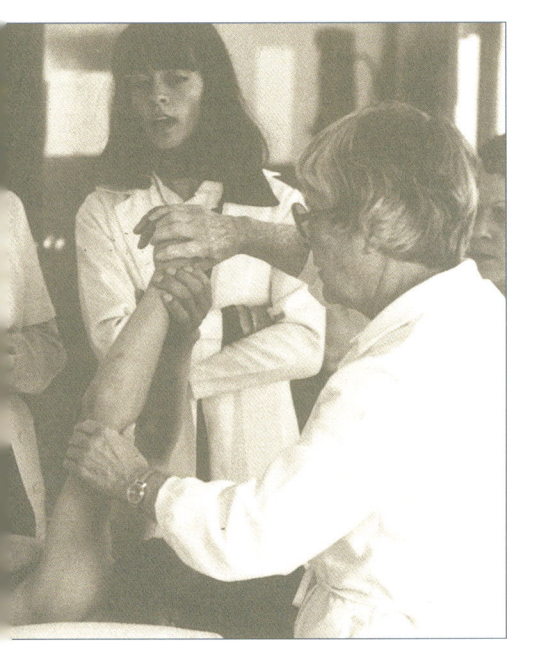

### Patients With Cerebral Palsy

Probably the most numerous group of clients to come into the purview of physical therapy in this era were the children and adults with cerebral palsy (CP), a non-progressive condition arising from CNS trauma before, during, or soon after birth. CP was an ancient disease, with England's Richard III believed to have been among the more famous individuals affected by this disease. Commonly identified as a "spastic" or "palsied" condition, CP had received considerable attention in the nineteenth century from British physician William J. Little. In 1862 Little presented a paper to the Obstetrical Society of London in which he described his observations on the 200 cases of spastic rigidity he had personally treated in his career. Little believed that the large majority were traceable to the effects of severe trauma and asphyxia at the moment of birth. As a result of his contributions, the condition was subsequently known as "Little's disease." Sir William Osler and Viennese neurologist Sigmund Freud also produced papers on birth palsies. But it was not until the 1930s that modern research into the syndrome had begun in earnest, and not until the early 1940s that a more or less uniform description of its causes and effects were put in place. (Remarkably, one finds in the April-May 1929 issue of the *Review* Lorena McPeek's paper on physiotherapy for spastic paralysis, including what appears to be the first functional evaluation form for the child with cerebral palsy.) Still, treatment was very much designed around the orthopedist-led model, with surgery the predominant approach. Physical therapists, though involved, were taught to work within a narrow range of therapeutic possibilities and to expect little of their patients in the way of improvement.

Leading the way to change were two physicians, Bronson Crothers and Winthrop Phelps. Crothers, a pediatric neurologist on staff at Boston Children's Hospital, established BCH's renowned neurological ward in 1930 where, with the assistance of Mary

*Dorothy Voss, shown here treating a patient, attended Knott's graduate course in 1951 and went on to become her teaching associate and co-author of the PNF text. Voss later joined the APTA staff and taught at Northwestern University, where she became intimately involved in formulating NU-STEP, the renowned study of motor behavior.*

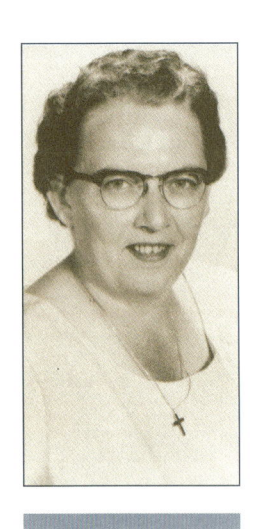

*Jane Carlin, head of the physical therapy program at the University of Pennsylvania, became the 19th president in 1956. A former officer in the WMSC, she had been the first woman to advance to the rank of Brigadier General.*

Trainor, director of physical therapy at the ward, youngsters with neurological birth injuries could be examined and treated with extensive physical therapy, including hydroexercise, ultraviolet light treatment, and a goodly dose of child psychology. (Trainor's expertise was so well known that Mary McMillan deferred to her in *Massage and Therapeutic Exercise*: "Miss Treanor [sic] has worked out some very helpful exercises. . . . Miss Treanor sings a little descriptive song to the child and . . . the child is taught by imitation to go through certain actions.") Trainor incidentally was one of the very first, if not *the* first, to use a homemade version of reciprocal-action skis in her CP clinic.

Phelps, who did his orthopedic training under Crothers, combined specialization in orthopedics and neurology, a unique combination in his time. He is remembered chiefly for his clinical classification of the major types of cerebral palsy, for his emphasis on the relationship between cerebral dominance and motor improvements, and for his highly selective application of different combinations of therapeutic modalities according to the type and severity of cerebral palsy. Perhaps his first and greatest contribution was in persuading the medical profession that cerebral palsy was not necessarily synonymous with mental deficiency and that efforts should be made to rehabilitate and mainstream youngsters with CP.

In 1937 Phelps opened his own Children's Rehabilitation Institute at Cockeysville, Maryland, as a multidisciplinary residential treatment center for CP. CRI became a mecca for educating physicians interested in cerebral palsy and for PTs and OTs and speech therapists who worked with patients with CP. His collaborators in developing effective physical therapy approaches were physical therapists Edna Blumenthal and Elizabeth Grayson. As the effectiveness of combining psychological, developmental, neurological, and surgical approaches to CP became ever more evident, professionals recognized the need for an ongoing forum to stimulate research and education specific to children with disabling conditions.

As Phelps's reputation grew, he wrote frequently about his findings, including two articles in the *Review*. He also held numerous demonstration clinics around the country, and this, in turn, gave rise to dozens of other cerebral palsy departments and centers. Adelaide McGarrett, a 1934 graduate of Harvard Medical School/Boston Children's Hospital, was another pioneer physical therapist to make CP her specialty. McGarrett ran a comprehensive physical therapy program at James Whitcomb Riley Hospital, Indiana University Medical Center, Indianapolis, during the war years. Blumenthal, who left her CP focus during the war years to serve in the USWMSC in Europe, returned to specialize in the care of infants with cerebral palsy, carrying on both clinical practice and teaching at North Carolina Cerebral Palsy Hospital (now Lenox Baker Children's Hospital) in Durham.

Funding for extensive research in cerebral palsy treatment was chronically inadequate until the late 1940s, when, as the *Review* put it, there was "a public awakening" to the need for better services. Then, in a few short years, great strides were made. The National Society for Crippled Children and Adults (the Easter Seal Society) established a Cerebral Palsy Division in 1946 with a Medical Advisory Council. In 1947 Phelps joined with Crothers and several other physicians interested in founding the multidisciplinary American Academy of Cerebral Palsy, which was conceived as a multispecialty professional organization dedicated to promoting research and education in the field of children with disabling conditions. Likewise, the National Institute of Neurological Disorders and Stroke became part of NIH, the United Cerebral Palsy Association was organized, and the first international conference was held, drawing 12,000 people. Jay Schleichkorn, after an early focus on polio, was another physical therapist to make CP his specialty. Schleichkorn spent 17 years with United Cerebral Palsy, working first as a therapist in a local center, then statewide as clinical and program director of UCPA of New York, and later as executive director of that organization.

### Kabat, Knott, And PNF

If Crothers and Phelps were the first modern leaders in CP treatment, they were soon joined in research and practice by other notable theoreticians and clinicians. One of these was Herman Kabat, a neurophysiologist and physician on the University of Minnesota's teaching staff. Kabat became interested in the problem of rehabilitating patients with neurological disabilities after having viewed firsthand the work of Sister Kenny in treating the paralysis of polio. Kabat came away persuaded that Kenny had some good ideas but convinced that her limited knowledge of the underlying neurological mechanisms kept her from truly effective treatments.

Kabat decided to take up the study of neuromuscular diseases himself. He started with the groundbreaking work of Sherrington and Pavlov, whose investigations had begun in the last decade of the nineteenth century. British neurophysiologist Charles Scott Sherrington had shown the integrative function of the nervous system and specifically of reciprocal innervation and inhibition as they relate to innate, stable reflex action arising in the spinal cord and brain stem. His Russian contemporary, Ivan Pavlov, had focused on conditioned reflexes, which, contrary to inborn reflexes, were located in the brain itself, were unstable, and could be lost through inaction, inhibited by stronger reflexes, or transformed. Pavlov had further shown that when nerve impulses were repeatedly transmitted across synapses by conditioning, synaptic resistance gradually decreased and new functional pathways were created in the cerebral cortex. To Kabat, this suggested that all kinds of deficient or pathological neuromuscular mechanisms and their resulting limitations of movement might be reversed through the facilitating effects of physical therapy.

Leaving his teaching post, Kabat went to Washington, D.C., in 1943, where he pursued a one-man clinical research effort while holding several medical posts, including that of consultant to the federal program for children with crippling disorders. The industrialist Henry Kaiser, whose son Henry Kaiser, Jr., had multiple sclerosis, came to see Kabat after reading an article the doctor had written that appeared in *Reader's Digest*. Kabat took the younger Kaiser under treatment, and when the young man

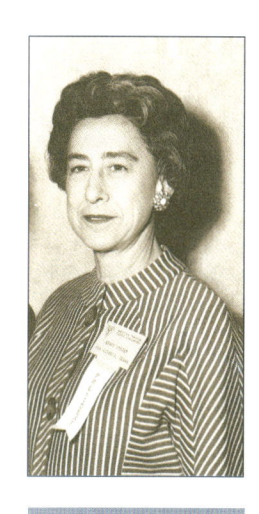

*Lt. Col. Agnes Snyder, AMSC, assumed the office of president at the APTA's 35th Annual Conference in Seattle, Washington, 1958. That same year, national dues were raised to $25.*

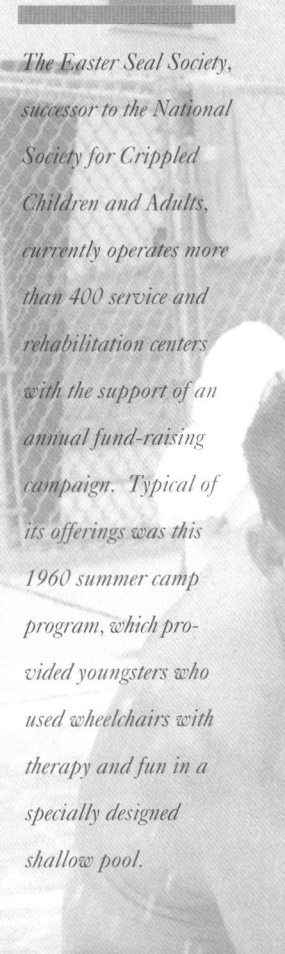

*The Easter Seal Society, successor to the National Society for Crippled Children and Adults, currently operates more than 400 service and rehabilitation centers with the support of an annual fund-raising campaign. Typical of its offerings was this 1960 summer camp program, which provided youngsters who used wheelchairs with therapy and fun in a specially designed shallow pool.*

showed improvement, the grateful father offered to fund Kabat's investigations by establishing the Kabat-Kaiser Institute for Neuromuscular Rehabilitation.

Kabat then went looking for a physical therapist to assist him and found Margaret (Maggie) Knott. Kabat was indeed fortunate in his discovery. Knott was a young woman of enormous energy, quick intelligence, warmth, and optimism. A physical education graduate of Appalachia State Teachers College in North Carolina, she left a brief stint teaching high school physical education to enter the training program for WMSC physical therapists at Walter Reed Army Hospital and then served at a base hospital in England until the close of the war. Less than six months after the Armistice, she joined Kabat in Washington.

Knott proved to be a dedicated partner in Kabat's research and later, as their work extended to a large clinical practice, a consummate teacher. Sue Adler, who became her student, says that no one could remain neutral regarding Knott because she was such a powerful presence, but that many found true inspiration in her work. "Over and over, she turned good technicians into dedicated professionals, helping us to find a way around our frustrations by giving us the essential tools to make us better therapists. She was equally capable of inspiring patients and staff to achieve levels of performance they had not imagined for themselves." (To the benefit of physical therapy, Knott also developed a passionate interest in the growth of her profession. Joining APTA, she became active in chapter affairs first in Washington, D.C., and later in California, where she would find time to serve as a member of the national

Board of Directors and as president of the California and Northern California chapters.)

Out of the Kabat-Knott collaboration came the first principles of proprioceptive neuromuscular facilitation (PNF), a therapeutic approach emphasizing the exercise of muscles in specific movement patterns. At the center of the theory was the phenomenon of "irradiation," by which was meant the exercise of stronger muscles first in order to assist or reinforce weaker groups in progressive steps. Their theories, initially called "Neuromuscular Reeducation," were among those presented in the May-June 1948 issue of the *Physical Therapy Review* on cerebral palsy. A second article, on "Application of PNF," followed in the October 1953 issue.

Through such articles, interest in PNF spread gradually through the physical therapy community. One who was profoundly impressed was Dorothy Voss, chief physical therapist at George Washington University Hospital, who attended a demonstration given before a District of Columbia Chapter meeting of APTA in 1950.

Voss applied to take a six-week education course with Knott and soon after left her post in Washington, D.C., to become Knott's assistant at Kabat-Kaiser. By that time, the center had moved its headquarters to the old navy hospital in Vallejo, California, and had some 30 qualified physical therapists handling as many as 200 patients a day, many of them industrial accident victims but others with chronic disabilities resulting from polio, cerebral palsy, multiple sclerosis, arthritis, and spinal cord injuries.

In their spare time, Knott and Voss developed a continuing education curriculum for PNF. They taught their first weekend workshop after the 1952 APTA Annual Conference in Philadelphia, followed by the first two-week course in Vallejo for attendees of the APTA Annual Conference in Los Angeles in 1954. Interest in their work led to additional presentations before the American Academy of Cerebral Palsy and two-week sessions in Vallejo, at Boston University, and elsewhere in the United States. On her own, Knott also was invited to demonstrate PNF at medical centers in South America and the South Pacific. During her more than 30 years of involvement with PNF, she personally taught more than a thousand individuals in continuing education courses at Vallejo and countless others in her travels. She was recognized for her generous contributions many times, not only by APTA but by the Chartered Society of Physiotherapy in England and by the Canadian Physiotherapy Association, both of which named her an honorary member.

Of broader import, Knott and Voss collaborated on writing the basic textbook on PNF. Titled *Proprioceptive Neuromuscular Facilitation*, this classic first appeared in 1956, the same year Voss moved to New York to become 11th editor of the *Physical Therapy Review*. The PNF text was updated and expanded in 1968, while Knott was still on staff at the renamed Kaiser Foundation in Vallejo and Voss was teaching at Northwestern University. Knott and Voss subsequently began work on a third edition, but when Knott died in 1978, her family inadvertently destroyed her portion of the manuscript. Voss then turned to Marjorie

Ionta, her friend and colleague since their early days at Massachusetts General Hospital, and together with occupational therapist Beverly J. Myers, an associate at the University of Illinois at Chicago, they wrote the third edition, published in 1985.

Myers had taken the first Voss PNF course directed solely at occupational therapists in 1974, but it was only after Voss had come to the Rehabilitation Institute of Chicago as a patient following back surgery that she and Myers came to know each other on a one-to-one basis. "Dorothy was a teacher's teacher," recalls Myers fondly. "Though I was her therapist, I was never sure which one of us was treating which." As both Voss and Ionta were approaching retirement, they invited the younger Myers to join them in the work with the idea of maintaining continuity for the future. Myers is now in the process of preparing the fourth edition of this classic with yet another physical therapist, Thomas Holland, who studied with Voss and worked closely with Ionta before setting up his own practice in LaCrosse, Wisconsin.

Knott, speaking about the evolution of PNF in her 1972 McMillan Lecture, said, "In our search for a more effective exercise program, our effort was concentrated on getting the patient to do all he possibly could do with the least expenditure of energy. The technique of exercise that I had been taught disturbed me." Here she refers to the practice of giving exercises the same way that the strength of an individual muscle was tested, by isolating it and focusing on weaknesses and disabilities rather than substituting other resources of strength. "Logically, more thought needed to be given to kinesiology and the actual functioning of normal muscular systems. Muscles do not work in an isolated way.... Muscles are spiral in character and rotation is a key to movement; therefore, functional motions are diagonal, not straight.... These motions are the same as [PNF's] patterns of facilitation.... Moving and exercising in these patterns makes the most logical sense."

Also making logical sense, as Dorothy Voss reported in her 1982 McMillan Lecture, was the developmental basis of PNF. But its logic was not apparent to her until she happened to read Arnold Gesell's *Infant Development: The Embryology of Early Motor Behavior.* Voss described her discovery of the connection to the pediatrician's analysis of the "sequence of the child's use of crayon: from scrawl, to vertical, to horizontal, to circular, to oblique (diagonal). Gesell pointed out that the same sequence applies in the development of visual behavior and percept-concept formation, as well as postural behavior. Everything was there before I discovered it!" In consequence, later editions of *Proprioceptive Neuromuscular Facilitation* introduced motor activities in accordance with their normal maturational sequences, a key advance in theory and practice.

At least four other therapists were also instrumental in developing innovative and influential approaches to CNS dysfunction in this era: Jean Ayres, Berta Bobath, Signe Brunnström, and Margaret Rood.

### Ayres's Sensory Integration

Anna Jean Ayres, a California-based occupational therapist with a doctoral degree in educational psychology, used her academic background in neuroscience and her clinical expertise as an occupational therapist as the foundation stones for an approach that came to be termed "sensory integration therapy." SI refers to the ability of the CNS to take in, sort out, and interpret sensations such as sight, sound, taste, smell, and touch, from which develop the skills of balance, stability, locomotion, coordination, and general body awareness. These in turn become the platform on which the refinements of perceptual-motor development — speech, reading, writing, and math — are erected. By Ayres's reasoning, infants and young children with cerebral palsy tend to have problems receiving and processing some or all of these fundamental sensations. Some have hyposensitivities to touch and movement; others have hypersensitivities; still others have combinations of the two.

Ayres's research began in the fifties at Kabat-Kaiser and UCLA and continued into the sixties while she was in private practice at the Ayres Clinic in Torrance, California. She came to believe that through engagement in purposeful activities, youngsters with central nervous system dysfunction could achieve greater degrees of spatial and body image integration and thereby develop effective adaptive responses. In furtherance of this concept, she developed a range of tools, standardized SI tests, and therapeutic techniques designed to improve the way the brain stem processes and organizes sensations, especially balance and fine motor coordination.

Ayres found a wide audience through lecturing, test manuals, instructional films, and the writing of two books and 56 articles, including one in the *Review*. While SI is still undergoing intensive clinical testing and while its genuine effectiveness remains to be proved, the basic arguments stated in Ayres's many published works have had a strong impact on many other contemporary therapies.

### The Bobaths And NDT

Berta "Berti" Bobath, a German-born physical therapist with a background in remedial exercises, and her husband, Karel Bobath, a neurologist, brought other kinds of innovations to cerebral palsy, not the least of which was their humanistic approach. Adopted citizens of England, they developed a reputation for success with "spastics" at Bobath Centre, their London-based clinic, that drew scores of professionals to observe and train. When some of those observers carried word of their work to the United States, the Bobaths were invited to give demonstrations at several American institutions, and in 1958 they traveled to this country to present their ideas.

The Bobaths' innovative system of therapy was, as with most innovations, countercultural and, to many, shocking. Indeed, in the opinion of one physical therapist, David Scrutton of Guy's Hospital, London, the Bobaths' teaching "single-handedly (or rather single-mindedly) turned the world of cerebral palsy — and with it much of developmental pediatrics — upside down."

As Scrutton explains it, despite the work of Phelps, Blumenthal, and a handful of others, the pervading view of cerebral palsy in the late 1940s and 1950s was dominated by what might best be described as "the immutable prognosis. The natural history was just that — a history — a future as unchangeable as the past." The therapist could help the child adapt to his or her disability with a certain amount of training and bracing, but there was a sense that no one, least of all the hands-on therapist, could alter the prognosis in any meaningful way. The Bobaths, by contrast, argued that early intervention, before the child had, in effect, "perfected his handicap," could open a wider range of possibilities. In particular, the Bobaths put physical therapists at the center of the rehabilitative process, making their human interaction with the child as important an element as any other part.

The Bobath approach evolved "quite by accident," according to Berta Bobath, beginning when she was asked to treat a 43-year-old patient with hemiplegia. "Instead of doing what I had been taught — exercises — I observed the patient," she said. "Slowly, by trial and error, by observation and deduction, I began relating things he was doing in response to what I was doing. It worked better than anything before." Essentially, she found that his spasticity was not unalterable, and that she could by stages help him achieve a high degree of freedom of movement. She later described the basis of her early treatment as "the inhibition of released and exaggerated abnormal reflex action, the counteraction of abnormal patterns, and the facilitation of more normal automatic and voluntary movements." In understanding these mechanisms, Karel Bobath was Berta's interpreter and research consultant, even while he maintained his own practice as a psychiatrist.

The Bobaths' first tour of the United States began in May 1958. It included a two-week-long course at the University of Pittsburgh's D. T. Watson School with Jessie Wright, a workshop at the annual gathering of the United Cerebral Palsy Associations of New York state in Syracuse, a workshop and lecture at the APTA Annual Conference in Seattle, an eight-week-long summer course at Stanford University, and three weeks of lecturing in the Los Angeles area. Instrumental in arranging the tour were Sarah Semans, a "Bobath alumna" and physical therapist on the staff of the Division of Physical Therapy, Stanford University School of Medicine, and Clara "Sonny" Arrington, who obtained partial funding for the tour through her work with the federal Social Security Agency's Children's Bureau. As Jay Schleichkorn would later observe in his 1992 biography of the Bobaths, "that first tour was to have everlasting effects on many people."

The system then known as Bobath, later renamed neuro-developmental treatment, or NDT, seemed to make perfect sense to many physical therapists who were able to see the couple in action. Leila Green, a physical therapist in private practice who attended the first Seattle workshop, decided then and there to enroll in the next extended Bobath course in London. "We watched [the Bobaths] create changes in the children's tone and posture that we knew we couldn't do," Green later recalled, adding that Berta Bobath handled her patients as one "molding a mound of clay into a figure." (Perhaps it was no coincidence that Bobath took up sculpture as a serious avocation in her fifties.)

Following Semans's example, Green became the second qualified coordinator-instructor of NDT in the United States, teaching the program from her base at the Kiwanis Children's Center, Milwaukee. With successive visits by the Bobaths and the training courses at Stanford and Milwaukee, the techniques of NDT became familiar not only to hundreds of physical therapists interested in CP but to physical therapists treating adult hemiplegia and other sensorimotor dysfunctions. (In 1964 the journal, the University of Pennsylvania, and the Children's Bureau co-sponsored the first symposium on "The Child with Central Nervous System Deficit." Sarah Semans, as sole author of one paper and senior author of a second, described her own adaptations of the Bobath approach.)

Pamela Mullens, who attended a Bobath-Green workshop in 1966 and was the third American to qualify in NDT, recalls the intense excitement she felt as she observed Berti Bobath assessing and treating children in a manner that was "more of an artistic experience . . . than a lesson in treatment. . . . I sat there watching the changes that took place in the children. Not only did their movement change, almost all children became more organized emotionally and socially. . . . There was a give and take about this therapy that reminded me of dance. Therapist and child were responding to each other, and the movement of both was very beautiful to observe."

Today there are more than two dozen coordinator-instructors in pediatric NDT, almost as many coordinator-instructors in adult hemiplegia, and an umbrella organization known as the Neuro-Developmental Treatment Association (NDTA), which held its first national meeting in Kansas City, Missouri, in 1988. The interdisciplinary NDTA certifies faculty, curricula, and course graduates, of which there are currently more than 4,400, including some 2,600 physical therapists. The concepts of NDT remain controversial. To some staunch critics in the profession, it is scarcely more scientifically grounded than rehabilitation at Lourdes; to others, it is truly "revolutionary." But few would argue that the Bobaths' contribution in helping to redefine the medical community's perception of cerebral palsy will stand forever. In June 1979 APTA's House of Delegates granted honorary membership to the Bobaths.

### Signe Brunnström's "Approach"

Signe Brunnström had made a considerable name for herself as an exercise therapist well before World War II and had gone on to make distinguished contributions in rehabilitating people with amputations and other casualties during the war. Still, it was only in the late 1940s that she found her true calling in the rehabilitation of people with hemiplegia, "the step children of medicine," whom she thought badly neglected by the rehabilitation community because they were so little understood.

Beginning in 1949, Brunnström signed on as part-time research assistant to Henry Kessler, her former navy commander at the Mare Island Amputee Center and founder of the new Kessler Institute of Rehabilitation in West Orange, New Jersey. Kessler, like Frank Krusen, Howard Rusk, and

George Deaver, is considered one of the pioneers of rehabilitative medicine, and he was very supportive of Brunnström's investigations. At the Kessler Institute, Brunnström plunged into the medical literature relating to stroke. Thanks to fluency in several languages, she was able to study seminal articles on postural reflexes and muscle tone, including Rudolph Magnus's monumental *Korperstellung* (Berlin, 1924), and the related clinical studies by his colleague A. Simons, originally titled "Kopfhaltung und Muskeltonus" in the German-language *Journal of Neurology and Psychology*. (She shared her findings with fellow APTA members, publishing summaries of both in the *Physical Therapy Review* in 1953.) In the process, she began to develop the methods which she would set forth in detail in numerous articles and in her major text, *Movement Therapy in Hemiplegia*, published in 1970. It remains the leading text on what is often referred to as "the Brunnström Approach," though the author always made it clear that her philosophy of treatment was never intended to be anything but a work in progress, open to change and improvement wherever and whenever better ideas were found.

Nonetheless, the Brunnström "approach" did have certain identifiable elements. For example, Brunnström's commentaries on rehabilitating the patient with stroke were based on the most detailed and precise observation of the sequential changes in motor function that typically occur following stroke, and they remain one of the best available resources for understanding that phenomenon. Also central to her theories and clinical practice was a thorough grounding in the basic reflex behaviors of the nervous system as they were then understood. Her observations on the action of muscles in health and injury were unparalleled for their time.

As her ideas of stroke therapy were beginning to form at Kessler Institute, Brunnström continued to consult and teach at Columbia University College of Physicians and Surgeons, at New York University's Institute of Physical Medicine and Rehabilitation, at the Burke Rehabilitation Center in White Plains, at the Veterans Administration Hospital in New York City, and at the New York State Rehabilitation Hospital in West Haverstraw. Brunnström also lectured frequently around the country, so that many hundreds of physical therapists in dozens of major teaching hospitals had an opportunity to benefit from her clinical workshops. She even found time to take up and carry forth Helen Kaiser's original work in establishing both a program for rehabilitation of individuals with amputated limbs and a physical therapy school in postwar Greece after accepting a Fulbright lectureship in Athens in 1950-51.

Brunnström's corpus of written works is astonishing. Early in 1935, only six years after arriving in the United States and in her newly adopted language of English, she prepared her first article, "Faulty Weight Bearing," for the *Physiotherapy Review*. Brunnström went on to write another 22 articles, numerous abstracts, and book reviews and to contribute chapters to three other collected works. In addition to *Movement Therapy in Hemiplegia*, she co-authored *Training of the Lower Extremity Amputee* with Donald Kerr in 1956 and was the sole author of *Clinical*

*Kinesiology* in 1962. One of the most popular books on the mechanics of body motion ever written, this classic is now in its fourth edition as *Brunnström's Clinical Kinesiology*, with a total of some 110,000 copies in circulation. Brunnström also participated in the preparation of three major research reports — one for the Committee on Artificial Limbs; one for the Office of Naval Research, Special Devices Center; and one for the NYU Institute of Physical Medicine and Rehabilitation. She had, as well, a major hand in the creation of five instructional films.

Although close and lasting friendships seem to be a particular mark of the greats of physical therapy, even here Signe Brunnström held some kind of record for the circle of friends and admirers she kept. Why this was so can be glimpsed from Mary Eleanor Brown's recollections of Signe, which appear in Jay Schleichkorn's biography of Brunnström, published in 1990: "I remember Signe as a vibrant woman full of energy, robust health, goodness, friendliness, good cheer, diligence, enormous motivation, high intelligence, and scientific fervor to find the truth, in order to help her students, her colleagues, her friends, and her profession.

"Athletically inclined, this friendly woman lived a physically active life to the fullest. She thought hard, read and studied hard, did her paintings, gardened, and built parts of her country place, solved problems, traveled, and worked zestfully in overwhelmingly complex conditions."

Brown admired Brunnström's frugality, which came of her decision to divide life between salaried work and the pursuit of new knowledge for its own sake. "[Signe] told me she had condensed her belongings, simplified her clothing, ate at the Automats or in her room, and literally lived for work at the hospital. She was, to me, an intellectual giant, the perfect scholar. Her classes and the libraries were home to her. She glowed with every new insight she gained and was an inspiration to all around her."

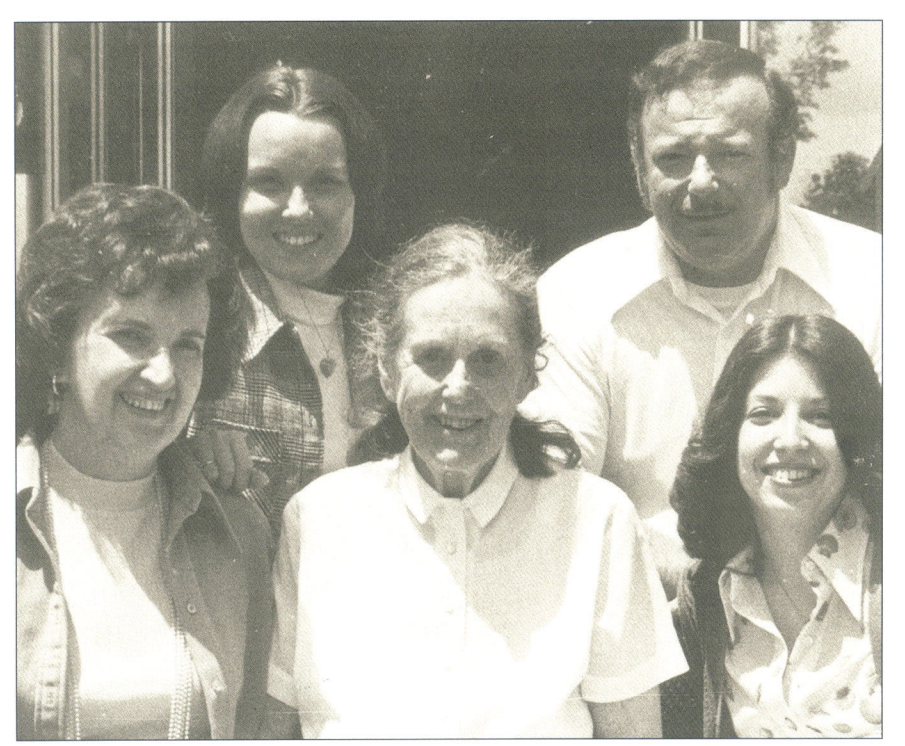

Brunnström was repeatedly recognized by APTA for her contributions to the profession. In 1965, on the occasion of the Annual Conference

*Signe Brunnström, center, is pictured here surrounded by admirers of her dedication to the scientific advancement of physical therapy. In addition to being one of the most prolific contributors to the discussion of physical therapy treatments (including authorship of* Clinical Kinesiology*), Brunnström was well loved by all, and her admirers often became friends.*

in Cleveland, she was presented with the first Marian Williams Award for her fundamental and significant contributions to the study of locomotion and exercise, of special value to patients recovering from stroke and those with amputated limbs. Overwhelmed by the honor, and perhaps frightened at standing before so large a group, the often shy 67-year-old Brunnström was momentarily so shocked that she whispered to Fran Tappan that she feared she herself was having a stroke. Perhaps that is why both times she was invited to deliver the prestigious Mary McMillan Lecture — first in 1967 and again in 1971 — she firmly declined.

In 1988, the Board of Directors of APTA paid a final tribute to Brunnström by attaching her name to the newly created Award for Excellence in Clinical Teaching. Their intent was stated in a resolution passed shortly before her death at the age of 90 in 1988, in which she was recognized as "an outstanding early pioneer in physical therapy . . . well-known author, educator, researcher, humanitarian, and clinician who has dedicated 50 years of her life to the profession of physical therapy." Brunnström, who was a naturalized citizen of the United States, was cremated and her remains interred in the Brunnström family plot in her native Helsingborg, Sweden.

### ROOD'S CONTRIBUTIONS

Margaret "Roody" Rood is probably the least known and least published among the postwar neurophysiological innovators, but she worked extensively in the treatment of persons with brain damage. Born in 1909 in Wisconsin, Rood received her certificate in occupational therapy in 1933. She worked for several years at the James Whitcomb Riley Hospital, Indiana University, supervising occupational therapists in the Cerebral Palsy Clinic. Here began her interest in treating neurological problems, a career she continued upon moving to the University of Southern California (USC), where she taught in one of the War Emergency Training Courses in occupational therapy.

After the war, Rood took a leave of absence to gain her master's degree and certificate in physical therapy at Stanford University. With the dual disciplines of occupational therapy and physical therapy, she went into private practice for a time and eventually returned to USC to chair the physical therapy department until her retirement in 1972.

"Always in motion, never finishing a sentence," according to her friends and admirers, Rood talked so fast and spoke so cryptically that her ideas as they have come down to us are chiefly known through the interpretations of other knowledgeable therapists, including Joy Huss, Margot Heiniger, Shirley Randolph, and Shirley Stockmeyer who studied with her. Asked to give the sixth McMillan Lecture at the 1969 Annual Conference in San Francisco, she delivered from brief notes a highly abstruse discussion of "Stereotyped or Integrated Response." The address was never written out, however, so it has the distinction of being the only McMillan Lecture never published.

Rood's significance to physical therapy is, nonetheless, considerable. Elizabeth Littel, writing in Scully and Barnes's *Physical Therapy*, noted, "Rood was one of the first therapists to emphasize the importance of the sensory half of sensory-motor behavior. . . . She also strongly emphasized the importance of autonomic function as a basis for normal sensory-motor behavior at a time when most therapists were scarcely aware that this was a factor worth considering."

Stated in the broadest terms, Rood's thesis was that inasmuch as motor patterns are developed from fundamental reflex patterns present at birth, and because these are gradually modified through sensory stimuli, it might be possible to bring about improvements in the child with dysfunction by overriding the abnormal stimuli with normal ones. Rood defined four guidelines to be considered in evaluation and treatment: controlled sensory input must be used to evoke muscular responses reflexively; as sensorimotor control is developmentally based, therapy must start at the patient's level of development and progress sequentially to higher and higher levels; each

*The second congress of the World Confederation for Physical Therapy, held at New York's Statler Hotel, drew more than 2,000 physical therapists from 34 countries.*

*This last formal portrait of Mary McMillan was taken following her attendance at the 1958 Conference in Seattle. McMillan died the following year, in October 1959.*

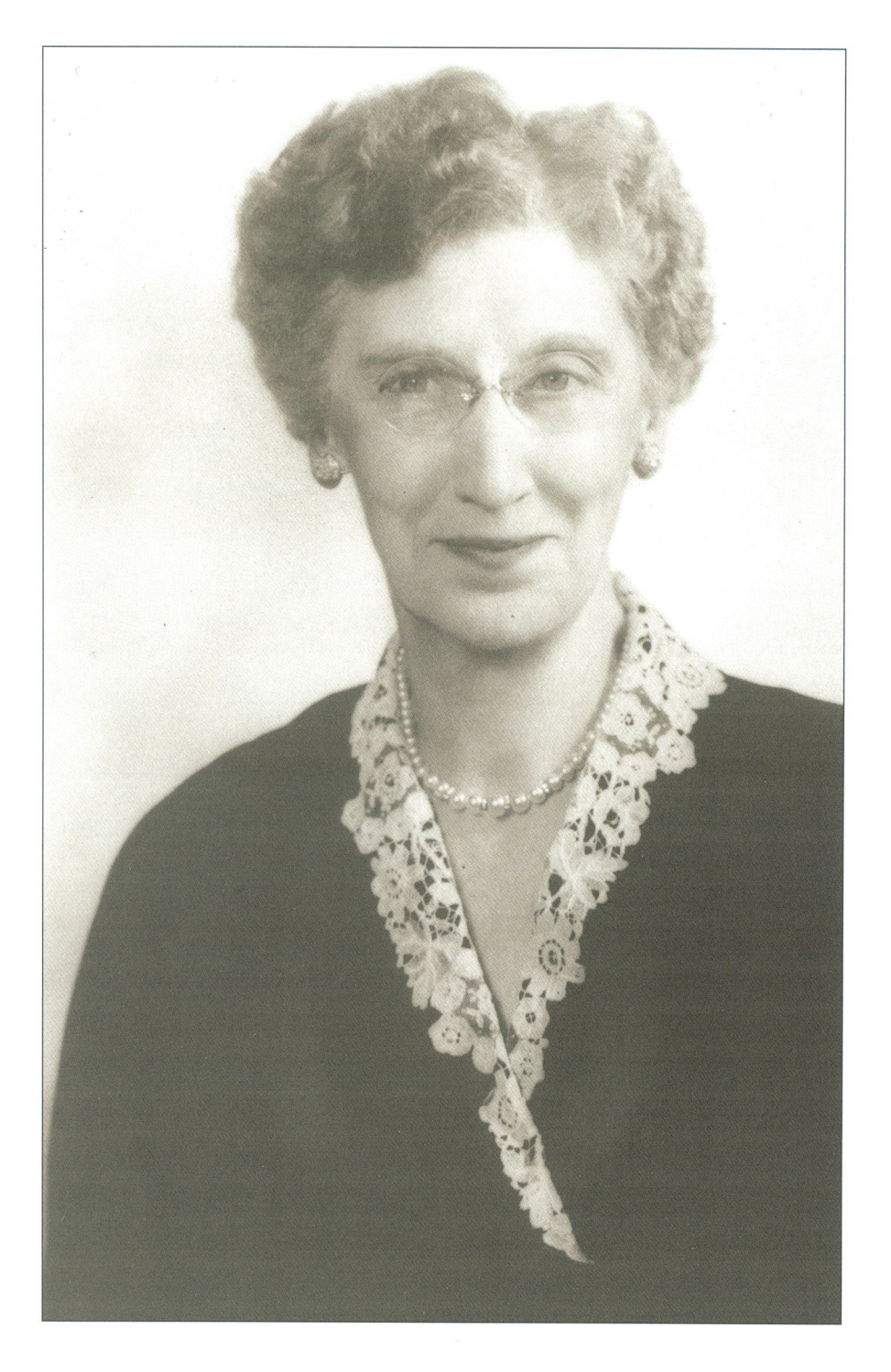

task must be designed around a purposeful activity, so that the movement produced is elicited by conscious attention not to muscle units but to the end-goal; and lastly, the best activities are those that lend themselves to repetition.

An avid golfer, Rood enjoyed a friendly rivalry with Maggie Knott on the greens for many years. Despite their considerable philosophic and professional differences, when Knott fell sick near the end of her life, it was "Roody" who became her most stalwart caregiver. Margaret Rood died in 1984 at the age of 79.

### MARY MCMILLAN'S LAST YEARS

"Progress is a relay race — one generation passes on to the next," Mollie McMillan once said. And in the years after her repatriation from China back into the United States, she was more than happy to acknowledge that the baton had passed to younger leaders. She did, however, maintain a lively interest in the Association through membership in the Massachusetts Chapter. In professional retirement, she rented a cozy apartment on Commonwealth Avenue in Boston, furnishing it with the many mementos of her travels, including many rare antiques and art works which she had been foresighted enough to ship home just before the war's outbreak. To her delight, she renewed old ties with her large and loving family, read her Bible daily, and entertained many of her old friends, some of them going back to the era of the reconstruction aides. Like many an old-time Bostonian, she cherished afternoon tea and conversation.

To the end, McMillan's humanity, humor, and dedication touched all who knew her. Mildred Elson later recalled that "to talk with Mollie was a tonic." With a twinkle in her eye, McMillan lifted everyone's spirits as well as their resolve. During the 1949 Annual Conference in her hometown of Boston, the membership gave her a special vote of appreciation to which she responded with characteristic modesty: "No, friends, it is not to me that credit or honor is due for the growth and development of the Association. It is to the chapter presidents, past and present, the national officers, past and present, . . . to your directors, standing committees, advisory committees, . . . to the years of devoted service . . . of the staff, to those in the army who throughout the years have fought and won military status for army physical therapists, . . . to those who gave their time and talents to make the *Physical Therapy Review* a success. It is to all these that I would like to do honor. The national Association has given to me so much, you have enriched my life exceedingly and made me very happy."

McMillan's interest in APTA was matched by her enthusiasm for the World Confederation for Physical Therapy. She was an important and popular participant at the second congress in New York in 1956 and had planned to attend the third congress in Paris had her health permitted. Unfortunately, the destructive effects of her wartime imprisonment resurfaced, making the last months of her life a time to test even her courage. She died of brain cancer in Boston on October 24, 1959, at the age of 78. Following funeral services at the Old South Church, Copley Square, her body was buried in the family plot in Brookline, Massachusetts.

Even after her death, Mollie McMillan's service to her profession continued. Throughout her working life, she had saved a part of her modest salary, passing it along to her brothers for investment. Over the years the funds had grown handsomely, and in her will she provided for the establishment of a trust fund to be administered by APTA. The fund, which came to be known as the McMillan Scholarships, was enhanced when the McMillan family made a second generous bequest in 1985 upon the death of Mary's sister. The fund provides assistance to worthy students in their final year of study for physical therapy careers. Between the first in 1963 and 1995, the scholarship fund has benefited more than 200 students with over a quarter of a million dollars in financial aid.

At her memorial, the Reverend Frederick Meek said of McMillan: "We Congregationalists do not canonize the outstandingly faithful for their deeds, but if we did, Mollie would be a likely candidate not only for what she did, but most of all, because of what she was in herself."

CHAPTER 6

# The Golden Years
# 1959 – 1979

*Lucy Blair held almost every senior staff post during her many years of service to the Association, culminating in her appointment as executive director from 1959 to 1969. So well loved was she that the 1969 Conference in San Francisco was designated "I Love Lucy Week."*

The sixties proved to be a stressful time for most Americans. After 15 years of postwar prosperity and government by consensus, the nation went through the throes of great cultural upheavals in virtually every sector, from social welfare and school integration to civil rights, sexual behavior, and miniskirts. Student protests, the 35-hour work week, manned space adventures, assassinations, urban riots, love-ins and walk-outs, psychedelic drugs, unisex hairstyles, and the involvement of the United States in a highly controversial war in Southeast Asia were just some of the events and forces causing Americans to reexamine their lives and their allegiances. On one subject, however, the public seemed to agree: high-quality health care was no longer regarded as a privilege. It was considered to be a right, and the institutions and individuals whose job it was to provide such services were scrambling to keep up with the demand.

The decade of the sixties also found upheavals and uncertainties within the American Physical Therapy Association. Annetta Cornell Wood's tenure as executive director in the national office lasted just 10 months before ending abruptly in the fall of 1959. Staffer Lucy Blair, who had held just about every other job in the national office, stepped in as acting director. Eight months later, after the Executive Committee and the Board of Directors had gone through the formal selection process, Blair was elevated to permanent directorial status, a job she would hold with distinction until her retirement in September 1969.

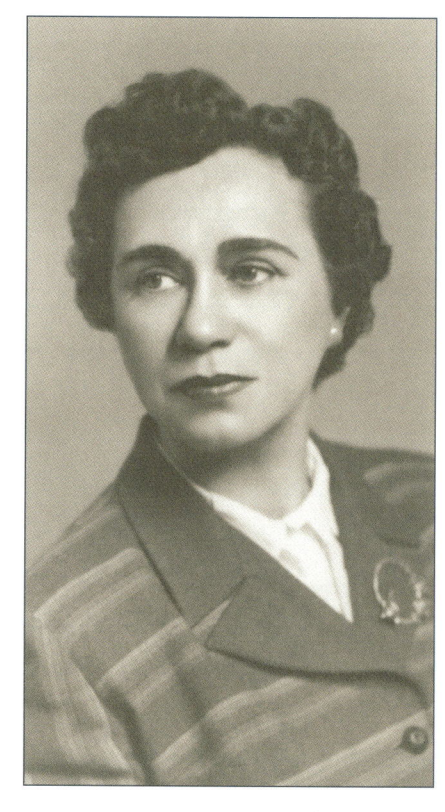

Blair brought to the job ideal personal qualities: infectious enthusiasm, a sharp wit and sense of humor, determination, charm, and an unflappable air that had carried her through many office crises. A New Hampshire "Yankee" through and through, she cared not at all for ceremony or for personal display. She wore her wrinkled tan raincoat in almost every sort of weather, and her habits of frugality were legendary. So was her gift for personal details. "She knew the names and ages of spouses, children, nieces, nephews, and grandchildren of every PT she ever met," recollects Eugene Michels, who felt himself privileged to have been an Association president during her era. "It was not for nothing that when she retired in 1969 the Annual Conference was an all-out 'I Love Lucy' festival," Michels observes.

Blair's professional qualifications were another strength. A graduate of Children's Hospital School of Nursing (a Simmons College affiliate located in Boston), she had received her physical therapy certificate from the Harvard Medical School Courses for Graduates in 1941, and her M.A. degree from Columbia University. She had gone on to serve as a physical therapist with the Visiting Nurse Associations in Boston and Milwaukee, the Wisconsin Bureau of Handicapped Children, the U.S. Navy (as a World War II WAVES lieutenant at three naval hospitals), and with the Joint Orthopedic Nursing Advisory Service. In 1950 Blair joined the APTA staff as senior consultant to the Department of Professional Services and was centrally involved in the polio emergency program, the gamma globulin studies, the Salk vaccine field trials, and the APTA program for foreign-trained physical therapists. In all these roles she traveled around the country constantly, becoming a welcome and familiar face at component meetings, physical therapy schools, and hospitals and rehabilitation centers from coast to coast. The new executive director knew far more people in the profession on a first-name basis than any other physical therapist in the country, a feature that helped preserve the cozy informality that still prevailed in the workings of the national office in the sixties.

Blair came into the executive director position at a difficult time financially. With the war on polio having come to a successful conclusion, the Association's principal benefactor, the National Foundation/March of Dimes, was in the process of withdrawing the financial support the Association had enjoyed for more than two decades. Much as the separation was reasonable and predictable, it came more quickly than expected, and the belt-tightening it precipitated at APTA was painful. With deficit budgets forecast, a comprehensive review of staff functions was ordered. Staff numbers were reduced, some committees were dissolved, and essential activities were shifted over to other already overburdened volunteer committees. Office supplies, postage, telephone, telegraph, and ordinary office maintenance work were curtailed in a further effort to balance the budget. Field visits by national staff to the chapters became less frequent. The printing of informational materials was also reduced, and those "handouts" that continued to be produced — recruitment and career information — were now offered with a price tag

*Mary Elizabeth Kolb, director of Pennsylvania's D. T. Watson School of Physiatrics, was APTA president from 1961 to 1967. During Kolb's two terms, the Association's journal took on a more professional tone.*

for the first time. In these various ways, income and outgo were wrenched into line.

Regrettably, some member development programs also had to be temporarily scaled back. Particularly at risk were the Professional Education program, the Professional Services program, and the Foreign-Trained program, all of which had been supported almost entirely by NFIP grants. If anyone was qualified to keep APTA centered on its primary mission and living within its reduced means, it was Blair, and she succeeded magnificently.

The presidency of APTA, in the hands of Agnes Snyder when Blair took over the executive director's job, passed to Mary Lib Kolb of Pennsylvania in 1961. Kolb went on to serve two terms. Her background included many years of involvement in Association affairs at the chapter and national levels. She was also director of the D. T. Watson School of Physiatrics, which was an affiliate of the University of Pittsburgh. Kolb's forceful personality and high-style appearance were in contrast to Blair's, but they worked well and accomplished much together.

### FROM REVIEW TO JOURNAL

Not long after Blair moved into the executive director's chair, Dorothy Voss began to wind down her nearly five-year involvement as editor of the *Review*; the pressure from her many other professional commitments had simply spread her too thin. Noticeable in the last months of her tenure is the frequency with which "guest" editors were invited to have their say on the editorial page and the rarity with which Voss spoke in her own editorial voice. The job of the managing editor, the day-to-day, hands-on person in the office, was also in flux, with the result that the *Review* felt obliged to apologize for the chronic lateness of issues, which sometimes appeared as much as three to four weeks after their appointed date.

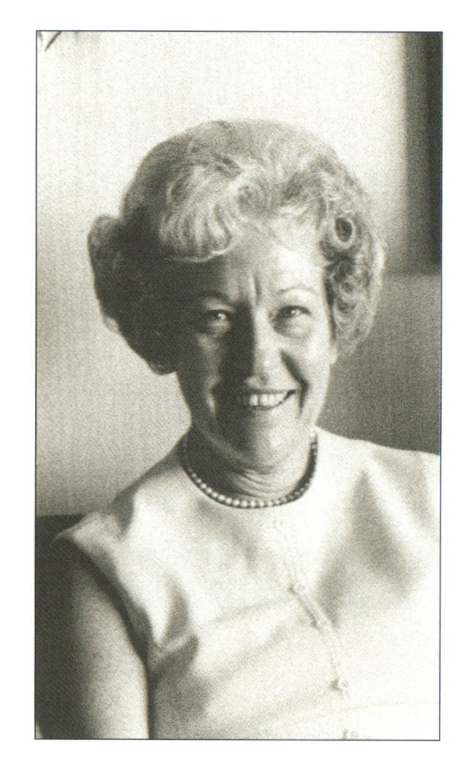

Another matter undergoing reexamination was the *Review*'s name. From time to time someone would suggest that a new name was needed, one that would include the designation "journal" and the name of the Association in its formal title, following the example of the *Journal of the American Medical Association*. The Executive Committee decided to poll the members, and with the majority's approval, the change to the new name, *Journal of the American Physical Therapy Association*, was formally made in 1962.

Voss resigned in late fall of 1961, and Helen Hislop, a member of the editorial board, was asked to take over as "acting editor," a title that was raised to "editor" in March 1963. Hislop's credentials were impressive by any standards. She had received her certificate in physical therapy at the State University in Iowa in 1951, had worked under Catherine Worthingham at the National Foundation for Infantile Paralysis, and had gone on to earn both master of science and doctoral degrees in physiology from The University of Iowa in 1960. At the time of her appointment she held dual positions as a staff researcher in the Department of Physiology, Albert Einstein Medical Center, Philadelphia, and at the School of Allied Medical Professions, Department of Physical Therapy, University of Pennsylvania. Along the way, she also managed to teach physical therapy at the University of Minnesota and at the D. T. Watson School and to participate in numerous symposia.

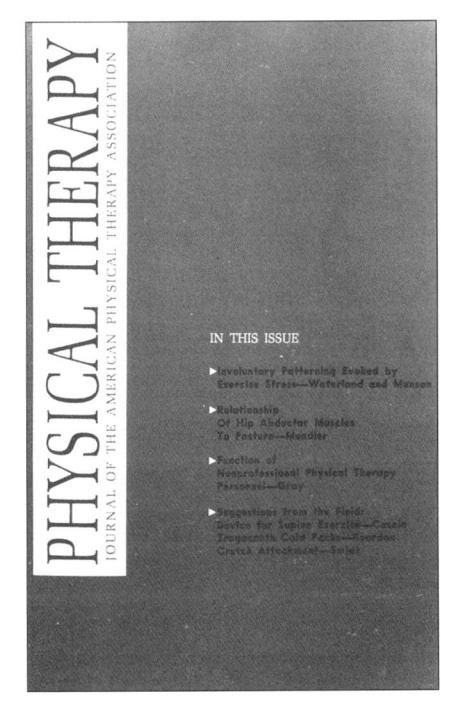

Hislop saw in the position of editor an opportunity to move the profession to a level that probably had never been fully visualized before. A woman of strong opinions, impressive intellect, high ethical standards, and tremendous output, she used the new *Journal* to spread her ideas on a broad range of fronts. Not a month passed during her eight-year tenure that her columns did not urge members in print to extend their reach in research, in professional development, in chapter and national service, as individual and collective voices for what was right and wrong. Never one to mince words, Hislop scolded slackers, chided hypocrites, and praised many unsung heroines and heroes of the Association for their valiant efforts.

Along with Hislop's monthly editorials, which touched on everything from the evils of medical quackery to the dangers of cigarette smoking, nuclear testing, and sloppy writing, she produced lengthy, foresighted articles. The new method of isokinetic exercise, described by Hislop and co-author James Perrine, and the role of modern biomedical instrumentation in physical therapy are just two of the myriad professional topics she tackled head-on. Regarding the latter, in the April 1964 issue of the *Journal*, she told readers that they must, as a profession, abandon their passive resistance to technological change and "accept responsibility for designing its methods and adapting these changing concepts to physical therapy's uses. . . . Our future technical success rests on our skill and boldness

*Helen Hislop, appointed editor of the* Journal *in 1963, examines her work. Under Hislop's aegis, the* Journal *not only took on a handsome new format, but greatly expanded the quality and breadth of its content.*

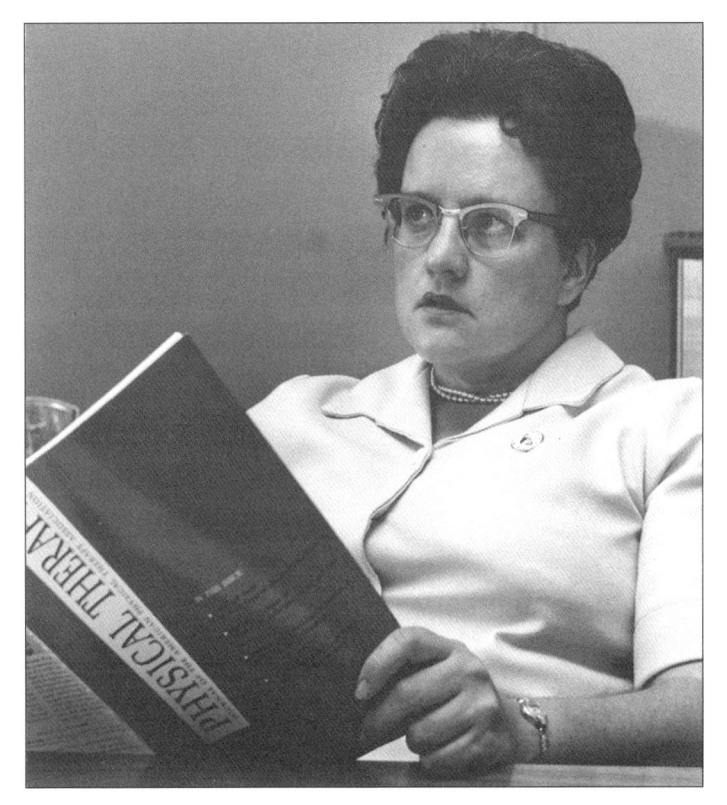

*This physical therapist treats a child on a tilt board, January 1974, a device used to facilitate adjustment to the upright position and to increase weight-bearing on the lower extremities.*

of mind to think through the interrelationships of modern technology and classical physical therapy without regard to habits and traditions."

The prescient Hislop went on to write at length about the burgeoning role of computers as tools to store, analyze, and synthesize data collected through clinical testing and to predict outcomes. "There can be no question that the road in the next 10 years is going to be a rocky one," she declared in the April 1963 issue. "It is time to take a risk . . . to use the implements and methods of scientific technology in the space age to broaden our profession."

Although the *Journal* was entrusted to her with a new name (a name that was to change again in January 1964 to *Physical Therapy*, with a subtitle of *Journal of the American Physical Therapy Association*), that change was only the first of many. Hislop introduced a new cover design, a new typeface, and several new editorial features including "Notes from Capitol Hill," which covered the fast-changing beat of legislative issues in Washington, D.C. The journal's length also grew considerably, from 816 pages annually when she began to 1,480 annually when she finished, and as a reflection of the new importance of the publication, the numbers of advertisers — and coincident advertising revenue — grew exponentially. (Finding companies to fill the space was relatively easy. Many of the major manufacturers and suppliers of equipment serving the needs of physical therapists came into the market about this time, including Burdick, Chattanooga Pharmacal, Cleveland Orthopedic, Cybex, Dallons, Everest and Jennings, G. E. Miller, Mettler, J. A. Preston, Teca, and Tru-Eze.)

As Hislop was able to demonstrate the value of APTA's communications arm to its membership, she helped to develop monographs and other reference materials from the journal that were then made available for use at professional symposia and in advanced coursework in physical therapy. Among these were the monographs on *Arthritis*, *The Child with Central Nervous System Deficit*, and *Principles of Lower Extremity Bracing*. This last is a classic collection of 14 articles from the September 1967 issue of *Physical Therapy*, which in 1995 is in its eighth printing. These experiences also provided the impetus to produce the *Style Manual*, an important tool to the profession at that time. Hislop also turned Mildred Elson's memorable 1964 Mary McMillan Lecture, "The Legacy of Mary McMillan," into a booklet that was broadly used in schools and clinics to introduce students to the history of the profession.

### FEAR OF FALLING

The 40th anniversary of the Association was observed at the 1961 Annual Conference held in Chicago, with 1,394 members registered for the five-day event. (The numbers registered represented roughly 16 percent of the then-current members, a level of participation that remained surprisingly constant for many years.) Six of the surviving 42 charter members attended a luncheon held in their honor. Although the occasion was meant to be festive, there was also a sense of poignancy and sadness in the fact that so many beloved figures were missing. Recalled posthumously at the gathering were Janet Merrill, first secretary-treasurer, who had died in 1951; Marguerite Sanderson, first director of reconstruction aides, 1954; and, of course, Mary McMillan, who had been gone just two years. Also remembered for their considerable contributions and friendship were John Coulter, who had died in 1949; Harold Corbusier, in 1950; James B. Mennell, in 1957; and Joel Goldthwait, in 1961.

Conscious of the passing of an era, APTA's Executive Committee invited past president Gertrude Beard to write a history of the first four decades for the membership. In "Foundations For Growth," the lengthy and spirited report that appeared in the December 1961 issue of the *Review*, Beard ended with a verbal snapshot: "As of February, the Association consists of 57 chapters [including two chapters each in California and Pennsylvania], representing all 50 states, the District of Columbia, and Puerto Rico. The membership nears 10,000. We believe this has been accomplished because the Association has fulfilled the important task as stated by Mary McMillan . . . 'To set a standard for physiotherapy, and neither in act, word, or deed, to lessen that standard.' "

One fear among physical therapists as they celebrated the Association's 40th birthday was that the call for their services would decline sharply with the end of the polio emergency. But health care was evolving across the board, and as soon became apparent, the demand for physical therapy services was not declining, only changing in its particulars.

Foremost, the nature of the conditions to be treated most commonly was changing. As polio, tuberculosis, and a host of other communicable diseases had come under control, the treatment of acute care patients and patients with chronic diseases and diseases associated with aging was gradually assuming a larger importance. This was evident not only in the clinical setting, but in the emphasis that large governmental institutions had placed on research funding in those areas. Surgeon General Leroy Burney, describing the Public Health Service's mission for the sixties, forecast, "The next great nationwide health efforts may be expected in . . . comprehensive health care . . . comparable with the great expansions of medical research and hospitals in the 1950s." Comprehensive care, he went on to explain, comprised a continuum of preventive, curative, and restorative services, which could be carried out only by allied health personnel with varied education, technical skills, and training.

Such a combination of services required the "team approach," in which many health care specialists had to work together harmoniously and according to plan. The Public Health Service, for its part, was becoming a huge grant-making agency, and this, in turn, was leading to a restructuring of the National Institutes of Health, the research arm of the PHS.

The public was changing, too. Not only had the proportion of elderly doubled in the fifties and sixties, but Americans across the board were far more health conscious than they had been in the past. Many had heeded President John F. Kennedy's alarm — that we were becoming a nation of spectators rather than athletes, a circumstance that endangered our health and our national security — and were taking better care of themselves. Kennedy made it a policy of his administration to promote physical fitness and called upon the schools to strengthen the health and fitness of youth through daily programs of vigorous activity. To assist schools in carrying out this mandate, the Department of Health, Education, and Welfare also prepared guidelines to measure physical ability and chart progress, ultimately establishing the President's Council on Physical Fitness and Sports. Similar efforts were made within the military, which found its recruits in need of better and more comprehensive conditioning.

Persons in need of specific health services were also demanding a voice in determining how their treatments were to be carried out. And they were increasingly likely to know something about the fast-breaking new technologies available — thanks to expanded news coverage in the popular press — and to expect the use of state-of-the-art methods and materials when treated. In consequence, health institutions were under constant pressure to stay current to attract and keep patients. Like virtually every other health profession in the sixties, the physical therapy profession and APTA found themselves far from ready for the rapid expansion of demands for their services.

That the change was already being felt is reflected in a survey reported by Captain Beatrice Thompson, staff physical therapist, Brooke General Hospital, Fort Sam Houston, Texas, in the June 1963 issue of the *Journal*. In an article entitled "Diagnoses and Procedures in Physical Therapy," Thompson began with the observation that the changes in physical therapy were coming about in response to such factors as an aging population, the development of increasingly sophisticated electronic equipment for research and treatment, and new insights into the nature of the bodily responses to acute injuries, arthritis, and cerebrovascular disorders. That practicing physical therapists needed to keep abreast of these changes through continuing education was implicit in being a good practitioner. However, Thompson reminded her readers, those physical therapists involved in designing the physical therapy curriculum and teaching the next generation had the additional obligation to "anticipate" what further changes might lie ahead and plan accordingly.

To aid in that process, Thompson surveyed five physical therapy facilities in San Francisco, Palo Alto, and surrounding Santa Clara County,

California, to ascertain how frequently particular diagnoses were made and to compare the numbers with those recorded in a somewhat similar study in 1948. Among the several shifts in referred conditions, she found that whiplash, brain damage, disc pathology, laminectomy, and spinal fusion were increasing markedly. Improved survival rates among the seriously injured together with the increasing frequencies of automobile-related injuries were chiefly responsible, although Americans' growing participation in high-risk sports was also a factor. Open-heart surgery provided another relatively new category of patients for the physical therapist. Thompson concluded that, at the very least, physical therapy education ought to be strengthened in the areas of pathology and the basic sciences. She also noted that several traditional therapeutic modalities had fallen out of use, among them Kenny hot packs, hydro-galvanism, long-wave diathermy, static electricity, and Sitz baths. Exercise, heat, and massage remained consistent favorites, as they had been from the early years.

### THE NFIP SAYS GOOD-BYE

Ironically, just as APTA was celebrating its 40th birthday, its relationship with the National Foundation for Infantile Paralysis was coming to an end. The very last financial tie — major support for the professional education program — was discontinued in 1962. In an editorial paying tribute to the NFIP's 20 years of assistance and encouragement, Helen Hislop reminded readers of just some of the more tangible evidences of the foundation's support: one in three of APTA's current members had received scholarships for their basic physical therapy education; thousands more had been helped to take continuing education courses; 100 members, comprising almost half of the current teaching faculty in schools of physical therapy, had received NFIP fellowships for advanced study that had made their academic careers possible. The Council of Physical Therapy School Directors had been born of NFIP sponsorship, as had student recruitment and guidance programs. The vision and foresight that had made all this possible, Hislop concluded, were attributable to the efforts of one person: former APTA President Catherine A. Worthingham, for 16 years director of Professional Education at the National Foundation.

Fortunately for APTA, the withdrawal of the NFIP did not signal the end of Worthingham's contributions, only a change of direction. Upon her leaving the National Foundation in 1962, Worthingham and APTA were given a grant by the Office of Vocational Rehabilitation to conduct an exhaustive "Study of Physical Therapy Education" centered around 42 currently active schools of physical therapy. When completed, the six-part Worthingham report proved to be one of those landmark documents in the evolution of a profession, comparable in its thoroughness and objectivity to the 1910 Abraham Flexner Report to the AMA that had led to reforms of medical education in America.

The first part of the Worthingham Report, which appeared in the January 1968 issue of *Physical Therapy*, compared the curriculum patterns for basic physical therapy education with those required for six other undergraduate fields, including the social sciences, engineering, and biological sciences. Worthingham's purpose was to assess the relative weight of major course requirements versus other general requirements and electives to determine whether physical therapy students might not benefit from broader undergraduate preparation or even a program taking five or more years.

Worthingham found cause for both encouragement and concern. She took as a positive indicator the ongoing efforts at many schools to continually revise and upgrade their programs. She also praised the levels of basic science preparation offered. But she was concerned to find a lack of opportunity for students to take humanities courses. One clear implication was that students with narrow education were likely to lack the flexibility, judgment, and vision to grow and adapt with a changing profession.

Later segments of the Worthingham Report appeared in *Physical Therapy* over the next two years as the author looked at every aspect of preparation for a career in academic and clinical physical therapy. She reported, for example, that physicians continued to dominate the direction and funding of physical therapy education, in part because most PT schools were the poor relations of medical schools whose limited resources favored the education of doctors, and in part because so few physical therapist instructors held the kinds of advanced degrees that garnered respect in the ranks of academia. Only 5 percent of faculty in physical therapy schools held doctoral degrees, of which not one was in the physical therapy field; of the 49 percent of faculty holding master's degrees, only half were in physical therapy studies.

Although faculty positions typically allow for and sometimes require ongoing research as part of the job description, Worthingham found only 28 percent of the instructors so engaged in these same schools of physical therapy. This disinclination to undertake original investigations deprived the profession of one of the traditional sources of new science as well as validation for current clinical practice. It put the majority of physical therapy faculty at a disadvantage in competing for leadership roles within academia and presented poor role models to the next generation of physical therapists.

Worthingham concluded her report with a series of broad-ranging recommendations designed to make physical therapy education more relevant to contemporary needs and standards. But perhaps her most lasting commentary had to do with changing the emphasis in theoretical and clinical curricula from one concerned primarily with "sick care" to one of "comprehensive, continuous, and coordinated health care." In this, she firmly predicted the trend to preventive health care and health maintenance.

### MAKING WAVES

Included in Worthingham's overview were data on the amount of time devoted to teaching various modalities. Several relatively new procedures had been added to the growing list of skills with which the physical therapist needed to be familiar. (None had appeared in Thompson's

1963 sample, presumably because they were still novelties.) One was ultrasound, a special form of kinetic energy distinct from light or heat.

First investigated in France after the turn of the century as a means of submarine detection, ultrasound was adapted to medical diagnostics and therapeutics in the 1950s. Its diagnostic capability was based on the ability of very high-frequency sound waves to penetrate the patient's skin and produce pulse-echo images or sonograms of soft and fluid-filled organs such as the heart, liver, and gallbladder. Another diagnostic form used Doppler ultrasound to record conditions of blood flow and heartbeat, with certain changes in pitch translatable into specific information such as the age of a fetus or blockage in an artery. The therapeutic use of ultrasound exploited the mechanical and thermal effects of still higher-powered sound waves to treat ligaments, tendons, and muscles by reducing inflammation and speeding healing.

The first paper on ultrasound therapeutics was presented at the 1954 Annual Conference in Los Angeles, the work of two Long Beach, California, physical therapists, F. Eugene Miller and James Weaver. Titled simply "Ultrasound Therapy," the paper made clear that though results of the treatment seemed very promising, much about dosage limits, clinical indications, and mechanisms of action remained a mystery. "Ultrasound massage," as it was sometimes referred to, was not touted as a specific cure for any disorder but had, they said, demonstrated usefulness in the symptomatic relief of the pain, soreness, and tenderness associated with such conditions as bursitis, tendinitis, and various forms of arthritis.

That the use of therapeutic ultrasound became widespread within a relatively short time can be deduced by a 1974 report in *Physical Therapy*, surveying the "Use and Performance of Ultrasonic Therapy Equipment in Pinellas County, Florida." The authors, a consortium of FDA and county health officers, found that in this small county's 40 facilities there were 58 separate ultrasonic units in use, consisting of 26 models from a dozen manufacturers. The authors also reported that ultrasound had grown in popularity until it exceeded in frequency of use for patient treatment both microwave and shortwave.

Other, still newer modalities to be introduced in clinical practice in the late 1960s were biofeedback and transcutaneous electrical nerve stimulation, or TENS. Biofeedback, which involved the use of relatively sophisticated electronic hardware — chiefly electromyographic instruments — to provide the feedback component of neuromuscular reeducation, was developed out of research in the 1960s showing that certain so-called involuntary functions could, with training, be brought under conscious control. The first use to be described in a physical therapy context was that of Edna Forward of Stanford University, whose 1972 *Physical Therapy* case report described successful use of a "muscle whistler" in teaching two patients, one with hemiplegia, the other with severe burns, to regain functional movement of a leg. Other therapists to become involved in the early years were Steven Wolf, Carmella Gonella, and Ruth Kalish, who worked closely with physiatrist J. V. Basmajian at Emory University's Rehabilitation Research and Training Center, where some of the most intense early investigations in biofeedback in relation to neurological impairment were carried out. (Basmajian was a supporter of APTA and a frequent contributor to the journal. He consistently urged physical therapists to take on a greater role in research.)

Somewhat later, growing out of studies conducted by Harvard cardiologist Herbert Benson and others regarding the relationship of stress, high blood pressure, and heart disease, biofeedback was also joined with relaxation training as part of a multidisciplinary biobehavioral program for stress management.

TENS was a rediscovered modality for use in pain management. A high-tech variant of the unwieldy nineteenth-century procedure known as galvanism, TENS won a new following after experiments in the 1960s by Ronald Melzak and Patrick Wall. In their now-famous gate-control theory, Melzak and Wall demonstrated that when milder electrical stimuli were properly applied to specific nerve endings, the transmission of more severe and persistent pain impulses could often be blocked. Out of this work had come a new generation of electroanalgesics, including dorsal column implants and transcutaneous electrical nerve-stimulating devices, with great potential in clinical physical therapy.

Given the novelty of the TENS notion and its potential importance to practicing physical therapists, *Physical Therapy* asked Steve Wolf to serve as guest editor of its December 1978 issue. Wolf, a highly respected educator, laboratory administrator, and researcher in neurological disorders at Emory, organized and coordinated the writing of an outstanding collection of articles on everything from the basic neurophysiological mechanisms underlying TENS to reports on appropriate use, specific TENS equipment, the placement of electrodes, clinical results, and a comprehensive search of the literature to date.

### COMMITTEE ON RESEARCH

Support for research had been a tenet of the Association's Bylaws from the very beginning, and not a year had gone by since then that someone in a leadership position had not urged members to take their research obligations more seriously. The House of Delegates regularly passed ringing declarations urging members to dedicate themselves to research, presidential speeches annually called on members to extend themselves, and Helen Hislop had used the pages of the *Journal* to literally teach the uninitiated how to design and carry out research. Yet nothing that fostered such activity in a practical way had been put in place. Indeed, when in 1964 the Association formed the Committee on Research, the committee's work was specifically limited to offering *outside* grantors objective and confidential reviews of grant proposals that dealt, however tangentially, with physical therapy; reviewing members' work was not considered an appropriate activity because it was thought to pose a conflict of interest. Served by Lorraine Lake, Lucy McDaniel, and Dorothy Briggs, this early review committee rendered its judgments almost entirely by mail, because there was neither budget nor time to assemble the reviewers in one place. (It should be noted that the committee's work went on quite independent of the activities of the Section on Research, which came into being in 1965 and which concentrated on meeting the research interests of Association members.)

By 1968 the Committee on Research's initial participants were ready to move on, and three new members — Carmella Gonella, Helen Skowlund, and Don Lehmkuhl — took their places. The new members had an ambitious agenda. They requested permission to revamp the committee's program with the specific intent of fostering research by giving members a more prestigious and stimulating forum in which to make their work known to their peers. The basic notion was to set up a formal review and evaluation process for original member-written papers, which it was hoped would be submitted for presentation at Annual Conferences. The screening process was set up in such a way that submissions could be considered objectively, without reference to authorship. Abstracts of papers accepted would appear in *Physical Therapy* for everyone to read, although it took some doing to persuade the editorial board to make the additional space available.

It should be noted here that in the first 40 years of Annual Conferences, little had been done to solicit original investigative (research) papers from members for possible presentation. In the words of Eugene Michels, "Conferences were largely something planned for members by the national office. . . . And the national office gave preference to invited speakers who, in distinction to members who competed to present their studies, were given honorariums, travel reimbursements, and space for their abstracts in the *Journal*. Of course, giving our members a more receptive forum, including publication of their abstracts beginning in 1979, turned out to be a dynamic idea, a key event in our history. It said to young research-minded PTs, who in the majority had moved on after gaining their Ph.D.s, that they had a home in our field after all. Promoting research in this way had a good effect on the educational system, too, in that faculty members with physical therapy backgrounds now had an opportunity to produce and present research as part of their credentialing in the same way that their peers in other academic fields had."

Michels himself became intimately involved in the committee's work. When the shift toward PT-generated research came, he was on the faculty at the University of Pennsylvania, whose noted School of Allied Medical Professions was being shut down because the university administration thought physical therapy offered insufficient intellectual content or scientific contributions to make it worthy of an Ivy League imprimatur. While Michels certainly did not share that view, he recognized his profession's vulnerability.

Leaving his position as the School of Allied Medical Professions' acting dean in June 1977, Michels began an 11-year stint on staff at APTA's national office. Michels soon became staff liaison to the Committee on Research. Over time, the committee evolved from one that merely selected members' papers for presentation and publication at Annual Conference into one that pursued the ambitious goals outlined in the influential "Plan

*This lapel insignia bearing an "S" has been worn by physical therapists in the Army Medical Specialist Corps since 1955 when the "W" from the days of the WMSC was replaced.*

to Foster Clinical Research in Physical Therapy." The plan, crafted by committee members Gary Smidt, John Echternach, and Steve Rose and adopted by the Board in 1978, would provide the focus for the Committee on Research in the years to come, its primary resource in keeping the research bandwagon moving.

A measure of how quickly that effort produced significant results can be seen in the fact that for the Annual Conference in 1979, a total of 61 research paper abstracts were submitted and reviewed by the committee. Two years later the number of submissions exceeded 100, and by 1988 it grew to more than 300.

### THE BATTLE OVER UNIONISM

For years the matter of how to achieve a fairer standard of pay and other security benefits for physical therapists had simmered at chapter and national meetings. By any measure, physical therapists continued to be undercompensated compared with other health professionals. (A Department of Labor survey of 321 selected occupations administered in 1959 and published in 1965 found physicians at the top of the income ladder with a median annual income of $14,561, followed closely by dentists, medical school professors, osteopaths, veterinarians, and optometrists. Pharmacists ranked 55th with $7,176, and the catchall category of "therapists and healers" was positioned at No. 146 with an average annual income of $5,406.) Concern about how to improve compensation for physical therapists made everyone a little testy and became a focal point of activity.

The security issue reached a flash point in late 1963 when the New York Chapter came to the defense of downstate members working in nonprofit hospitals. Under the provisions of the New York State Labor Relations Act, the right of hospital employees to organize and bargain collectively with employers was not only protected by law, but employees not otherwise represented were forced to join such hospital union shops as a condition of employment. Consequently, when Local 1199 of the Drug, Hospital and Health Care Employees Union launched a campaign to become the official bargaining agent for a large segment of hospital workers in the state, physical therapists found themselves exposed and vulnerable. Although housekeeping and maintenance staffs were the main object of the campaign because they were the most numerous and the least organized component of the hospital work force, specialty groups such as physical therapists, occupational therapists, dietitians, and a few others were also targeted. By reason of their relatively small numbers, these professionals were neither automatically excluded (as were physicians) nor otherwise organized for collective bargaining (as hospital nurses had become through the American Nurses Association).

Although the majority of southern New York physical therapists wanted no part in union organization, they viewed the creation of an alternative, legally recognized organization as the only option that would allow them to remain independent. Barbara Cossoy, Anthony DeRosa, Sam Feitelberg, Hy Dervitz, and Bob Bartlett, all active in the leadership of the New York Chapter, led its membership in a strategy to make the chapter the collective bargaining agent for the state's physical therapists. Feitelberg, who in his professional life was the chief physical therapist and coordinator of physical therapy and occupational therapy at Columbia-Presbyterian Medical Center, enrolled in a series of training seminars at the Cornell University School of Industrial and Labor Relations, and the New York Chapter voted to change its articles of incorporation to allow it to act as a collective bargaining agent.

It took no time at all for the news to reach APTA national headquarters and the Executive Committee, which viewed the chapter's activities as a concession to the very forces that were inimical to the profession. President Mary Lib Kolb fired the first salvo of opposition in the February 1964 issue of *Physical Therapy* under the banner headline "Unionism or Professionalism." She reminded readers that "through its 43 years APTA has struggled constantly to assume the role of an organization which truly represents a *profession* with its inherent responsibilities." Collective bargaining in the manner of a trade union, she said, could only destroy individual initiative and endanger the ideals of service on which the American Physical Therapy Association was founded. While the New York Chapter might feel that it operated in a unique environment and that an exception should be made, Kolb insisted that a change of this magnitude would inevitably have repercussions for chapters across the United States, that such actions could not be taken independently, and that the good of the majority must prevail.

The editorial and the issue stirred up a storm of correspondence and enlivened the House of Delegates meetings at Annual Conferences for three years. The large and powerful California and Pennsylvania chapters were particularly opposed, and according to Feitelberg, the 20-odd delegates from New York found themselves all but ostracized during the opening debate. Some members suggested that physical therapists caught in the union squeeze resign their jobs rather than involve themselves in collective bargaining, and the meeting adjourned with a policy statement declaring APTA opposed to any and all activities resembling unionism.

The New York Chapter, for its part, was unshaken in its resolve, and in the months to come, it sent members out to a score or more of "swing" chapters to argue its case at length. By 1965 the tide had begun to turn. Chapters in Massachusetts, Illinois, Michigan, Connecticut, and New Jersey saw "the writing on the wall" and declared their support for the New York Chapter. When a second attempt was made at the Annual Meeting to force the New York Chapter to cease its activities or leave the Association, Board member James Zimmerman rose to say, "the winds of change are blowing," and the motion was rejected. The following year, a somewhat less judgmental

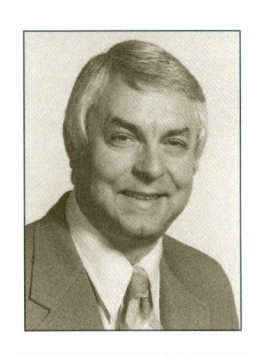

*In a remarkable (and largely unsung) achievement, physical therapy was explicitly included in Medicare legislation for both outpatient and private office services. APTA had no formal lobbying arm in the mid-1960s, and it was the individual efforts of physical therapists Clem Eischen of Oregon (shown here), who was chair of the Private Practice Section's legislative committee, and John Pellow of Oklahoma in influencing their members of Congress that led to the favorable legislation.*

House of Delegates called for the formation of a special committee "to study the socioeconomic conditions related to the practice of physical therapy" in all the states and to prepare for the Association such information as members might need to better understand collective bargaining, standards of employment, and the state and federal laws relating to such issues.

The Board of Directors named Feitelberg and Dorothy Pinkston to undertake an objective evaluation. The two returned several months later with an extensive document which, among other things, represented a radical change of perspective on Pinkston's part. The report began with a detailed historical review of the Association's involvement in socioeconomic issues. It showed, contrary to general belief, that the Association had, from the very beginning, taken positions on the welfare of its members. These ranged from informal lobbying efforts to gain appropriate recognition and pay raises for reconstruction aides in 1921, to periodic salary surveys designed to guide employers in personnel policies beginning in 1944, to the formal creation of the Division of Professional Services in 1953.

The study went on to recommend that inasmuch as the socioeconomic pressures driving unionization were certain to vary dramatically from state to state, such concerns and responsibilities should be left to individual chapters, as in the example of New York State. Pinkston and Feitelberg thought, however, that the national office could play a critical role as a clearinghouse for information and education on socioeconomic security issues related to the profession. Their recommendations carried the day, ending what Feitelberg believes was "probably the most significant floor fight in the history of the Association over a political issue." As for the New York Chapter, it did not waver from its purpose. Despite strenuous opposition on the part of Local 1199, including some not-very-subtle efforts to dissuade Feitelberg from competing with the union, he and his team successfully negotiated a series of excellent contracts, substantially improving local physical therapists' salaries and benefits for several years thereafter.

### THE GREAT SOCIETY

Among the many social initiatives launched during Lyndon Johnson's presidency, none had a greater impact on physical therapists than the enactment in 1965 and 1966 of the Medicare and Medicaid programs, the first steps toward national health insurance. Medicare (which was appended to the 1935 Social Security Act as Title XVIII) provided federal funding for many of the medical costs of older Americans and the disabled. It overcame deeply entrenched resistance to what had been perceived as "socialized medicine" by making benefits available to everyone over 65, regardless of financial need; by linking payments to the existing private insurance system; and by allowing patients to choose their medical providers in the open market. Medicaid extended the insurance concept to welfare recipients of all ages and was administered by the states with a combination of federal and state funding.

The effects of the two programs were far-reaching. Many millions of people previously receiving little or no health care suddenly gained virtually unlimited access, with the result that the market, and the dollars available for health services and for expensive medical technology, expanded dramatically. Compared with statistics from 1950, when some form of insurance covered 11 percent of the nation's health care costs, the expanded coverage now carried 32.4 percent of costs. Hospital costs also soared. In the two decades between 1946 and 1966, the cost of an average hospital stay per day increased 359 percent, from $12.50 to $44.88, with no end in sight! There was, as well, an unprecedented demand for home health care services as a result of the Medicare legislation.

As Catherine Worthingham noted at a symposium at the 1964 Annual Conference in Denver, "The dilemma with which physical therapy is faced is that there are not enough physical therapists to perform the [current] essential physical therapy services." With national insurance legislation on the verge of going into effect, she warned, the problem might well become so severe that others could decide to solve it for them if physical therapists persisted in "playing ostrich with their collective heads in the sand." Among those organizations and professional groups known to be waiting in the wings were the U.S. Departments of Labor and Health, Education and Welfare; vocational schools and junior colleges; physician groups; nursing homes; and state health departments. None of these outsiders could be expected to look for solutions that made sound physical therapy principles their first priority.

### PTAs: To Be Or Not To Be?

Energized by the remarks of Worthingham, Hislop, and others that were subsequently published in *Physical Therapy*, members began pushing for new approaches to extending physical therapy services in the expanding market. The most obvious solution was one that had been rejected repeatedly in previous decades — the development of uniformly trained nonprofessionals as aides or assistants. It must be noted that aides, both paid and volunteer, had been assisting physical therapists in some hospitals and clinics for a very long time, taking care of equipment and supplies, accompanying patients to and from treatment, and carrying out other general housekeeping tasks. But there was a key difference between the old practices and the proposed innovation: under the older, informal arrangements, job descriptions and follow-up training were handled within each clinic on a case-by-case basis. Many aides had little or no education beyond high school, nor did their responsibilities require such. One rather extensive aide program had been instituted in the early sixties at Rancho Los Amigos Hospital in Downey, California, under the leadership of physical therapist Viola "Robbie" Robins. There, each physical therapist was teamed with a noncertified helper. Another program was thriving at St. Joseph's Mercy Hospital, Detroit, Michigan, where Charles Dorando was director of physical therapy services. The Institute of Reha-

*Uniforms and patches have been the subject of controversy over the years as physical therapists have wrestled with the issue of how best to identify themselves "on the job." By the late 1980s, members were sharply divided on this issue. At about this time the patch was dropped due to the prevailing belief that it connoted technical rather than professional status.*

## The Politics of "Allied Health"

Sources of funding and organizational expediency have always exerted some pressure on the shaping of professional curricula. Nowhere was this more evident than in the virtual explosion of Schools of Allied Health beginning in the mid-1960s.

The term "allied health" was not new. It had been used by the medical profession as an umbrella term to distinguish the "thems" from the "us" for decades. Included in the definition of allied health providers were physical and occupational therapists, medical technologists, public health officers, medical illustrators, dental hygienists, health care administrators, and dietitians, to name only the most prominent. Though some physical therapists chafed at what they considered the subordinate status implied, APTA long took the position that the physical therapy profession stood to gain more benefits than liabilities in living with the designation. However, before the 1960s relatively little was done to affirm the alliance in the form of educational programs. Indeed, up until 1963 only four schools followed such a model.

The first school to experiment with a full-fledged allied health program was St. Louis University, which opened the School of Nursing and Health Services in 1929. Another two decades were to pass before the interdisciplinary idea was tried again, this time at the University of Pennsylvania, which put together its own program in 1950. These schools were followed in turn by programs at the University of Florida (1957) and Indiana University (1958). With considerable variation from place to place, they offered a hodge-podge of baccalaureate and two-year certificate programs with the physical therapy "major" typically being the "flagship" department, boasting the most distinguished faculty and the most rigorous academic requirements.

Then in the 1960s the passage of the Great Society's Medicare and Medicaid programs greatly expanded the need for skilled personnel in virtually every sector of health care. This led in quick succession to the Allied Health Professions Training Act, an inflow of government funding to college and university teaching programs, and the rapid spread of the "team approach" to many new and existing schools. Under the terms of the Allied Health Professions Training Act, the disbursement of federal financial assistance was to be carried out by the Bureau of Health Manpower within the Public Health Service. By implication, the government intended to do all within its power to discourage what it saw as the increasing fragmentation of the health care system.

Anticipating the changes, nine additional schools of allied health were formed. Subsequently, 13 directors drawn from these institutions – Boston University, Indiana University, Loma Linda University, Northeastern University, Ohio State University, St. Louis University, SUNY-Buffalo, Temple University, and the Universities of Florida, Illinois, Kentucky, and Pennsylvania — together formed the Association of Schools of Allied Health Professions (since renamed American Society of Allied Health Professionals).

In the new health care environment, ASAHP grew by 1980 to encompass some 126 schools of allied health, in two-year colleges, four-year colleges and universities, and health science centers, as well as 25 national professional associations and close to 1,600 individual members. With this kind of strength, it came to play an influential, if not always welcome, role in the direction of physical therapy education. Though APTA initially hoped that ASAHP would become a counterbalance to the medical profession, such representation did not materialize as APTA members had envisioned. Indeed, ASAHP's leadership—the people who rose within the academic community to run the schools — were seldom drawn from the professions represented within the schools. This "Dean's Club," as it has been dubbed, seemed to some to be taking the separate entities of allied health out of the frying pan only to put them squarely into the fire. Particularly unwelcome over the intervening years have been ASAHP's attempts to control accreditation and certification and to discourage occupational specialization in favor of more generalized approaches to education and practice.

Citing the submergence of many PT programs within allied health schools and the continuing control of the profession by organized medicine and the federal government, Geneva Johnson expressed "serious doubts" about the survival of her profession unless the Association mounted its own counteroffensive. Writing in the January 1974 issue of *Physical Therapy*, Johnson said she was particularly jolted by the term "allied health professional," because it put physical therapists into the same pot as a host of supportive personnel. While the latters' existences were traceable strictly to the needs of physicians, nurses and dentists, Johnson went on, physical therapists came into being "in response to the needs of patients," a fundamentally different route.

If the profession allowed its members to be lumped with "supportive personnel" as a matter of educational efficiency or expediency, Johnson warned, then the time would come soon when the "distinct and unique service" provided by physical therapists would be devalued both in the education required and in the spheres of health care set aside by others for them.

In the early 1980s APTA resigned from associate membership in ASAHP, citing differences over many issues, not the least of which was APTA's desire to maintain the hard-won autonomy and distinct identity of the profession.

bilitation Medicine at New York University also had an extensive on-the-job aide training program.

By contrast, under the newer proposals, formal education programs at new or existing academic institutions (instead of hospitals) were suggested, along with some kind of certification process. But such a proposal raised a multitude of concerns among many physical therapists. Worthingham thought she saw historical reasons for the resistance: "The early days of the development of physical therapy in this country were depression years. Also, it was difficult to obtain recognition for a new treatment service. Physical therapists became protective of every aspect of their field because of fear for their economic security." This historic memory, Worthingham suggested, triggered old fears whenever the topic of nonprofessional assistants was raised, however different the circumstances had become. Other physical therapists bridled at such comments, saying that the endorsement of nonprofessionals by APTA might appear to formalize a two-tiered level of service. Ironically, the latter concern had been raised by some physicians during debates on the use of physiotherapists 40 years earlier!

In 1964 the Board of Directors appointed an ad hoc committee consisting of Helen Blood (chair), Thelma Holmes, Beth Phillips, Martha Wroe, and Charles Dorando, all of them, at the very least, open to bringing nonprofessionals into some kind of formalized relationship with physical therapists. For three years the group worked on a policy proposal that covered every conceivable ramification, from what to call nonprofessionals to how they should be trained, supervised, and accounted for in patient billing procedures. The committee addressed concerns regarding the extent to which the nonprofessionals' presumably lower fees might give them the edge in being hired in physicians' offices and to what extent the public's understanding of the profession might be undermined by a new category of health care worker. They also faced squarely the possibility that failure to act might inadvertently encourage other allied health groups to take over some facets of physical therapy practice. The committee finally concluded that the positive implications of developing the assistant role would far outweigh any perceived negatives.

On the one hand, said Dorando, "Getting physical therapy services to people in need was always our underlying goal, and the physical therapist assistant offered us the opportunity to do that." On the other, the PTA also seemed to provide a modus for the physical therapist to become more professional. As Thelma Holmes put it, "We saw a change in the performance of [our] job; we could become more focused on higher levels of decision making, problem solving, and management."

As a result of the committee's favorable findings and despite the unanimous opposition of the Board's Executive Committee, APTA in 1967 adopted a policy statement that set the foundations for the birth of the physical therapy assistant (PTA) program. (Two years later the term would be changed to physical therap*ist* assistant to underscore the fact that the PTA assisted the individual physical therapist rather than the more global field of physical therapy.) That same year, Miami-Dade Community College in Miami, Florida, and St. Mary's Campus of the College of St. Catherine, Minneapolis, Minnesota, were the first to enroll students in their programs, and just two years later the first 15 PTAs graduated with associate degrees. By 1970, there were nine PTA education programs up and running, thanks in part to federal legislation enacted in the mid-1960s that provided financial assistance to junior colleges offering manpower training in the allied health fields. With funding from a Kellogg Foundation grant, PTA educators formed the Physical Therapist Assistant Education Group (PTAEG) and held their first meeting in St. Petersburg, Florida. Among the initial participants were such strong proponents of the PTA concept as Bob Patterson, Bella May, Nancy Watts, Barbara Bradford, Shirley Asklund, Hazel Adkins, Barbara White, Bob Harden, and Helen Blood.

The ad hoc committee had recommended that the Association establish a membership category specifically for PTAs that would give them both recognition and prescribed opportunities to participate in some APTA affairs. In 1970 the House of Delegates took the first steps toward bringing PTAs into APTA by offering temporary affiliate membership. This status was formally mandated in 1973 by a one-vote margin in the House of Delegates. Eligible PTAs were admitted to limited participation in national Association affairs, which, according to amendments of the Bylaws, included a half vote, the right to speak and make motions, the right to hold committee appointments, and the right to chapter representation in the House of Delegates. PTAs could not, however, hold elected office. Dues were levied at proportionately reduced levels.

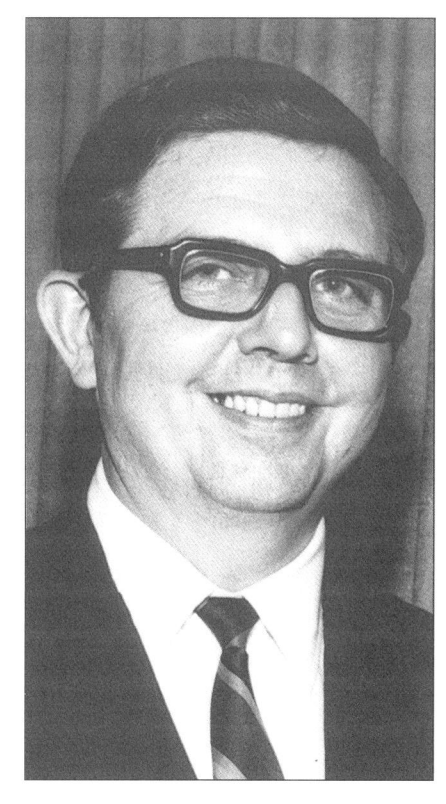

Meanwhile, Mary Lib Kolb had passed the gavel to her fellow Pennsylvanian Eugene "Mike" Michels, who became the first of a succession of five men to occupy the president's chair between 1967 and 1985. Michels, who had carried out both his entry-level physical therapy education and graduate work at the University of Pennsylvania, had been both a clinician and a member of his alma mater's faculty. He was well known to the membership through the numerous chapter positions he had held in Pennsylvania and through service to the national organization as APTA treasurer and chair of the Finance Committee. With a deep attachment to the furthering of clinical research as well as education, Michels brought to his two three-year terms not only strong leadership skills but the convictions of a fire-

*Eugene Michels enjoys the distinction of being the first male physical therapist to be elected president. Serving in that capacity from 1967 to 1973, he broke precedent again in 1984, when he became the first man to deliver the prestigious Mary McMillan Lecture.*

brand, and he continued APTA's long strides toward professional maturity.

### TOWARD SPECIALIZATION

With widening access to health care and momentous advances in medicine and medical technology, a new health care environment was emerging. One of its more notable features was the explosion of information, which was rapidly overwhelming the capacity of most generalists to keep even nominally informed in all areas. Whether by desire or by practical necessity, many in the medical profession were being drawn into specialization. The same pressures were felt, albeit with less urgency, within the physical therapy community, in which the aura of "technician" had never been fully shaken off.

At first, the trend was expressed within APTA's membership in the growing importance of special interest sections, which had proliferated to a dozen by the mid-seventies: the Section on Research, formed in 1965 (John Brake, first chairperson); State Licensure and Regulation (Robert Ayers) as well as Administration (Clara Bright) in 1970; Sports Physical Therapy (Ronald Peyton) in 1973; Pediatrics (George DeHaven) and Clinical Electrophysiology (Dean Currier) in 1974; Orthopaedic (Stanley Paris) in 1974; Cardiopulmonary (Scot Irwin) in 1975; Obstetrics and Gynecology (Elizabeth Noble) as well as Neurology (Mary Anne Rinehart) in 1977; and Geriatrics (Osa Jackson-Wyatt) in 1978. Each had its own leadership, each its unique professional and legislative agendas; and many, such as the older Self-Employed (later Private Practice) Section, found themselves caught up almost immediately in complex reimbursement issues brought on by the new Medicare/Medicaid legislation.

But sections were and are, by definition, rather independent groups. Individuals were free to join one or more sections on the basis of interest and the desire to keep abreast of current developments through continuing education programs and informal networking. Membership in a section carried no formal professional recognition; outstanding physical therapists at work in every professional venue in those years, received recognition only through the admiration of their peers. The only practical way for a physical therapy clinician to improve his or her status at the time was to move up through the management hierarchy. However, overseeing other physical therapists and acting as a liaison to other parts of the health care team inevitably took the managing physical therapist away from direct involvement with patients. For many physical therapists, this was not a satisfying alternative.

There was also the unpleasant fact that individuals outside the profession were often able to claim "specialty" status by virtue of narrowing their focus and developing *less* versatility. Certainly respiratory therapists, athletic trainers, exercise physiologists, and physicians' assistants were encroaching upon aspects of physical therapy practice, and physicians' assistants were gaining more and more ground in the orthopedic cast rooms and amputation clinics.

Recognizing these limitations on physical therapy career development, some section members became prime movers in the seventies in leading

APTA toward formal recognition of clinical specialization. In 1973 the House of Delegates charged the Board with studying the feasibility of establishing mechanisms for specialty certification, the most likely means of identifying the "experts" among them. While broad-based interest was initially difficult to discern, the issue of specialization grew into a "hot topic" by the time the first midwinter Combined Sections Meeting was held in Washington, D.C., in February 1976.

The Association's leadership nonetheless approached specialization with more caution, seeing it as both a blessing and a curse. On the one hand, specialization prepared the way for higher levels of clinical competence and scientific expertise, which had the obvious potential of benefiting patients with special needs. But it also raised the possibility that the profession would become fragmented. Physical therapy specialists could become isolated in their own separate compartments, having less and less to do with the general foundations of physical therapy, at the risk of viewing their patients only in a narrow context and not as the complex human beings they really were.

Helen Hislop gave voice to these concerns in her McMillan Lecture delivered at the Anaheim, California, Annual Conference in 1975, but she went on to declare that specialization, together with advanced academic opportunities, offered the only realistic means to generating better clinical science. "After 50 years, the *science* of physical therapy is entering its infancy," she told the group. "The determination of the profession to retain a viable place in the health care system . . . and to improve the quality of patient care must, for an indefinite future, necessitate a large, continuing research and development enterprise. . . . To convince others of our aptitude, we must prove to ourselves that our methods work."

She claimed that so long as the profession lacked doctoral

*Wearing a hip action brace and a smile, a youngster at Ranchos Los Amigos Hospital, Downey, California, practices crawling with his therapist.*

199

programs of its own and a corps of clinical specialists focused on expanding the science of physical therapy, physical therapists would never be better than "mental pickpockets" trading upon the exploration and hard thinking of other professional groups. Hislop called upon her colleagues to shape the destiny of the profession by creating structured programs to train and certify clinical specialists. She also warned against creating too much dogma or too many rituals, which would discourage the best candidates from applying.

APTA's House of Delegates took up the challenge, establishing a task force that in 1978 produced a specialist certification program designed to give formal recognition to individuals with advanced knowledge, skills, and abilities in a special area of clinical practice. The task force, made up primarily of section leaders, initially identified four areas of specialization based on existing patterns of practice: cardiopulmonary, neurology, orthopedics, and pediatrics. At the same time, it developed "Essentials for Certification of Advanced Clinical Competence in Physical Therapy." The House of Delegates then appointed a Commission for Certification of Advanced Clinical Competence, which evolved into the American Board for Certification and later the American Board of Physical Therapy Specialties.

According to the "Essentials," each specialty area was to operate under the supervision of an APTA-supported Commission for Certification, and to develop its own criteria for eligibility. As Carolyn Crutchfield, one of those closely involved, said, "the certification process had to be valid, legally defensible, attainable, and fair." This meant that before each committee could prepare its extensive test items it had first to agree upon what constituted an advanced body of knowledge and then validate those premises. As Crutchfield said, without exaggeration, "This was no small task."

Meanwhile, the rules for seeking certification were made explicit. Candidates would have to present written evidence of at least two full years of clinical practice in the designated specialty, experience in administration or consultation, and some measure of research productivity; it was presumed that each area of specialization would have additional requirements specific to its own practice patterns. No additional academic credentials were named beyond those required of all APTA members.

Seven years later, with the commission retitled "board," in conformity with the American Medical Association model, and the mechanisms for financing and administering the examinations settled, specialty certification was ready for a road test. (As they had from the beginning, the sections continued to be the chief force in keeping the specialization process alive and well.) Henceforth, board certification could be won only through successful completion of a written examination consisting of 200 multiple-choice questions. Such status was granted for a period of 10 years only, after which applicants had to apply for recertification. Pioneers in specialty certification the first year were Linda Crane, on the teaching staff of the University of Miami School of Medicine and chair of the Cardiopulmonary Section; Scot Irwin, on the faculty of Georgia

State University and Director of Physical Therapy and Rehabilitation at Clayton General Hospital; and Meryl Cohen, a member of the adjunct faculty, Institute of Health Professions, and Coordinator of Cardiac Rehabilitation Physical Therapy at Massachusetts General Hospital, Boston. Along with gaining the stature of trailblazers, this trio could add the designation "Cardiopulmonary Certified Specialist (CCS)" to their list of professional credentials.

### CASE WESTERN RESERVE: A NOBLE EXPERIMENT

The earliest effort to launch a two-year graduate program for the basic education of the physical therapist appeared at Case Western Reserve University (formerly Western Reserve University) in Cleveland, Ohio, in 1960. As with so many other innovative notions in the education arena, Catherine Worthingham's name is associated with the initial proposal which she brought before the university's president, John Millis, and which Case Western's Graduate Council accepted in 1958. Worthingham approached the university because it already had established graduate programs in other health professions, including speech pathology, social work, and medicine. Physical therapist Louise Suchomel recruited an outstanding faculty, beginning with physical therapists Geneva Johnson, Dorothy Pinkston, Agnes Connor, Marian Russell, and Don Lehmkuhl. In 1962 Norman Taslitz, a physical therapist with a doctoral degree in anatomy, replaced Marian Russell, and the following year, Mary Eleanor Brown came on board as well to direct a new continuing education component.

The curriculum, which was designed and periodically revised with the close involvement of local clinicians, was experimental by nature. Along with thorough education in the fundamentals of anatomy, physiology, and physical therapeutics, it sought to bring to the student a wider view of health care. From the first semester onward, the program exposed students to the world of scientific inquiry and research and culminated in preparation of a thesis under the supervision of a thesis committee that included a scientist, a clinician, and a faculty member. Students were also given close personal contacts with established clinicians in the field through clinic work and through opportunities to meet and observe visiting lecturers of unusual distinction.

Through regular forums, they were exposed to vital issues affecting the profession, part of the faculty's larger plan to develop attitudes of professional involvement and participation. As it was hoped that many of the students would go on to give some part of their career to teaching, instruction in the principles of teaching and in communications skills, including poise in oral presentations, was also integral to the program. (In one particularly notable example of this requirement, every member of the graduating class in 1965 and each member of the faculty presented a paper at APTA's Annual Conference that year.) Courses in administration and supervision, aimed at preparing graduates for leadership roles in the clinical setting, were scheduled in the latter months of the program. Finally, graduates were required to accept employment imme-

## NYU: A Legacy Of Innovation

New York University has rightly been called a trailblazer in the history of physical therapy education. It holds the distinction of having started not only the first four-year bachelor's degree program for physical therapists, but also the first postprofessional Ph.D. program for physical therapists.

The program leading to the B.S. degree opened to students in September 1927 as a unit of the Department of Physical Education, Health and Recreation. Shailer Lawton, a psychiatrist and internist on the faculty, was both educational and medical advisor, and after helping to develop the PT curriculum, he became the department's first director. Candidates for the baccalaureate degree in physical therapy took their specialty education during the senior year; however, it was also possible to earn a certificate by taking the same nine-month-long physical therapy curriculum. Responsibility for the professional aspects of this specialized segment was shared initially with the Hospital for the Ruptured and Crippled (now the Hospital for Special Surgery). Later students attended some classes at either Lenox Hill or the Hospital for Joint Diseases, and carried out clinical practice at any one of eight different hospitals in the city.

In 1932 George Deaver, the noted rehabilitation leader, succeeded Lawton as director, and it was during his 14-year tenure that the master's program (1942) was established. (Part of that time Deaver served simultaneously as medical director of the Institute for the Crippled and Disabled.) When Deaver retired in 1946, the curriculum consisted of anatomy, pathology, physiology, psychology, physics, electrotherapy, radiation therapy, hydrotherapy, ethics, massage, and therapeutic exercise (the latter two taught by physical therapist Mary Eleanor Brown); four components in which the specifics of physical therapy in medicine, orthopedics, neurology, and surgery were paired; and clinical practice, with physical therapists Barbara White and Mary Eleanor Brown sharing the teaching load with M.C. McGuinness and George Deaver of the medical school. (Teaching pay in these years was $8 per hour for MDs, $5 for instructors, and $100 per semester for teaching assistants; tuition for the 36 points and 400 hours of clinical practice required to complete the regular course of study was $432.) Class size varied considerably from year to year, with as few as one graduate in 1944 and 29 the following year. While most physical therapy schools still did not accept men, NYU was proud to say it was open to all; indeed, seven of the eight graduates in 1942 were men.

Deaver was succeeded as NYU's physical therapy program director by Elizabeth Addoms, a 1945 graduate. Under Addoms the program was extended by stages to 12 months, clinical practice hours were increased to 450, and academic standards generally were raised still higher. With the opening of Howard Rusk's Institute of Physical Medicine and Rehabilitation nearby, some theory courses were switched to this very innovative facility. Edith Buchwald Lawton, who developed the widely used Activities of Daily Living, was on the faculty, along with physician Donald Covalt.

In the years since, NYU's PT program has continued to grow and diversify. Upon Addoms' retirement in 1970, Arthur Nelson (NYU '54) succeeded as program director and developed the nation's first postprofessional Ph.D. program in physical therapy in 1973. The following year the Physical Therapy Program became a department within the newly designated School of Education, Health, Nursing and Arts Professions (SEHNAP) and plans were set in motion for the development of two additional postprofessional master's degree programs—cardiopulmonary physical therapy (1975) and developmental disabilities (1984). Further evidence of the growing complexity of PT education came in 1980 when the 14-month postbaccalaureate certificate program was phased out and 74 credits became the minimum requirement within a four-year professional baccalaureate program. The department submitted its proposal for a professional doctorate program in physical therapy to the New York State Board of Regents in 1984. In 1995, the State of New York authorized NYU to begin development of a professional doctorate program in physical therapy.

The real measure of the quality of NYU's program remains in its roster of faculty and graduates, the latter now numbering well over 3,000. In addition to the already named notable physical therapists who have been on the faculty are Signe Brunnström, Jack Hofkosh, and Marilyn Moffat. Among the graduates who have gone on to serve the profession in leadership roles are two APTA presidents (Robert Bartlett '57 and Marilyn Moffat '63); three members of the Board of Directors (Roger Nelson, Fred Rutan, and Stanley Siegelman); four Catherine Worthingham Fellows (Brown, Moffat, Arthur Nelson, and Jules Rothstein); two editors of *Physical Therapy* (Moffat and Rothstein); seven Lucy Blair Service Award recipients, and numerous chapter presidents, chairs of PT education programs, and heads of hospital departments and practices. Among the many outstanding graduates of the doctoral program, several international students have returned to their homelands in Nigeria, Egypt, and Kuwait to teach physical therapy along the NYU model. And in another more direct instance of internationalism, NYU works cooperatively with Yang Ming Medical College in Taiwan to provide education for the physical therapy faculty there.

*The Mary McMillan Lecture Award, the highest honor the Association confers, has been awarded virtually every year since 1964. Recipients deliver a major address at the Annual Conference, at which time they receive this commemorative medallion.*

diately following graduation in a hospital department approved by the faculty so that clinical training and professional growth could be guided in the initial years of practical work.

Case Western's program, fine as it was, was slow in getting launched and lasted scarcely a decade. In the first year of operation, with the program not yet accredited and its existence little known, the program attracted just one student, Elaine Bradford, who graduated two years later in 1962. The next graduates, just two, received their master's degrees in 1964, and in the following years, class size rose until it reached a top enrollment of 16 entrants in 1969. But just as the program was hitting its stride, financial problems intervened. Student tuition, even in the best of times, covered only a fraction of the costs of educating a physical therapist, and when federal funding to universities was sharply reduced as a corollary of the escalating costs of the Vietnam War, the reverberations were felt throughout Case Western's departments. Ironically, one of the few areas in which grant funding was not directly affected was in physical therapy, but other programs with larger enrollments and longer traditions at the university suffered severely. In a triage decision, the university leadership selected the physical therapy program for termination, and it was phased out following the graduation of the class of 1971.

The legacy of Case Western is nonetheless substantial. Its faculty initiated what they chose to call the Mary McMillan Lecture in 1962, anticipating by two years APTA's own celebrated lecture series. CWRU's first guest lecturer was, fittingly, Catherine Worthingham, who spoke on "The Future of Physical Therapy Education" in 1962. She was followed by Helen Hislop, Jacquelin Perry, Sarah Rogers, Ruby Decker, Carmella Gonnella, and Margaret Moore, all renowned names in the profession. In a larger sense, the Case Western program also provided a standard against which newer programs have since been able to measure themselves. Lehmkuhl has called it "the Camelot of its time." Its time of troubles proved a foretaste of problems at the University of Pennsylvania's School of Allied Medical Professions and at Stanford University.

## VIETNAM

With John F. Kennedy's inauguration as president in 1961, the U.S. military involvement in Vietnam began to grow, culminating in the deployment of American ground troops in the spring of 1965 under President Lyndon Johnson. That commitment ultimately grew to 500,000 troops during Johnson's presidency and ended in March 1973 when the last military forces were withdrawn.

The first physical therapist on the scene was Army Medical Specialist Corps Colonel Barbara Gray, a 14-year veteran, who volunteered to go over in March 1966 to assess staff and equipment needs. Gray's arrival marked the first time a physical therapist and commissioned officer had been assigned deliberately to an active combat zone. As a result of her study and the direct requests of on-site hospital commanders, physical therapists were assigned to all army surgical, field, and evacuation hospitals in the country.

In all, some 47 physical therapists did tours of duty, every one of them volunteers in what turned out to be fierce competition for relatively few berths. Most were single women, although at least three men were in the group. Once assigned, they treated not only U.S. personnel, but Vietnamese military and civilians brought into U.S. Army hospitals. They also trained numbers of their Vietnamese counterparts in techniques that were then put to use in Vietnamese hospitals.

Colonel Sue Ozburn, who served at the 36th Evacuation Hospital, about 30 miles from Saigon, during the Communists' Tet and May offensives in 1968, recalls that physical therapists worked extraordinary hours to handle the large caseloads, using "terrible" equipment. "At my hospital, 300 beds were set aside for Vietnamese civilians, all of them burn patients. We saw 250 patients a day; the nurses and I routinely worked 12-hour shifts seven days a week. Most of the casualties were from the Viet Cong's white phosphorous grenades. We'd put the wounded into the whirlpool immediately, because their skin would often still be burning when they came in. When, as sometimes happened, they were coming in faster than our two whirlpools could take them, we took to hosing them down as the only practical solution. The water wasn't

*The importance of early intervention with physical therapy was recognized as never before in the Vietnam conflict. To assist in recruiting additional therapists for field service,* Physical Therapy *ran this recruitment advertisement in the November 1969 issue. In all, 47 PTs were sent overseas.*

205

*Royce Noland was executive director from 1969 to 1985, an era that saw the Association grow from a small, informal organization in New York to a major professional force in health care in the nation's capitol. Here, Noland talks to his executive assistant, Rita Ruskin.*

drinkable, but it worked all right for the purposes."

Ozburn says that she learned to make do with minimal equipment. "We had to wash our own towels and sheets and make our own weights and parallel bars. I did have two diathermy machines, but as the temperature was often upwards of 110°F, I couldn't use them. Mostly I used ice." Ozburn recalls that physical therapists in Vietnam were also given unprecedented responsibilities for patient care. "We rarely saw a doctor. They were in surgery all the time dealing with surgical orthopedic conditions. Consequently, the nonsurgical neuromusculoskeletal problems were usually evaluated and treated by the PT team. With our own military casualties, we saw a lot of delayed primary closure due to fragment injuries, and we developed protocols to keep them moving until they could be closed up and evacuated to Hawaii or Japan or the [mainland] U.S."

No physical therapists were injured or killed in Vietnam, but the work took its emotional toll. Ozburn says of the experience, "I don't remember my last four months there or my first month back home." Joining a veteran support group, she found that her nightmares were shared by many others. She remained in service for six more years but could never shake the burden of those harrowing months, and she retired early. "Seeing difficult and disturbing cases has always been a part of our work, but the experience of seeing desperately wounded patients day after day, literally within minutes of having sustained their battlefield wounds, and of having numbers of them die while in our care, was something none of us was prepared for."

### THE ROYCE NOLAND YEARS

More or less coincident with the winding down of U.S. involvement in Vietnam, Lucy Blair, APTA's longtime executive director, decided it was time to reconnect with her roots in Peterborough, New Hampshire. In 1969, she informed the Board of her intention to resign. A search for a successor was launched immediately, and some 25 applicants asked to be considered. Although many members regarded Mary Lib Kolb, who had come on staff as associate executive director following presidential service, as Lucy's heir apparent, Royce Noland of California was eventually selected.

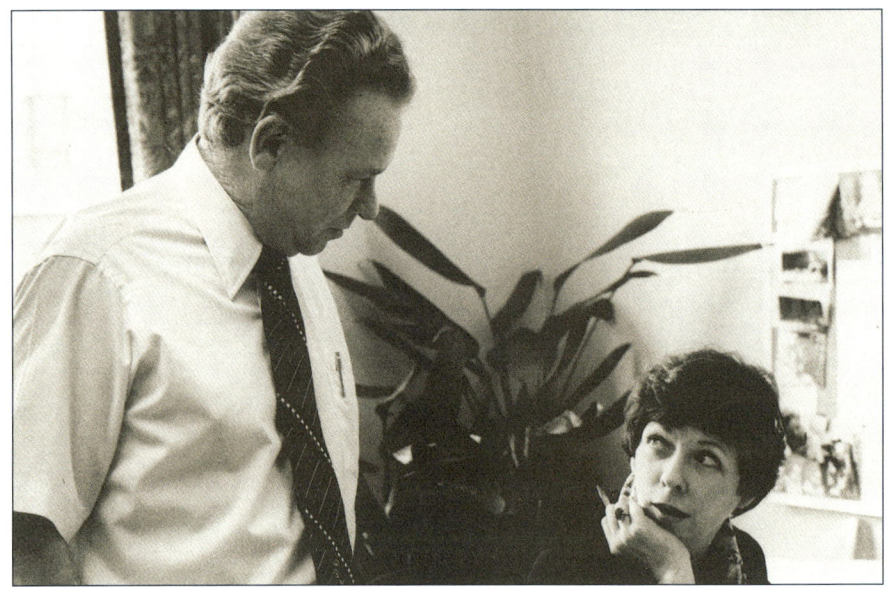

206  *Healing The Generations*

Noland inherited a substantial organization. By this time, the national office was in the Mutual of New York Building at 1740 Broadway, two blocks south of its former address at Columbus Circle. Its staff of 25 was divided among four divisions: education (liaison with education agencies and schools, school accreditation, faculty placement, student recruitment materials); professional services (chapter affairs, professional practice issues, foreign-trained program, PTA program, placement); conference services (a part-time position to oversee the work of a professional conference manager and to work with committees in planning programs, exhibits); and the journal division (editorial and production responsibilities, circulation, advertising, as well as the planning of symposia and seminars that generated manuscripts). Overseeing all functions was the executive division and its director, responsible for working with APTA's Board of Directors, various committees, and legal and judicial affairs, as well as maintaining liaison with government agencies and keeping the organization prudently within its budget.

Lucy Blair's wide popularity with the APTA staff would have made her "a hard act to follow" under any circumstances. The self-effacing Blair had never been one to make heavy demands of others or delegate tasks easily. Whenever the Board needed an extra duty carried out, Blair's first instinct was to take on the additional assignments herself. She would rather work evenings and weekends to get the job done than require more effort from her colleagues.

Blair and Noland were about as humanly different as two people could be. Royce Noland was not only the first man to assume the pivotal role of executive director, but he came from the opposite coast, with as many of the "laid-back" qualities associated with denizens of the Golden State as Blair had the quintessential characteristics of the New Englander. Noland brought both a new style of executive leadership and a solid grounding in business principles and financial management that would pay dividends in the Association's growth for many years to come.

Noland had in-depth experience as a physical therapist, in both the public and private sectors. Educated in physical therapy at Stanford University, he did his military service at the U.S. Public Health Service Hospitals in New Orleans and San Francisco, then went into private practice in Santa Cruz. (It was during these years that he and his associate, F. A. Kuckhoff, had invented the celebrated knee-strengthening N-K Exercise Table.) Active in Association affairs through his four years as executive director of the California Chapters, his chairmanship of the Self-Employed Section from 1964 to 1966, his position on the Judicial Committee, and a host of other appointments, Noland had demonstrated talents in administration. In his new assignment he proved himself eminently suited to assuring that the Association's executive arm would meet the evolving needs of the profession in the future. Staff members would be accountable to the Board of Directors, from which policy directions would flow.

Noland's transition became more difficult when he began to carry out his first major directive from the Board — to move headquarters from New York to Washington, D.C. The decision had been arrived at only after lengthy deliberation and with full knowledge that many longtime employees would be dislocated. But the move was part of a larger strategy to reduce office operating expenses and to increase the influence of the organization with government policy makers and other health-related organizations, many of which were already settled in the national capital for the same reasons. (The Washington move had, in fact, been under discussion for several years.)

The closing days in New York were reportedly very difficult. The transfer was ultimately made with a skeleton staff. Marilyn Moffat, who had been editing *Physical Therapy* part-time for nearly two years, remained behind for personal and professional reasons. Soon to be wed, she was also a new instructor at her NYU alma mater while completing her doctoral degree and developing her own private practice. For lack of an immediate successor, the journal was put under the temporary trusteeship of the Board of Directors, after which Lieutenant Colonel Elizabeth Davies, AMSC, took over.

The only employee from the Blair era to go south was Muriel Kelly, who had survived a bout of polio and had been a loyal worker in the membership records department for many years. Executive Assistant Rita Ruskin and Director of Management Services Don Magee, recent Noland appointees, became the core of the new Washington staff, which took over leased space at 15th and M Streets, within walking distance of the Capitol, early in June 1970. With the move, many organization records were lost. Lucy Blair volunteered countless hours reconstructing records after the move. Even so, the disruption left a legacy of problems that continues to hamper the full historical record of APTA to this day.

Further complicating matters for APTA at the time was the fact that the 47th Annual Conference had coincidentally been scheduled for Washington that same June. The local chapter leaders who might ordinarily have taken charge of organizing the conference were simultaneously trying to help Noland's people get settled in their new location and hire a new staff. The Board and various committee members consequently found themselves recruited for emergency duty in many aspects of conference planning and execution.

Within months, however, it became increasingly clear that the decisions to hire Noland and to move to Washington had been good ones for the long-term development of the Association and the profession. And the new staff began to grow. Among the new faces appearing at the national headquarters that first summer were physical therapists Elizabeth Fellows, Department of Professional Services, and Nancy Ward, Department of Educational Affairs. Physical therapists Frank Allender, Program Development, and Robert Teckemeyer, Government Relations, signed on soon after.

Eugene Michels, who was president from 1967 to 1973, summarized Noland's contributions in a letter he wrote in support of the former executive director's nomination for the Lucy Blair Service Award in 1990. Michels said that within two years of assuming the office, Noland had led the organization "from an inward-looking, largely insulated organization to a dynamic force at the national level in health care, health care legislation and regulation, health professional education, and accreditation. . . . It was as if APTA had 'turned a corner.'" Michels recalls Noland as an "amazingly resourceful, innovative and visionary individual. He ruled with a gentle hand, yet he seemed to know everything that was going on."

In all, Noland's career as executive director spanned the presidencies of five presidents, and while many others, both elected and on staff, share in the credit for what was achieved, Noland was a major facilitator throughout. A brief run-down of some of the highlights is in order. During Michels's watch, Noland inaugurated the *Government Relations Bulletin* in 1970; developed the Association's progressive position paper on "Priorities in the Health Care System" (1971); developed *Progress Report*, a monthly newsletter edited by Frank Allender that covered ongoing Association business in a timely fashion (1972); created the Component Services Desk at headquarters to assist chapters and sections; and established APTA's political action committee (1973). During the presidency of Charles Magistro (1973-1976), Noland launched the *Chapters* (later *Component*) *Bulletin* (1974); oversaw the first formal professionally managed Combined Sections Meeting in Washington, D.C. (1976); and helped to terminate an APTA/AMA collaboration in favor of APTA's own accrediting program (also 1976). Coincidentally, the Association's income and expense budgets exceeded the long-anticipated $1 million mark. President Robert Bartlett's term (1976-1979) was also marked with notable progress, including the start-up of APTA's Information Central (1978) and the transformation of the Physical Therapy Fund into the far more ambitious and effective Foundation for Physical Therapy (1979).

Noland also knew how to make APTA's voice heard when federal legislation affecting the Association's interest was in the making. Perhaps the most dramatic example of this was his organization of members in successful efforts to get APTA-proposed amendments regarding private practice written into law. Medicare, when initially enacted, contained no provisions for covering the services of physical therapists in independent practice. The profession not only saw the law changed to include the services of private practitioners, but as the decade closed, it also saw the ceiling limitation of $100 raised to $500, an astonishing change of heart on the part of Congressional watchdogs.

Economic consequences accompanied this time of change. Between 1966, when the dues had last been raised, and 1972, the cost of doing business had increased 33 percent. The general economy was dismal, with the result that advertising revenues in *Physical Therapy* dropped by some $50,000 in a single year; at the same time, printing costs rose sharply. Then-treasurer Charles Magistro recalls, "As treasurer, I had the difficult task of presiding over our first deficit budget in many decades and of figuring out how to meet not only the expected budget items coming out of our growing list of activities, but several unanticipated items. 1972 will surely go down as one of our more challenging years ever!"

That Magistro and his Board colleagues succeeded in meeting the challenge is evidenced by his election to serve as APTA's 23rd president in 1973. A 1950 graduate of Columbia

*This golden anniversary medallion was handed out with the program to attendees of the 1971 Annual Conference, after which the mold was broken.*

University's physical therapy program, Magistro had gone on to establish a private practice in the Pomona-Upland area east of Los Angeles, to teach as clinical associate professor at the School of Physical Therapy, University of Southern California, and to play an active role in the governance of APTA at local and national levels. Magistro has been variously described as "the patient-oriented social conscience" of the profession and as a "statesman-clinician" who showed by powerful example the value of thoughtful, deliberate examination of all sides of key issues.

### EMANCIPATION

Among the "unanticipated items" causing strains in APTA's budget were surely the Association's efforts to gain a measure of autonomy. The remarkable social and economic changes wrought in society in the sixties and seventies were more than matched by changes within the profession's standards and practices, which had to a significant degree been under the control of outside agencies and other organizations. Now, in a series of conscious and well-orchestrated moves, the leadership brought APTA several critical steps along the road to independence.

The first hurdle to be breached was APTA's relationship with the American Registry of Physical Therapists and the parent American Congress of Physical Medicine. In June 1960, with prompting from President Agnes Snyder, the House of Delegates issued a resolution regarding changes demanded in the management and design of the American Registry. The House called for the creation of an independent national board for physical therapy certification to evaluate the competency of physical therapists. Replacing the autocratic rule of the physiatrists, the new board would be composed of five physical therapists and four others to be drawn from the medical specialties that commonly rely on physical therapy services, physiatry being but one of them.

The resolution sent waves of alarm through the various physician groups. In the *Bulletin of the American College of Physicians*, it was implied that physical therapists were becoming unruly, that they had basked in the sun and glory of the medical profession, only to break away like so many headstrong youths upon achieving a measure of status. The physiatrists' leadership asked the Council on Medical Education and Hospitals to intervene as a supposedly neutral third party in bringing the physical therapists back into line. A representative of the council came before the House of Delegates with a counterproposal at the January 1961 meeting. Finding the counterproposal unacceptable and sensing an impasse, the House set in motion plans to discontinue APTA's official relationship with the American Registry, and it redoubled its commitment to achieve national certification through legally binding state licensure in every state.

The AMA and other agencies of organized medicine raised alarms among themselves that physical therapists had as their ultimate goal operation outside of the traditional prescriptive relationship with physicians. The House, seeking to allay fears, restated its firm commitment to leave diagnosis and prescription to the doctors. And Helen Hislop underscored the point in an editorial declaring, "We seek stronger, not weaker, ties with medicine. We seek cooperation, coordination, and communication with *all* branches of medicine. [But] we still affirm the basic right to govern our own affairs." Although the ARPT continued to exist for several years thereafter and to offer "registration" to qualified applicants, its imprimatur became increasingly irrelevant, and it was dissolved by its parent organization in 1971.

Similar assertions of independence were made in regard to the hospital standards that tended to interpose the physiatrist between physical therapists and all the other primary referring physicians whose patients might require their services. The issue, which had been simmering for two decades, came to a head in the spring of 1972 when the Joint Commission on Accreditation of Hospitals proposed to revise its procedural manual by substituting the term "Physical Medicine Services" for "Physical Therapy Services." To the House of Delegates, which met on the matter in June, the change was a clear and bold attempt at usurpation of power. By its terms, referring general practitioners, orthopedists, cardiologists, and other primary care physicians would be required to take their requests for physical therapy treatments to a physiatrist, who would then instruct the physical therapist as a technician regarding an already-agreed-upon plan of action. In a strongly worded position paper, the House declared, "Such interposition increases the cost of physical therapy services, disrupts the necessary consultation between the referring practitioner and the physical therapist, and, in some instances, poses a barrier to timely and appropriate referrals to physical therapy." APTA demanded that the terminology and the implied procedural policy be rescinded. After considerable backing and filling, the JCAH removed the new wording, and physical therapists were assured direct two-way access with all referring physicians.

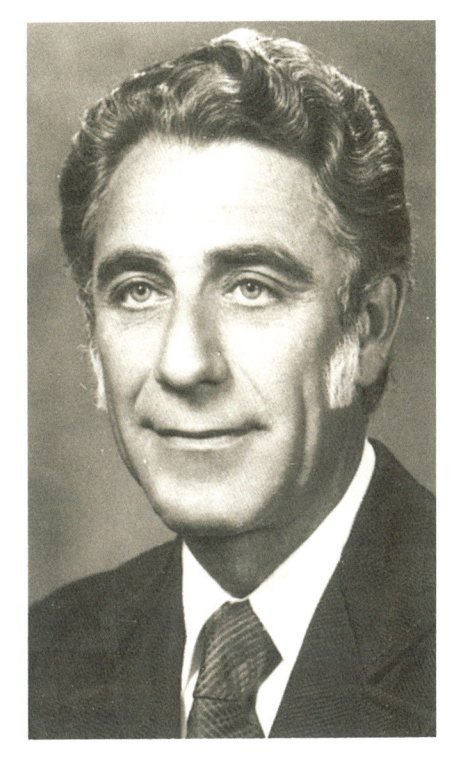

Standards of education and training also underwent evolutionary advancements in response to pressures from APTA. In 1960 the House of Delegates adopted a resolution "that the American Physical Therapy Association consider attainment of a baccalaureate degree the minimum education qualification of a physical therapist." Between 1965 and 1975, the number of institutions offering baccalaureate degrees had swelled from 35 to 63, with just 13 still at the postbaccalaureate certificate level.

With such progress, APTA's leadership was emboldened to raise the hurdle once again. The task of convincing the membership fell, quite

*Charles Magistro, director of physical therapy at Pomona Valley Community Hospital in California, was APTA president from 1973 to 1976.*

*The Golden Years 1959 – 1979*   211

*Robert Bartlett, former president of the New York Chapter, rose to lead the national organization in 1976. During his presidency, APTA thoroughly examined educational standards and accreditation processes.*

naturally, to the experienced educator and professional leader Robert Bartlett, who succeeded Charles Magistro as president in 1977. Graduate of the physical therapy certificate program at New York University, class of 1957, Bartlett had gone on to head the physical therapy programs at the State University of New York Downstate Medical Center and at Duke University Medical Center, Durham, North Carolina, all the while playing an active role in local, state, and national physical therapy affairs.

Bartlett called upon the House to examine education standards and to seriously consider raising minimal requirements to the postbaccalaureate degree, which he said "is universally accepted as the appropriate entry level of education for a profession." After much lively debate, and in full recognition that setting such a goal would by its nature seriously challenge the status quo, causing political turmoil in the process, the 1979 House adopted the policy. It gave all concerned 11 years to implement the changes, which it hoped would be in place no later than the end of 1990.

Recognizing that standards of education were meaningful only if educational institutions were held to them through an on-site accrediting process, APTA also took on the difficult issue of accreditation in these years. The collaborative arrangement for accreditation of physical therapy education programs that had been worked out between the AMA's Council on Medical Education (originally the sole accrediting agency) and APTA in 1959 had not proved altogether satisfactory. Michels recalls that members "became disenchanted when they found that APTA was doing practically all the work and making the decisions, and the CME was rubber-stamping the results."

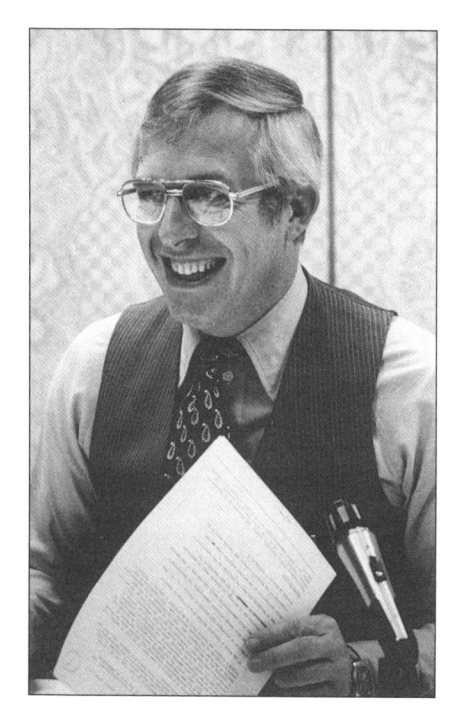

The CME was also dragging its heels on the matter of changing certain features of the basic accreditation standards that APTA felt were needed to keep the profession current. Sarah Rogers, APTA's long-time Education Consultant, was one of the prime movers in persuading the membership of its responsibility for — and long-term interest in — bringing the process out from under the domination of the medical profession. Finally, in 1976, APTA unilaterally adopted a revised set of "Essentials of an Acceptable School of Physical Therapy" and referred them to the CME for adoption as a joint venture.

When the CME failed to do so promptly, APTA announced its decision to terminate its collaborative association and to seek independent recognition as an accrediting agency of physical therapy schools. Against strong opposition by the AMA, the American Hospital Association, the American Society of Allied Health Professionals, and the Association for Academic Health Centers, the APTA leadership forged bravely ahead. Thanks to an unprecedented effort on the part of the national office and the Association's volunteer committees, in both the academic and clinical arenas, APTA was able to present convincing testimony as to its fitness as an accrediting agency. After lengthy review, the Council on Postsecondary Accreditation (COPA) granted recognition in April 1977. Four months later, the U.S. Commissioner of Education followed suit. The AMA stood its ground, however, for six more years, continuing to offer accreditation to those institutions that sought it. Then in 1983 it withdrew, leaving APTA as the sole accrediting agency in the U.S. for physical therapy education programs.

### The Many Faces Of Membership

Another issue that APTA began to address in this decade was minority participation. Other than the NFIP-sponsored effort to recruit African-Americans to work in the polio emergency, little in the way of active encouragement had been offered to young minority candidates in regard to entering the profession. Their numbers, although not officially recorded in these years, are presumed to have been small, but a cadre calling itself the Coalition for Health Advocacy and Recruiting of Minorities (CHARM) formed in the mid-1960s to see what could be done to change the situation. They gained the attention of APTA's Board, which in 1971 charged the Department of Educational Affairs with developing cooperative programs with interested physical therapy schools to provide appropriate recruiting materials. The Board also established an annual institutional award of $500 to be given to schools actively recruiting minority students. *Physical Therapy* took up the matter in a written colloquy that same year, and contributors came out strongly for affirmative action at every level. All of this set the stage for the Association addressing affirmative action and minority affairs in the 1980s.

Another sign of professional maturation within APTA was the establishment of a succession of Association awards, which began in 1963 and now number some 17 tributes all told. (Student scholarships given out to promising candidates with monies earmarked by McMillan in her will also began in 1963.) The earliest and still the most prestigious prize is the Mary McMillan Lecture Award, which was established in 1962 by the Board of Directors in memory of the Association's beloved first president and physical therapy trailblazer. Its stated purpose is to acknowledge and honor a member of the Association who has made a distinguished contribution to the profession in administration, education, patient care, or research. The award carries an honorarium, and the recipient is expected to prepare and deliver an address at the Annual Conference. With the exception of the years 1970, 1974, 1988, 1994, and 1995 (years which coincided with the World Congress and other special circumstances), the award has been conferred annually since Mildred Elson became the first lecturer in 1964.

The Marian Williams Award for Research in Physical Therapy was established in 1963 to commemorate the work of Marian Williams of Stanford

University. Williams's professional life combined superb teaching skills and extensive writing with research in the areas of kinesiology, electromyography, and muscle testing. Signe Brunnström was the first recipient, receiving the bronze medal in 1965.

The Golden Pen Award, for outstanding contributions to *Physical Therapy*, was first given in 1964. Jacquelin Perry, a physical therapist and orthopedic surgeon, and Ronald Lamont-Havers were the first recipients. Lamont-Havers was an infrequent contributor, but Perry went on to produce some 45 well-conceived contributions during her career, including the landmark article "The Contribution of the Physical Therapist to Medicine," published in the journal's November 1965 issue.

The Lucy Blair Service Award, established in 1969 to honor the long and dedicated service of Lucy Blair, is given to one or more members each year for contributions of exceptional value to the Association. Blair was the first recipient in 1969, and service pins were awarded to 20 members in 1971, the first year in which the award was truly activated.

The Dorothy Briggs Memorial Scientific Inquiry Award was created in 1969 to commemorate the work of Briggs, a physical therapist and active member on many national Association committees, as well as an outstanding educator and an active investigator at the University of Wisconsin. The award recognizes student members who have demonstrated the ability to develop well-conceived, suitably designed, and clearly expressed experimental investigations suitable for publication in *Physical Therapy*. The first recipient was Major Mary Elizabeth Lucas, a master's degree candidate at Stanford University, whose article on "Perceptual Disorders of Adults with Hemiparesis" appeared in the October 1969 issue of the journal.

The Jack Walker Award was established in 1978 with funds donated by the Chattanooga Corporation of Chattanooga, Tennessee, to honor the former president of one of the leading manufacturers of physical therapy equipment. The award recognizes work published in the Association's journal that makes a significant contribution to clinical practice or research. The first recipient was Mary Baker of Atlanta's Emory University Regional Rehabilitation and Training Center, for primary authorship of "Developing Strategies for Biofeedback: Applications in Neurologically Handicapped Patients," published in the April 1977 issue of *Physical Therapy*.

New in 1974 was the Award of Excellence for Minority Recruitment and Services, which carried a monetary award of $500 as well as a citation plaque. The inaugural award went to the Department of Physical Therapy, Georgia State University, Atlanta, whose efforts on behalf of minority recruitment were led by faculty member Lynda Woodruff.

### BUILDING A FIRM FOUNDATION

The Foundation for Physical Therapy, which emerged in 1979 from the 22-year-old Physical Therapy Fund, and was actually a joint effort involving many hands, provides an excellent example of the growing professionalization of the organization and its supporting structures in these years. The organization's new beginnings are directly traceable to Charles Magistro, who by his own description conceived the plan while flying to a PT Fund board meeting in 1977 shortly after stepping down as APTA president. The PT Fund, which in its first two decades had managed to disburse less than $80,000 in grant funds, had never been well-supported by the membership. If the year 1964 is any guide, contributions were coming in at a rate of seven cents per member.

The PT Fund's diligent board worked constantly to keep it from the brink of financial collapse. Periodic rescue efforts, however, had proved to be temporary solutions at best, said Magistro, "like going out in the rain with an umbrella: you don't get too wet, but it's still raining."

Magistro, who recognized that "our failure to scientifically document the efficacy of services could pose a serious threat to our profession in the years ahead," conceived of a broader-based, wholly independent, tax-exempt foundation that would attract substantial funding from external sources. To be effective, he foresaw that it would need its own executive director, trustees, staff, and budget. With the help of Noland, who was also secretary-treasurer of the PT Fund; Robert Hickok, a PT Fund board member; and others, the details of the reconstituted foundation were fleshed out. The House of Delegates gave its enthusiastic go-ahead in 1979.

To provide the Foundation for Physical Therapy with operating capital until it could become self-sustaining, a period anticipated at three years, the HOD levied a special, one-time $15 assessment of each active member. Despite the eloquent words of leaders like Helen Hislop, who declared that each member had "an immense moral obligation" to support physical therapy research, the levy met with substantial resistance from a minority of members, some of whom resigned from the organization rather than pay. But in the end, the Foundation launched with roughly $350,000 in seed money. The Foundation's nine-member board of trustees was elected by APTA chapter presidents representing the entire membership at that year's Annual Conference in Atlanta. The trustees in turn chose Magistro as first chairman and later hired Dan Ruskin as the Foundation's first director.

The new organization got off to an impressive start, granting more in scholarship and research aid within its first year than had been given away by the PT Fund in all the previous years combined.

It was, by any measure, a promising omen for the eighties — and beyond.

CHAPTER 7

# The Diamond Jubilee Years
## 1980 – 1996

*Don Wortley, a private practitioner in Salt Lake City, Utah, served as president of the Association from 1979 to 1982. Under Wortley's leadership, APTA prepared to meet a new era of health care regulations and practices.*

In the last two decades, health care in the United States has changed at a rate that has astonished even the most imaginative prognosticators. Among the dominant forces in those changes have been quantum advances in health sciences and technology, increasing efforts to control health care costs, and the shift of patient care from hospital inpatient settings to ambulatory clinics and home care. The patient profile has also changed dramatically. Due to better health care and altered social attitudes, patients with increasingly complex problems, such as the sick elderly with multiple system involvement, those with chronic neurological diseases, and persons with severe impairments due to trauma and substance abuse, are all receiving the benefits of physical therapy care.

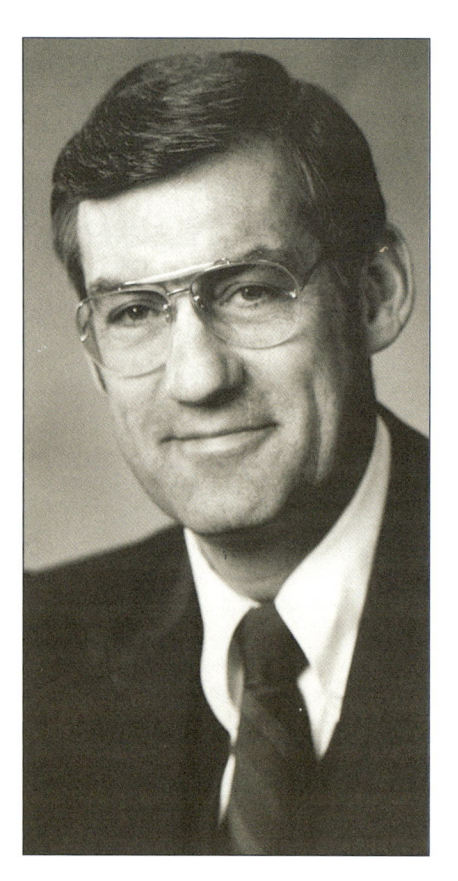

To keep pace with these changes, APTA and the profession of physical therapy have gone through unprecedented development and self-analysis in recent years. Through it all, the values and goals of the founders — to enhance human movement and function and thereby positively affect the quality of life of each patient — remain very much at the core of the profession and in the hearts and minds of its practitioners.

### KEEPING FIT AT THE ORGANIZATIONAL LEVEL

In his final presidential address Don Wortley, APTA president from 1979 to 1982, said that the Association reminded him of Alice in Wonderland. It often seemed more intent on moving ahead than on figuring out where it wanted to go. Whether it was business before the Board or the staff, all too often problems were addressed in isolation and only when solutions were needed immediately. Under such

216  *Healing The Generations*

circumstances, little was done to measure the long-range economic consequences of policies or to review interim results and make midcourse corrections.

In 1979, with Royce Noland's guidance, the Board committed itself to beginning the process of implementing strategic planning in its classic sense. Thenceforth, the Board, with the support of the House of Delegates, the ultimate policy-making body, was to set long-range objectives for the Association with budgets, task forces, and staff personnel to carry them out. In this way, the Board could allocate the finite resources of the organization over time with reasonable assurance that it would have the money to carry them out as intended. Wortley, summing up his three years in office in 1982, called the introduction of strategic planning the "crowning achievement" of his presidency. Eugene Michels concurs: "Having been on the Board before strategic planning was introduced and on staff after its implementation, it was clear to me that we had finally found the secret to success. Now we had a means to plan and budget whatever programs were needed to carry us forward, and that made the organization far more powerful and effective in virtually every one of our endeavors."

Among the first fruits of strategic planning was the reorganization of the Association into three divisions — Administration, Professional Relations, and Research and Education — each with its own associate executive director and programs. At the same time, the various panels of the Board of Directors were reconfigured and renamed to correspond with these functions. (A new office — Minority Affairs — was subsequently added to Administration under this table of organization, with Brenda Dowtin as its first coordinator.)

Strategic planning was given a further tweak in 1988, when the House of Delegates charged the Board to refine its priorities by setting a number of formal goals and objectives each year and presenting them for a vote by the membership. As former Governance Office director Margot Daffron recalls, the Board groaned collectively at taking on this added task. But they changed their attitudes later that fall as Executive Committee members and executive staff began the process during an unforgettable weekend retreat at Executive Committee member Marilyn Moffat's Long Island home.

"We were all in New York City to attend the East Coast dinner for the Friends of the Foundation for Physical Therapy," Daffron relates. "The 'goals' thing was very much on our minds, time was running out, and Marilyn suggested that since we were all in town anyway, we steal some time away to brainstorm at her house where there would be no distractions. Late that evening eight or nine of us, part Board, part staff, piled into two cars and drove out to Locust Valley in a downpour. To no one's surprise, Marilyn led us on a high-speed chase along wind-

*APTA's Department of Minority/International Affairs maintains a directory of minority members with 20 or more years of experience. Each year a list, published in booklet form as shown, is updated to reflect the growth of this group within the Association. As of 1995, the list had grown to 122.*

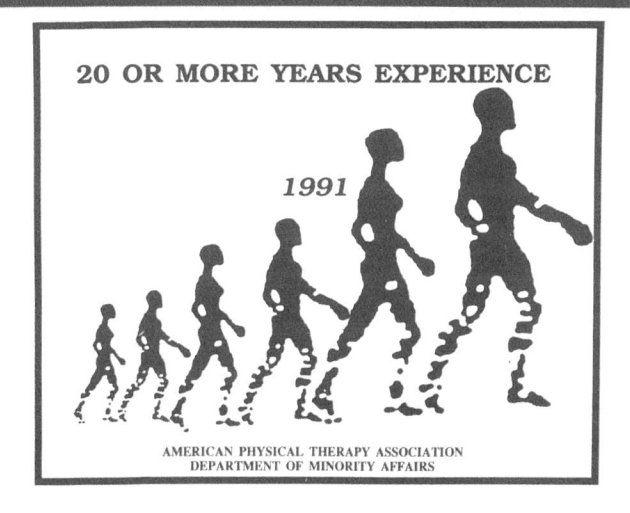

ing, slippery roads through the darkness. The rest of us, half-terrified, did our best to follow!" Daffron says that after a good night's sleep the group settled in for nearly two days of intensive discussion, finally hammering out eight goals. The list then went to the full Board in March and to the House of Delegates in June 1989, where it was enthusiastically adopted.

Working through the process, almost everyone agreed, had proved to be far more valuable than anticipated in that it mapped the road that a consensus of APTA members wanted to travel. Since 1988, the setting of goals and objectives has become an annual part of Association business, though accomplished with considerably less drama. The goals, which were seven in number for 1995, consistently speak to the areas of practice, education, research, and public awareness. Each goal is intended to have an outreach of three to five years when first implemented, although modifications in wording are often made in subsequent years. Each goal is accompanied by a series of specific objectives by which progress can be measured.

## PUTTING THE HOUSE IN ORDER

Continued growth of the membership and chapters made it advisable in 1980 to amend the Bylaws to set some limits on the size of the House of Delegates, APTA's principal policy-making body since 1944. The number of chapter delegates was fixed at 400, although by a complex apportionment formula designed to assure representation for affiliate members as well, the actual number of delegates brings the total somewhat higher. (In 1994, under 1992 modifications in the formula, 438 individuals were recognized as voting delegates.)

Another piece of House of Delegates fine-tuning implemented in the eighties was the rescheduling of the annual House session. In its early history, House sessions coincided with the Annual Conference in June. Thus delegates and interested observers were forced to miss much of the educational programming. Beginning in 1980 the session was advanced so that all legislative activities could be carried out between Friday and Sunday; by 1985, the session was scheduled between Saturday afternoon and Monday midday, leaving delegates free to join the conference thereafter.

The House is managed from the dais by three officers, each of whom holds office for a term of three years: the Speaker of the House presides over the meeting and guides debate; the Vice Speaker, who also oversees elections and registration, acts as timekeeper during floor debates and functions as the Speaker when she or he is absent; and the Secretary records the minutes. An appointed parliamentarian sees to it that *Robert's Rules of Order* are strictly enforced. In addition to the officers and the voting delegates, there are many other non-voting individuals who participate in floor discussions and caucuses, acting, in effect, as consultants; these include APTA Board members, section delegates, representatives from the Affiliate and Student Assemblies, designated APTA staff members, and members of a host of appointed committees and task forces. All participants are seated at predetermined locations within the hall according to their affiliation.

Most motions proceed according to a standard pattern. Initiated variously by a chapter, a section, one of the assemblies, an individual member, or the Board of Directors, they are first submitted to the House Reference Committee many months in advance of the June session. Each motion is reviewed in committee for clarity and wording, assigned a Reference Committee or "RC" number, and given a position on the official agenda, according to content. (Amendments to the Bylaws go to the top of the agenda, followed by amendments to the standing rules, with main motions coming after.) A packet containing all issues on the agenda — as many as 40 to 50 per year — along with information on candidates running for election and the annual HOD Handbook, is then prepared and sent to the delegates for review some two months in advance of the meeting. Delegates then take the motions to their component groups to solicit feedback so that when they attend the actual House session, they are prepared to act on behalf of the people they represent.

The conduct of the House was enhanced significantly in the late 1980s with the introduction of computer technology to the House floor, due in large part to the efforts of Board member Jane Walter. Computerized scanning simplified the balloting process, and floor debate on motions was streamlined as proposed revisions were projected onto two very large screens on either side of the dais. (Since 1989, with Dorothy Pinkston the initial coordinator, the proceedings have also been broadcast on closed-circuit television to the "Gallery Extension," an informal observation room off the House floor. Members of APTA's Prime Timers group act as hosts and interpreters in the gallery, providing anyone interested in becoming a future delegate an excellent opportunity to learn how the House operates.)

The assemblies within the House of Delegates are a relatively recent development that came about as a means of allowing physical therapist assistant members a structure through which they could meet their unique needs. In 1983 several "affiliate members," including Virginia May, Cheryl Carpenter, and Tricia Garrison, petitioned the House for recognition as a non-voting component, hoping to gain the chance to participate in debates in the same way that sections were recognized. When section status for affiliate members proved incompatible with the Association's Bylaws, the Affiliate Special Interest Group was developed. Over the next few years, the ASIG grew in size and volubility but still lacked a formal mechanism for representation within the House.

In 1989, as one result of a House-mandated study of the Association's organizational structure, the Bylaws were amended to allow the creation of "assemblies" as a third type of component. At the same time, the House approved the formation of the Affiliate Assembly, composed entirely of PTA members. The amendment is regarded by PTAs as a turning point in their history: it gave them a formal way to come together and discuss issues that directly concern them — which they now do three times a year at Annual Conference and at open Affiliate Assembly board meetings in spring and fall.

In 1992 the delegates voted to allow PTAs to hold office at the chapter and section levels. Cheryl Carpenter,

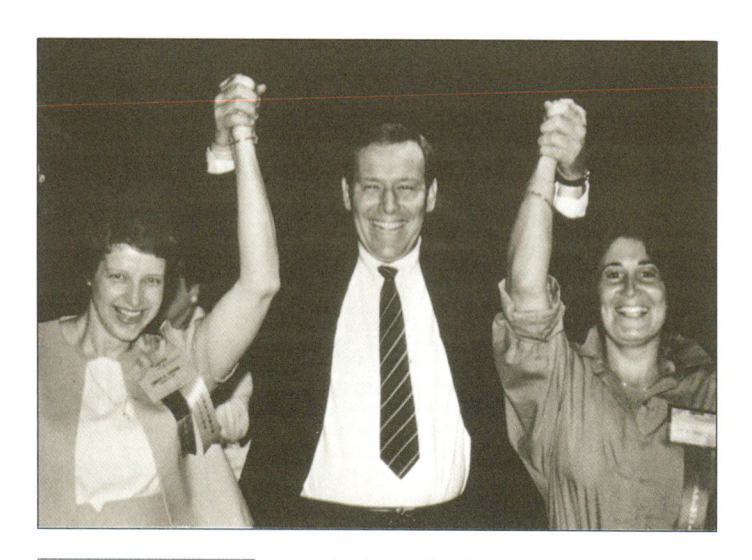

*Following specialty certification, recipients are awarded certificates of advanced clinical competency. The first three recipients are pictured above. Left to right, Linda Crane, Scot Irwin, and Meryl Cohen celebrate at the recognition ceremony, now an annual event during the Combined Sections Meeting.*

who is credited by many as the spearhead of this 20-year-long drive for recognition, became the first chair of the Affiliate Assembly. With the success of the Affiliate Assembly established, the Student Assembly was formed in 1991. Each assembly is allowed two delegates in the House who may speak and make motions on behalf of their component but may not vote.

### Growth Of The Sections And Specialties

The rapid expansion of the physical therapy profession into areas of specialization continued to express itself in the eighties as special interest sections and their subsidiary special interest groups, or SIGs, proliferated. As in the past, the formal recognition of each section raised concerns among many members that the Association itself might become dangerously fragmented. But there was no arguing that APTA could not, on its own, meet all the specialized needs and interests of its membership, and by the mid-1990s the House of Delegates had sanctioned 19 sections, each with its own internal structure, programs, and publications. Further evidence of the viability of sections: some 66 percent of members (more than 40,000) were active in one or more of them.

Recent additions include the Veterans Affairs Section, 1980 (Margaret Lambert, first chair); the Section on Hand Rehabilitation, 1982 (Henry Boutros, first chair); the Oncology Section, 1983 (Jeri Walton, first chair); Acute Care/Hospital Clinical Practice Section, 1992 (Marcia Pearl and Jim Dunleavy, co-chairs); and Aquatic Physical Therapy, also 1992 (Judy Cirullo, chair). Other sections of earlier vintage changed their focus sufficiently to merit name changes. Community Health thus became Community Home Health in recognition of the growing importance of physical therapy care for the homebound; State Licensure and Regulation became Health Policy, Legislation and Regulation; and Obstetrics and Gynecology became the more inclusive Section on Women's Health.

With each addition, the importance and vitality of the Combined Sections Meeting has grown apace, and the annual four-day gathering each February now draws nearly 3,000 participants. So, too, APTA has gained additional resource bases of experts from whom it can draw guidance on particular issues and activities. One group that was proposed for section status, though tongue-in-cheek, comprised life members and other retired members of APTA; in 1982 Fred Rutan made the suggestion that these seniors form the "Honorary Section." Inez Peacock revived the idea five years later when she led the successful drive to create the "Prime Timers." This unique group within APTA, which dates from 1987, is an informal "club" of retirees and life members who meet periodically as friends while providing the benefits of their experience to the organization. Among their many contributions have been efforts to preserve the Association's history.

A natural outgrowth of the sections has been the continued growth of the specialist certification process. The complex process of creating the appropriate mechanism for voluntary certification, which began in the mid-seventies, began to bear fruit in 1985, when the first three candidates achieved specialist certification in cardiopulmonary physical therapy. Added in subsequent years were the Clinical Electrophysiologic and Pediatric Specialty areas in 1986; Neurologic and Sports Physical Therapy, in 1987; Orthopaedic, in 1989; and Geriatric, in 1992. Altogether more than a thousand candidates have achieved certification in the decade since the system was introduced. Of these, more than a third have sought and earned the OCS (Orthopaedic Certified Specialist) designation. Still other special interest groups, among them Women's Health, Oncology, and a group seeking advanced certification for General Physical Therapy, are currently investigating the feasibility of advanced specialist certification. In an effort to make the examination procedure more accessible to busy practitioners all over the country, the American Board of Physical Therapy Specialties (ABPTS) instituted electronic testing in 1994 and offered it at nearly 100 regional test sites rather than at the centralized CSM meeting site. Incidentally, the numbers of candidates applying rose 51 percent from 1993 to 1994.

### Home, Sweet Home

When the time came to assess the Association's future housing needs, the strategic planning process provided the Board with the necessary tools. There was no disputing that moving headquarters to Washington in 1970 had been a good decision, but the office lease in the District of Columbia was to end in 1985. Rents were sure to rise steeply with renewal and, in any case, the existing space would soon be inadequate. With membership approaching 30,000 and continued growth virtually guaranteed, the Board thought the Association could prudently purchase its own office building. The search began in earnest in 1982 under new APTA President Robert Richardson. (Richardson would serve from 1982 to 1985. A specialist in the treatment of arthritis, he had served as president of the Pennsylvania Chapter, was coordinator of rehabilitation services at St. Margaret Memorial Hospital in Pittsburgh, Pennsylvania, and had been a long-time participant in national Association business.)

After looking at some 60 prospects, the Board finally focused on Building #4 within the newly constructed TransPotomac Plaza complex. Rising on the west bank of the Potomac, the 1111 North Fairfax Street address in Alexandria, Virginia's Old Town was just a short drive to Capitol Hill, even closer to National Airport, and convenient to a host of health care agencies and associations with which APTA has frequent contacts.

Frank Mallon, who had joined the staff as legal counsel and associate executive director for professional relations in the wake of the 1981 restructuring, recalls that Royce Noland once again proved his remarkable range of talents in overseeing the move. "Not only did he handle most of the real estate search," Mallon comments, "but

*Robert Richardson, director of physical therapy and rehabilitation services at St. Margaret Memorial Hospital, Pittsburgh, and a specialist in the treatment of arthritis, succeeded Wortley as president in 1982.*

he orchestrated space allocations. Deciding which staffers got which windows and how much square footage, while taking into account everyone's relative status and seniority, was no easy matter. It took a real planner and politician, and he did a masterful job."

On a Saturday in May 1983, the seven-mile move was accomplished with relatively few hitches. By the following Monday, some 65 staffers were at their new posts, albeit many of them sitting on the floor or perched on boxes as they awaited the sorting out of desks and chairs and telephone extensions. Before a couple of days had passed, everything was up and running — with virtually no interruption in any department's services.

Strategic planning was once again the agent of change when the Association weighed the notion of purchasing a second building. The staff had initially occupied only the second and third floors of the four-story building in the TransPotomac complex, renting out the rest, but by 1990 almost all available space had been taken over by the Association, and there was a reasonable prospect that more would be needed in a few years. After a careful study of options, the Board decided that with the real estate market and interest rates at an all-time low, it was time to purchase adjoining Building #3, which was formally dedicated in November 1992 with Marilyn Moffat, a strong advocate of the purchase, presiding.

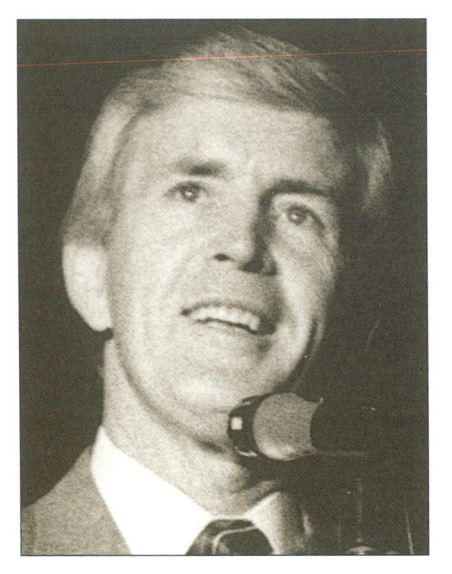

APTA currently has some 145 staffers on site and occupies all of 1111 North Fairfax and about a third of its neighbor, with room to grow as needed. One beneficiary of the expanded space has been the Association's archives. Little more than a basement room supported by a handful of members and staff in 1981 when first started, the collecting and organizing of early documents, photos, memorabilia, textbooks, and recordings has gradually grown in seriousness and professionalism over the years. Today, the archives are a budgeted item, with a director, a program, a library, and a room open to the public. An activity of ongoing urgency to the archives is the recording of oral histories. Created through audio- and videotaped interviews, they focus on selected physical therapists whose long and noteworthy careers contain the seeds of the profession's history. Among the more than 40 interviews collected to date are those of Leon Anderson, Helen Blood, Lucille Daniels, Mildred Elson, Adelaide McGarrett, Margaret Rood, Rosemary Scully, Sarah Semans, Fran Tappan, and Elizabeth Wood.

### HEALTH CARE FINANCING

During the late seventies, the Carter administration had launched a federal legislative effort to contain spiraling payouts in the Medicare system by curbing the percentage of annual increases. The attempt ultimately failed, and by 1982 there were dire predictions that Medicare would soon go bankrupt. Congress, in its frustration, sought draconian measures through an amendment to Title XVIII (Medicare) of the Social Security Act of 1965. This amendment, which called for a fundamental restructuring of the method by which hospital inpatient services for Medicare beneficiaries were financed, was put on the legislative fast track. After only four months, it arrived for signature on President Ronald Reagan's desk just before the Easter 1983 recess.

Extremely complex in its details, HR 1900-PL 98-21 was scarcely understood by anyone, including those who voted for it, according to APTA's Frank Mallon, and its premises were barely tested in a one-year pilot project in the state of New Jersey. The legislation turned upside down the mechanism for paying hospitals under Medicare. Instead of reimbursing actual (or retrospective) costs on the traditional fee-for-service, free-market basis, a prospective payment system was established in which diagnosis-related groups (DRGs) were introduced. Under the DRG system, each hospitalized patient was classified into one of 467 diagnosis-related categories. A rate based upon past audits of similar cases was set, and hospitals were then reimbursed according to the diagnosis category. If the costs of a patient's care exceeded the fixed rate, it was the hospital rather than the third-party payer that had to absorb the shortfall. If the hospital's costs were less than the cap-

*On the occasion of APTA's purchase of Building #3, William Coughlan, APTA executive director, shakes on the deal with Wout Couster, representing the property's seller. To mark the occasion, Couster brought a "housewarming gift," a lovely porcelain vase, now a permanent fixture in APTA's offices.*

*APTA's headquarters at 1111 North Fairfax Street, Alexandria, Virginia, provide offices for some 145 employees, along with the recently improved archives, which have taken on increasing importance as the Association nears its 75th anniversary. APTA moved into the first of its two Trans-Potomac Plaza buildings (middle building in the photo) in 1983. By 1990, more space was needed for staff and programs, and the Association expanded into the adjacent building (far right).*

itated rate, on the other hand, the hospital pocketed the surplus. In theory, the system created incentives to manage inpatient care with maximum efficiency. In actual practice, however, this kind of cost containment frequently tended to reward poor service and to move the Medicare patient out of the hospital and into a lower, less-intensive level of treatment as soon as possible, which was sometimes sooner than it should have been.

APTA did not oppose the legislation on reimbursement in a broad sense because fee schedules for physical therapists were so embedded in the system as to be virtually impossible to isolate. However, Association members and staffers, along with outside counsel George Olsen, of Williams and Jensen, did become involved in gaining exempt status for rehabilitation hospitals and separate rehabilitation departments within acute care hospitals. "The basis of our argument," Mallon remembers, "was that there were no reliable data to support the development of a prospective payment system for rehabilitative care. The variability of conditions, services, and patient progress was too great to allow development of a pre-set payment cap." Mallon adds appreciatively, "Our advocate on this critical exemption was Massachusetts Representative James M. Shannon, who served on the House Ways and Means Committee, which had — and still has — jurisdiction over the entire Medicare program. Following its enactment, the exemption was periodically considered for repeal, but studies commissioned by Congress to determine a basis for a prospective system failed to produce results that could justify such action. The rehabilitation community owes a big 'Thanks!' to Jim Shannon."

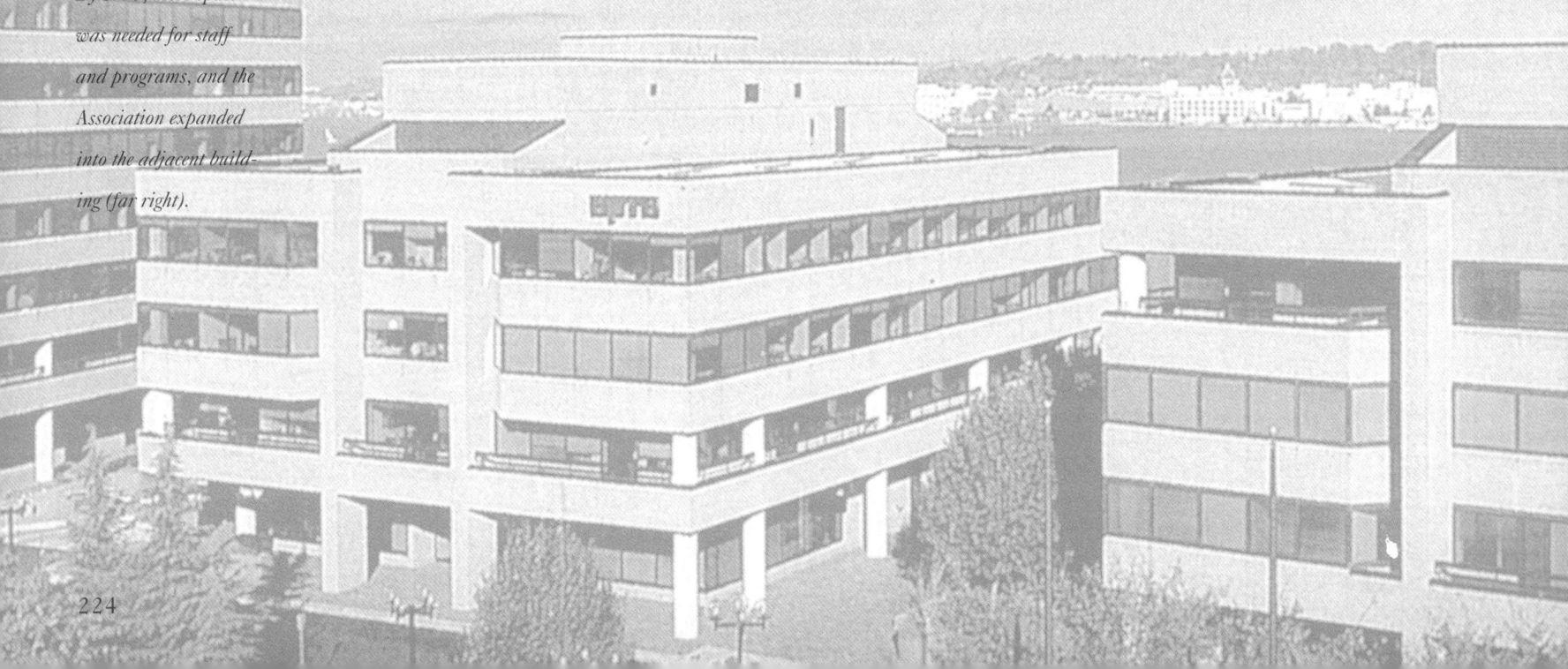

As the new DRG-based system represented a major shift in payment methods, hospitals were given three years to implement it fully. The effects became apparent almost from the start: hospital admissions of older patients, which had been rising steadily for years, declined slightly, and the average length of hospital stays was reduced sharply. At the same time, physical therapy referrals of both hospitalized Medicare patients and outpatients increased significantly, a good indicator that physicians and hospital administrators recognized physical therapy as an effective, efficient means of rehabilitating patients within Medicare's new time and cost constraints.

From the practitioner's point of view, however, increased use of physical therapy services for Medicare patients was not a simple solution. All too often, patients were leaving their hospital beds "quicker and sicker," only to return for readmission when problems recurred, as many had predicted. Teaching hospitals also found their patient profiles changing; a far larger percentage of clients had acute illnesses, which worked to limit students' exposure to the kind of diverse acute and short-term rehabilitation cases that clinical instruction is supposed to provide.

The changes brought by prospective payment reforms also raised new questions concerning the process by which the decisions to treat or not to treat patients were to be made. What role would physical therapists have in assessing treatment need? Assuming they should be intimately involved, were they sufficiently prepared to participate in the fiscal and management processes? Upon what evidence could they assert the cost effectiveness of one therapy over other alternatives? Aside from cost, were there other advantages/disadvantages to the creation of a whole new array of ambulatory health care centers to treat these patient groups, and would not some form of prospective payment control soon be demanded by all third-party payers in the private insurance sector as well? Lastly, what new ethical questions might be introduced to physical therapy education, research, and practice by all these changes in the health care environment?

As the rest of this chapter will relate, these and many other conundrums continue to engage the Association and its membership.

### THE FOUNDATION SETS ITS COURSE

The newly constituted Foundation for Physical Therapy entered the eighties with high ambitions and a much-improved financial base from which to act. Charles Magistro had since been succeeded as chair in turn by Bob Bartlett, Jim McKillip, and Marilyn Gossman; more recent CEOs were Steve Seater and Fred de Gregorio.

As a result of stepped-up fund-raising efforts, the Foundation was able to institute several categories of grants and to disburse aid at levels previously unimaginable. Initiated in the very first year was the General Research Grant, which was designed to fund original research by emerging investigators. From its beginnings, the General Grant has grown to offer a maximum of $30,000 annually for two years; in 1994, the Foundation awarded 12 such grants. Among the many outstanding figures in physical therapy research who were thus supported in the early phases of their careers are Stuart Binder-Macleod, Suzann Campbell, Rebecca Craik, Chukuka Enwemeka, Michael Emery, Stephen Haley, Fay Horak,

*Linnea Yurick, a physical therapist in the premature ward of Cleveland Metropolitan General Hospital, treats her tiny patient with a mix of movement and play. The photo originally appeared in the 1986 APTA calendar.*

Mary Moffroid, Michael Mueller, Mark Rogers, John Scholz, Richard Shields, and Anne Shumway-Cook.

Added in the second year of the Foundation's existence were the Doctoral Research Awards. These were made possible through the generous bequest of Phoebe Romberger, a physical therapist and lifelong member of APTA. Romberger had received her B.S. at Purdue in 1935 and took her physical therapist training under Jessie Wright at the D. T. Watson School in Pennsylvania, graduating in 1940. Romberger went on to establish and direct the physical therapy department of Woodstock Memorial Hospital in northern Illinois. An avid outdoorswoman and breeder of English bull terriers, she is remembered for her indomitable spirit and joie de vivre. Forced to retire in 1975 on account of a series of small strokes, she moved to Florida. The 67-year-old Romberger suffered her last and fatal incident in 1979 while jogging near her home. In her will, she designated that her entire estate, nearly $160,000, be given to advance research in physical therapy, and this generous sum was used to establish the Foundation's Phoebe Romberger Fund. Additional bequests from other donors have since extended the reach of the program, which assists doctoral candidates in furthering their research investigations. The committee that oversees this award had, by the mid-1990s, disbursed more than $1 million to assist more than 200 doctoral candidates and their research in progress. Janet Gwyer, Leonie Nelson, Tom Seether, and John Scholz were first-year recipients. The following year found Jules Rothstein among the grantees. He received $3,000 in 1981, while a Ph.D. candidate at New York University, to complete his study "Muscle Defects Associated with Long Term Steroid Therapy." Twenty-five doctoral students received funding in 1994.

Additionally, the Foundation has offered since 1988 a number of undergraduate scholarships. Among the groups especially targeted for this assistance are outstanding minority students (Minority Scholarship) and students with a special commitment to a career in clinical rehabilitation (Campanella Scholarship Fund).

The Clinical Research Center Grant is a more recent program created to fulfill a Foundation aim of establishing independent, interdisciplinary clinical research centers under the direction of physical therapists. The overarching goal of such research centers is to isolate the actual effects of physical therapy interventions as a component of the multidisciplinary rehabilitation process. The first such grant — $600,000 over three years — was awarded to The University of Iowa in December 1990. The university's award-winning proposal focused on developing the processes and methodologies necessary to research and produce scientifically valid outcomes using both theoretical research cores and specific clinical projects involving physical therapists, neurologists, orthopedists, cardiologists, and administrators.

As the Foundation approached its 15th anniversary, it initiated a series of consensus conferences intended to identify specific areas in which additional research was urgently needed. The first such conference, whose costs were underwritten by a special $50,000 grant from APTA, was held in late August 1993 and focused on work-related injuries. A consensus conference modeled on this first highly productive experience followed on geriatric disabilities (1994), and more are scheduled on sports-related injuries and rehabilitation from catastrophic injuries.

The original member assessment, along with contributions from individual physical therapists, corporate benefactors, and other private-sector

*Outpatient physical therapy has grown into a $6 billion-a-year business. Physical therapist and APTA member William Lee Day works with a patient at Professional Sports Care, a firm that provides amateur and weekend athletes with the same level of physical therapy that million-dollar players from professional sports teams receive.*

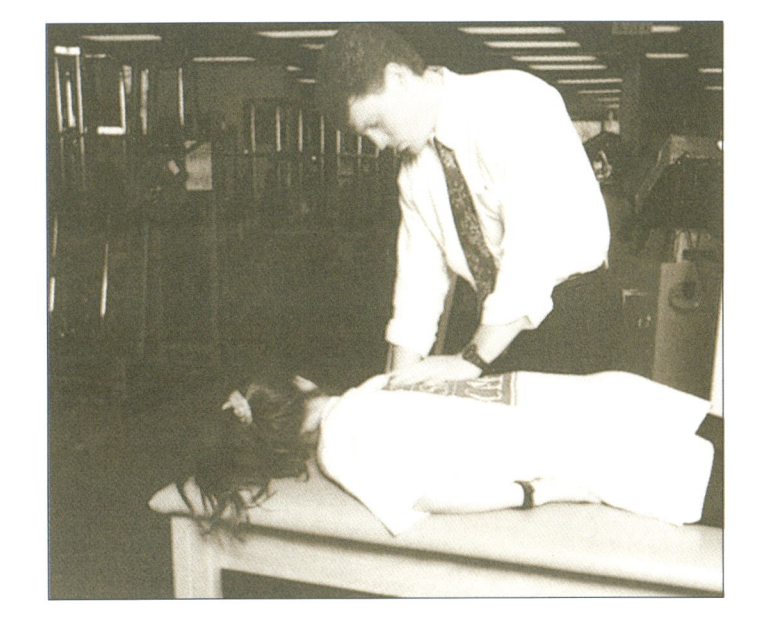

*Beth Little, a physical therapist at the Charlotte Rehabilitation Center, North Carolina, is shown here in the early 1980s using tennis strokes to instruct a patient with an amputation in balance and weight-shift skills. For children and adults alike, therapy is made more interesting and understandable when it takes the form of a familiar game, exercise, or sport.*

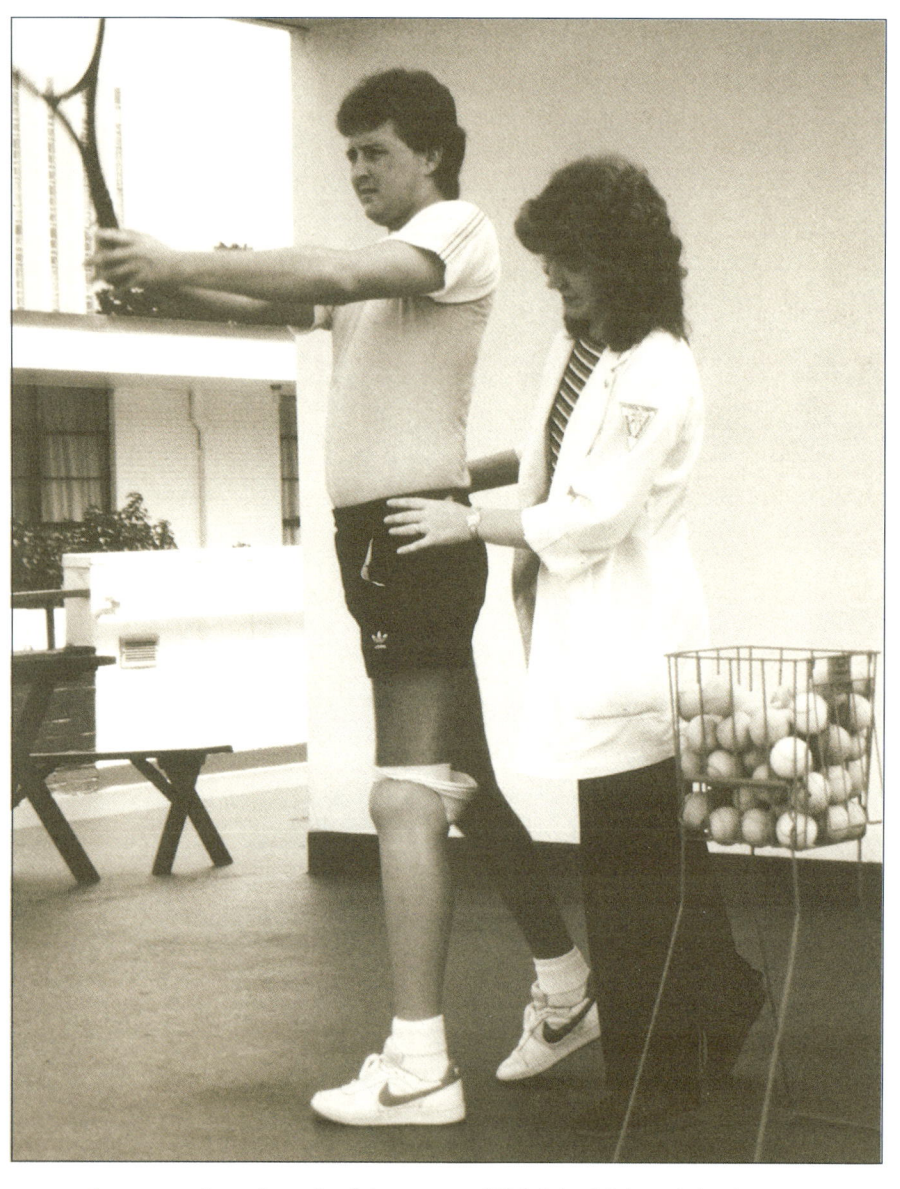

sources have constituted much of the Foundation's funding. An outstanding case in point is the Clinical Research Center Grant, the funding for which was initially established when CEO John Maley of the Chattanooga Group, Inc., threw out the "Chattanooga Challenge" to the APTA membership with an offer to match all contributions. Since its inception, the Foundation has managed to raise and disburse more than $4 million, the long-term effects of which are already showing up in the clinical setting.

### THE RESEARCH AGENDA

The Foundation has always had a legal and financial reason to operate separate from APTA by dint of its tax-free status, but because it shares the same general goals and interests with regard to research as the Association, the two groups have generally been supportive of each other. Coincidentally, the Association's "Plan to Foster Clinical Research," initiated through the work of the Committee on Research (now the Advisory Panel on Research), began to bear fruit at about the same time that the Foundation received its initial seed money.

In addition to an exponential increase in research paper abstracts, other benefits flowed from implementing the Association's "Plan to Foster Clinical Research": goals and objectives for the development of theory in physical therapy, the presentation of theory papers at Annual Conference, open forums on research topics each year at

Annual Conference, guidelines on ethical and scientific integrity in physical therapy research, manuals on clinical research design and data analysis (including design of surveys), the Association's "Standards for Tests and Measurements in Physical Therapy Practice" (developed by a task force headed by Jules Rothstein) and the *Primer on Measurement: An Introductory Guide to Measurement Issues*, authored by Jules Rothstein and John Echternach and published by APTA in 1993.

In 1992 the House of Delegates voted to further enhance the Association's research efforts through creation of a Resource Center for Research and Learning. Described as a series of services rather than a place, the Center is intended to integrate and strengthen selected information programs within APTA that are related to research and professional development. Among the services anticipated are state-of-the-art data bases on physical therapy research, practice, administration, and related health care issues; interactive self-assessment and instructional programs; and updated guides to designing and presenting research projects.

## THE WORLD TURNS

By the mid-eighties, APTA seemed to be settling into a fairly comfortable routine of growth and professional development at the state and national levels. In 1985 Jane Mathews of Massachusetts succeeded Robert Richardson and began her two-term presidency. (Mathews was the former director of graduate studies of the Department of Physical Therapy at Duke University, with a doctorate in the area of health services and human resource development. At the time of her election, she was chairperson of physical therapy at Sargent College, Boston University.)

Shortly after Mathews took office, Royce Noland ended his 17-year tenure as executive director of the Association. It had been, by Mathews' description, an extraordinary run, a career "of exceptional service" to the profession. During Noland's years as CEO, the membership had tripled and the annual budget increased from $600,000 to $7 million. (In 1990 the Association would recognize his contributions by awarding him the Lucy Blair Service Award.) While the Board searched for a replacement, "Mike" Michels, associate executive director, stepped in as interim director. In February 1987, William D. Coughlan was named APTA's chief executive, the first non-physical-therapist to hold the post. Coughlan brought to the assignment some 21 years of experience in health agencies, much of which was in management positions, including the American Medical Association, the U.S. Department of Health and Human Services, and the American College of Cardiology.

Coughlan's nearly eight years with the Association brought a number of important additions to the services offered by the national office. Notably, he initiated the Marketing Department, which focuses on recruiting and retaining members through ongoing market research, membership surveys, and other forms of interactive evaluations, as well as the development of products and services to meet member needs. He oversaw an increase in non-dues revenue from $4.8 million in 1987 to $11.6 million in 1993, and an increase in membership from 47,500 to more than 61,000 during the same period. Coughlan also enlarged the menu of contract services available to chapters and sections, and he oversaw the internal reorganization that took place in 1992 when the tripartite structure at headquarters was further separated into seven divisions to increase efficiency and visibility.

Heading up the new divisions was the office of the CEO, or Executive Division, and six senior vice-presidents reporting to the CEO were responsible for communications; education; finance and administration; governance, components, and meetings; health policy and practice; and research, analysis, and development. Many smaller departments were also added or enlarged, and in this Coughlan made a special effort to enhance the cultural diversity of the staff and the membership. And the growing globalization of the profession was recognized by the addition of International Affairs to the responsibilities of the Department of Minority Affairs.

With Coughlan's arrival, Michels was able to turn his attention more fully to his staff liaison role on a project that had started as a charge from the House in 1986: the formal study of APTA's organizational structure. The study had been ordered in response to an assertion that despite tremendous changes in the environment in which physical therapy was being practiced and in the growth of the organization and its constituencies, APTA's governing structure was scarcely different from that which Mary McMillan and the other founders had brought into being in 1921. A Board-appointed task force, chaired first by Carolyn Hultgren and later by Jerry Connolly, was charged to consider whether and what changes were needed. Documentation of the history of APTA's organizational structure, produced early in the study, showed that, contrary to general belief, the structure had changed in many ways over the years.

Hearings were held at every level, and scores of suggestions were entertained each year from 1986 through 1989. The task force also factored into its decision-making process the various alternative forms of organization to be found among other roughly comparable associations. The final judgment was that APTA's structure and system of governance were remarkably good, needing only minor adjustments and improvements to meet the needs of the future. Michels worked with the task force to complete its report and recommendations to the Board and House in 1989, a year after his own retirement in July 1988.

### A Dollar Short and a Day Late

One change that not even strategic planning or structural fine-tuning could effect in the time frame specified was the 1979 decision to raise entry-level education from the baccalaureate to the postbaccalaureate degree by the end of 1990. As stated in the original resolution, "the rapidly expanding boundaries of physical therapy practice and the exponential expansion of relevant knowledge evoke demands [that we] expand the content . . . and broaden the general or liberal education of the physical therapist." Most delegates voting in the affirmative assumed that what was meant by "postbaccalaureate" was a master's (M.S. or M.P.T.) degree, although some fought not to designate the degree because the professional doctoral degree in physical therapy (D.P.T.) was seen as the appropriate degree.

From the moment the postbaccalaureate challenge was thrown down in the House of Delegates, there had been a strong minority undercurrent of caution in moving forward. Much of it had come from people who feared that raising requirements would put an impossible strain on the supply of skilled faculty. At the same time, universities responsible for making changes in their curricula were generally opposed to any mandatory change, for they found themselves under financial assaults from the twin horsemen of rapid inflation and federal and state funding cutbacks. Although the Association became the sole recognized accrediting agency for physical therapy education programs in 1983, its accrediting commission, CAPTE, was specifically mandated by the House of Delegates to take a neutral role on the issue of raising the level of the professional degree. To maximize its credibility, the accreditation process was thus, by design, kept at a discrete, some would say "pure," distance from APTA.

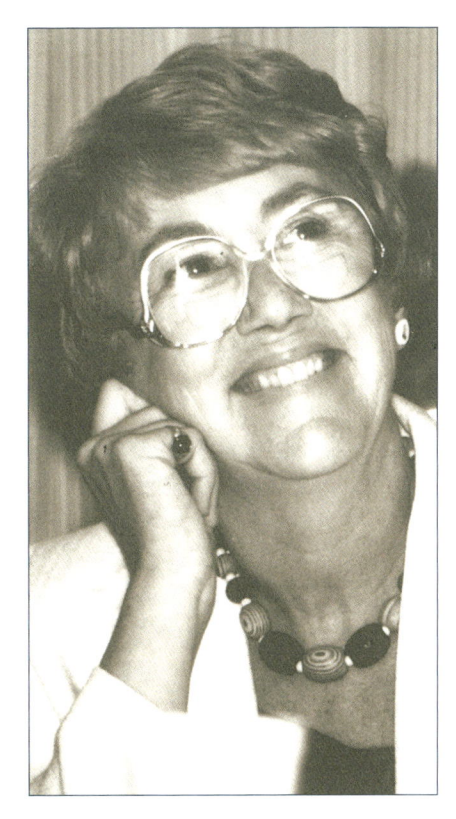

Also looming was the question of whether a more rigorous curriculum, requiring more months to complete, would have a negative effect on the chronic shortage of professionals in the field. If people were discouraged by the difficulties of the current professional (entry-level) programs, surely even greater numbers of potential candidates would shy away from the proposed requirements. Topping it all off, there was the issue of reimbursement. Persons with more extensive professional education would command higher financial rewards once in practice, but would third-party payers and patients be willing to foot the higher bills?

By 1988 it was clear that the minimum postbaccalaureate goal was not going to be met on schedule, and perhaps not even by the year 2010, unless the profession could reach a consensus on just what kinds of education and preparation were essential.

APTA formed the Task Force on the Content of Postbaccalaureate Entry-Level Curricula and, in 1991 and 1992, the Association held a series of "IMPACT" conferences at which 178 physical therapists — clinicians and academicians — convened. One important consensus that came out of these proceedings was that curricula were already so overloaded with content that students and instructors were often stretched beyond their capacities to cover the required materials adequately. Marilyn Moffat, who succeeded Jane Mathews as president in 1991, speaking from her own experience as professor in New York Uni-

*Jane Mathews, director of Boston University's physical therapy program, held the president's chair from 1985 to 1991. She is shown here enjoying a 1989 student conclave.*

# The "Postbacc" Debate

The profession's efforts to enhance postbaccalaureate education in physical therapy are at least as old as the mid-1940s, when Stanford University pioneered the first post-professional (or post-entry-level, as it used to be termed) master's degree program in physical therapy. Other schools soon followed, notably at Boston University, the University of Southern California, New York University, and Texas Woman's University. All began offering advanced degrees of this order in the 1970s. Another educational benchmark was reached with the launching in 1970 of the first post-professional doctoral program uniquely designed for physical therapists at NYU.

Also factoring into the pressure to enhance professional education back in the 1960s and 1970s was the growing desire on the part of some physical therapists to practice independently. When Florence Kendall and Ernie Burch of the Maryland Chapter shepherded the passage of legislation to permit autonomous practice within their state in the mid-1970s, some members of APTA wondered aloud if such practice did not breach the Association's ethical boundaries. Following significant study of this issue by the Board and its taskforce, the House of Delegates ultimately determined that autonomous practice was appropriate in principle, and the membership voted to revise the Code of Ethics to remove any lingering ambiguities on the issue. At the same time the House reached general agreement that physical therapists of the future needed better educational preparation if autonomous practice was to become widespread. This became a persuasive argument in favor of making the post-professional degree a fundamental educational requirement.

Concern that natural evolution toward this goal would take too long led the House to charge the Board with finding methods of accelerating change. The Board's report to the 1979 House led to a long and heated debate and, ultimately, a resolution calling for all entry-level (now professional) education programs for the physical therapist to be raised to a minimum of the postbaccalaureate degree by December 31, 1990. RC 14-79, as it was designated, was passed by a vote of 369 yeas to 147 nays. A task force consisting of Jane Walter (chair), Bob Bartlett, Sam Feitelberg, and Marilyn Gossman (Board liaison) was given the job of studying the impact of the resolution and coordinating its implementation.

As the task force soon recognized, the well-intentioned resolution presented a set of problems that made raising entry-level education within the intended timeframe well-near impossible to achieve. The first glitch was in the initial wording of the resolution. Accreditation of school programs, it declared, would henceforth be contingent upon their administrators' "Declarations of Intent" to comply with APTA's new requirements. As a number of deans and chancellors quickly countered, APTA's newly gained power of accreditation was a public trust, not to be used to leverage change unilaterally. Then there were the still more intractable problems of recruiting sufficient faculty and funds to make a sweeping redesign of curricula possible. Would students be drawn to these programs, or was the already severe shortage of candidates for physical therapy education likely to grow worse as standards were raised? Lastly, even if these barriers were removed, where was the consensus on what would constitute the optimal postbaccalaureate degree program?

Long before the deadline, it was clear that RC 14-79 was destined for trouble. So opposed were members of the Association of Schools of Allied Health Professions, which by the 1980s represented the majority of deans of schools preparing physical therapists, that ASAHP and APTA parted company. The level of mutual trust that had existed was severely compromised. At one point ASAHP went so far as to question APTA's continued recognition as an independent accrediting agency, a challenge that was eventually dropped.

In the wake of so much controversy, APTA has not changed its belief in the desirability of raising "entry-level" education as a future goal, but it has come to recognize that the road to success is smoother when the travelers carry a map. In September 1993, Joseph Black, Senior Vice-President of APTA's Education Division, spearheaded a consensus-building process whose explicit purpose was development of a new consensus-based model of physical therapist professional education. Unlike previous approaches, this model as Black has explained it is not to be descriptive (explaining what is), nor prescriptive (mandating what should be), but *normative*, intended as a voluntary standard for programs. Such a model not only must reflect future directions and aspirations for the profession, but it must articulate a set of values currently shared by the profession. This normative model also must be responsive to changing expectations, the expanding body of knowledge, and the physical therapy practice environment. And it should never be regarded as finished, but rather a work subject to yearly review.

By the spring of 1995 progress toward making the post-professional degree the normative educational model was substantial. Fifty member-consultants representing the education and clinical practice communities were brought together twice in 1994 as a "Coalition for Consensus" to hammer out a new paradigm for a practice-based model of education that would serve communities of interest both within and outside APTA. As this history went to press, Black and his staff were presenting their draft proposal to some 40 forums around the country at which more than 1,000 members participated in discussions and revisions.

The final report and recommendations are scheduled to go to the Board of Directors at the end of 1995 and to the House of Delegates for approval in 1996. Even before this is completed, however, the gradual shift toward higher standards of professional education continues on its own. By 1995 well over half of the schools were already at the "postbacc" level, with many more in development. According to Black, "This voluntary change is one more demonstration that the decision made in 1979 was a good one, only now we are getting there through cooperation rather than confrontation."

versity's Physical Therapy Program, suggested that "both our baccalaureate and master's entry-level programs . . . actually rival doctoral levels when one gives appropriate credit units for the [content level of] courses taught."

Conferees also agreed that physical therapists of the future had to be prepared educationally to tackle whole new areas of responsibility not yet taught in conventional curricula. In addition, they needed a knowledge base in "transcurricular" areas, such as behavioral science, to become "reflective therapists" capable of understanding the social and psychological aspects of illness and aging. Lastly, those at the conference concurred on the need to do more to recruit and retain both academic and clinical faculty, with particular emphasis on gaining tenure for academicians so that they would be inclined to make long-term commitments to teaching.

Coincident with the IMPACT initiatives, an APTA Task Force on Clinical Education began drafting voluntary guidelines to assist academic and clinical educators in establishing and improving clinical education sites.

(Clinical education today comprises some 28 percent of the total entry-level curriculum. It is carried out in a variety of practice settings representing the diversity of physical therapy practice options. There are currently nearly 5,500 such facilities offering intensive "real world" experience in patient care, as distinct from the didactic part of the curriculum.) In the late eighties a focused effort was made to arrive at some kind of consistent level of experience.

Today, not one but three levels of degrees are used at the professional level. The four-year bachelor's degree continues to be offered, but slightly more than half of the current 148 programs around the country are at the professional master's level and, including time spent in pre-professional education, take five to seven and one-half years to complete.

Very new to the scene is the "professional" D.P.T. Creighton University in Omaha, Nebraska, is the pioneer of this degree program, which was inaugurated in September 1993 with an entering class of 48 students. Talks began in 1986, when a broad spectrum of academicians and practitioners were consulted as to the feasibility of such a program. Geneva Johnson served as primary consultant, and after two more years of planning, the decision was made to proceed. Gary Soderberg, director of the physical therapy program at Creighton University, was hired as the first director and chair of the new eight-semester professional D.P.T. program.

The post-professional doctorate in physical therapy is available at a relative handful of institutions, with the oldest being New York University. Established under the leadership of Arthur Nelson in 1970, the program graduated its first "doctors" — Mary Moffroid and Dorothy Shattner — in the mid-1970s.

**GETTING THE WORD OUT**

After nearly 10 years as full-time in-house editor of *Physical Therapy*, Marilyn Lister left in early 1988. The Board of Directors decided to use the opportunity to reexamine the entire editorial set-up. Of prime concern was the issue of editorial independence. The practice of having a staff editor ran counter to prevailing standards within the scientific community, where "out-of-house" editors were the rule. While the Board debated next steps, Robert Lamb, one of the journal's associate editors, stepped in as interim editor, even as he continued to carry a heavy teaching load at Virginia Commonwealth University in Richmond. The smoothness with which Lamb and the APTA editorial staff managed the transition demonstrated that it was possible to direct the journal from a distance, and in June 1988, the Association named Steven Rose to a five-year term as its new out-of-house editor.

Rose, who was a 1983 recipient of APTA's Lucy Blair Service Award as well as a Catherine Worthingham Fellow of the Association (1985), brought to the appointment eminence in all three facets of the profession — clinical practice, education, and research — with particular emphasis in neuroscience, in which he held a doctorate from Albert Einstein College of Medicine. At the time of his appointment, he was associate director of research and graduate studies in the Division of Physical Therapy at the University of Miami. With the APTA leadership's full support, Rose and his new staff managing editor made a number of changes designed to give *Physical Therapy* a more contemporary appearance, including its now familiar bright blue cover. Rose, who has been described as a "consummate generator of ideas . . . and a world class provocateur," also revived the tradition of thought-provoking editorials. In them, he decried inertia and worked tirelessly to bring to the profession movement, change, and growth through research. His formula for success was, to quote one of his colleagues, "unique . . . one part candor, one part charm, two parts logic, and an occasional pinch of acrimony."

Tragically, Rose served for less than a year before succumbing at the age of 49 to a rare and particularly aggressive form of cancer. Interim editor Bob Lamb, joined this time by his colleague in research Rebecca Craik, came forward again to guide editorial content while the search for a permanent editor-in-chief of *Physical Therapy* resumed. In October 1989, Jules Rothstein, then associate professor of physical therapy at the Medical College of Virginia in Richmond and subsequently head of the Department of Physical Therapy at the University of Illinois at Chicago, took over, and he continues to serve with distinction.

Ironically, as the academic rigor of the journal increased over the years, topics of a more newsworthy and hands-on character were inevitably displaced. The monthly *Progress Report* had been created back in the early seventies to cover news and ongoing topics of national and component business, and this publication continued to thrive in the eighties. But other gaps in coverage widened, leading to the launching of *P.T. Bulletin*, a national weekly, the first issue of which was mailed on February 12, 1986. The *Bulletin* has proved invaluable in its ability to give late-breaking reports of legislative initiatives at the state and national level, and it has also become the prime billboard for professional recruitment ads. Ten years after its charter issue, nearly 110,000 readers inside and outside the Association are on the *Bulletin*'s mailing list. Unique among APTA periodicals, this one is published by an

*APTA's publications are the lifeline of the organization. Shown in the background is* Physical Therapy, the Journal, *which is the scholarly descendant of the* PT Review *begun in 1921.* PT Magazine, *shown in its premiere issue, January 1993, is a lively new publication, designed to cover topical issues relating to the profession.*

independent contractor under a royalty agreement with the Association.

Still lacking, however, was a general magazine with hands-on practice advice to meet the continuing education needs and interests of practitioner members, and to fill this niche, *Clinical Management in Physical Therapy* was introduced as a quarterly in 1980. *Clinical Management* lasted a dozen years, then was merged in January 1993 with *Progress Report* into the monthly *PT — Magazine of Physical Therapy*. *PT Magazine* has proved to be a vigorous and colorful addition to APTA's periodicals line-up, with many of the best features of its predecessors plus distinctive qualities of its own.

With more hands available, *PT*'s editorial staff of six has the time to develop in-depth clinical feature stories along with legislative and industry news, monthly Association news, the globally oriented "World View" report, and news items relating to the activities of individual PTs and PTAs. Regular columns provide another outlet for discussions of ongoing professional issues in practice, reimbursement, technology, and other topics. *PT*'s monthly "Habits of Thought" column on ethics, coordinated and often written by Catherine Worthingham Fellow Ruth Purtilo, is one of the magazine's most distinctive offerings.

Not surprisingly, *PT Magazine* has received numerous national awards for excellence in its young life, including the prestigious 1994 Gold Excel Award for Overall Magazine Excellence from the Society of National Association Publications.

### LOBBYING CONGRESS

Gaining the ear of state and federal policy makers on behalf of physical therapists is an ongoing activity that goes back to Marguerite Sanderson's day, if we include efforts to maintain and finance the reconstruction aide program. But it is made all the more urgent by the current environment of change. Beginning with the reorganization of the Association in the 1980s, this important work has been centralized in the Association's Health Policy and Practice Division (formerly Professional Relations) and its Government Affairs staff.

During that time, this office has coordinated the efforts of countless member-volunteers and has represented APTA members on many thorny practice issues. Among its notable successes have been two revisions of the salary equivalency rates used by Medicare to reimburse facilities for contracted physical therapist and physical therapist assistant services. Another was persuading Congress to raise the limit on yearly Medicare services provided by private practitioners from $500 to $750 in 1988 and to $900 in 1993. The latter was won only after a strenuous fight in which the Government Affairs Department roused thousands of member-volunteers in key states to participate in a week-long letter-writing and phone blitz to their congressional representatives.

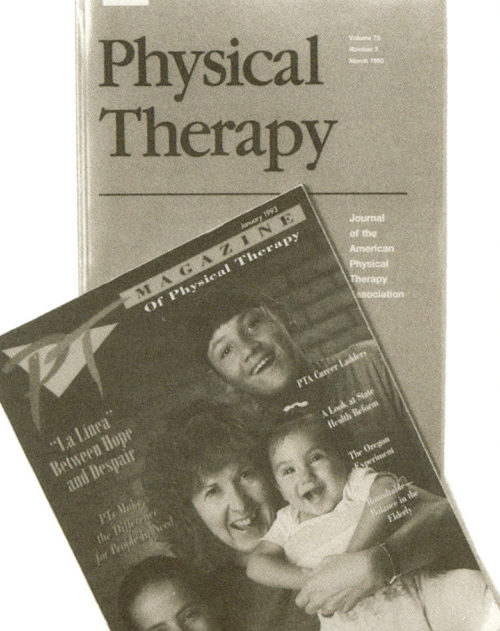

Direct access has also generated continuing debate. Direct access entails the freedom of the therapist to evaluate and treat patients without physician referral. It also implies the freedom of the patient to choose a practitioner other than a physician as a primary care provider. The long-standing prohibition against physical therapists treating without physician referral began to crumble in 1974. That year, the U.S. Army, faced with a severe shortage of physicians and a very high level of musculoskeletal injuries due to the demands of military training, solved its problem by permitting PTs and OTs to become "physician extenders" in army hospitals. Physical therapists thus assumed initial contact roles for musculoskeletal evaluations, and they have continued in this capacity ever since.

In the late seventies APTA revised its code of ethics to permit evaluation of patients within the scope of physical therapy practice without referral wherever state laws did not expressly prohibit it. This important change led many chapters to press for changes in their state practice acts, and the Professional Relations Division of the Association often provided major assistance to such efforts. By 1989 practice without referral — in effect, direct access — had become legal in 20 states; by 1994 the number had climbed to

*When treating children, both passive and active exercises often are incorporated into play and recreational activities. This child wears her back support with a smile as she practices balance and correct posture atop a pony.*

237

*The issues of practice without referral and the relationship of physical therapists to other health care practitioners made for lively House of Delegates debates during the eighties. This button was one popular way to declare a position.*

30, with Delaware and Oregon the latest to enact the change.

Still other issues before Government Affairs have been federal funding for physical therapy education programs, independent contractor status, a ban on referral for profit, and enhanced support for rural health care. Unquestionably, the overriding issue as the profession faces the late 1990s is the impact of changing ideas and initiatives of the health care environment—and particularly managed care—on the provision of physical therapy.

### THE RISE OF INDUSTRIAL PHYSICAL THERAPY

In 1976 General Motors made headlines by spending more money on health benefits for its employees than on rolled steel for its auto assembly lines. In the next two decades, this story echoed throughout American business and industry, as companies large and small found themselves scrambling to keep up with the rising costs of maintaining healthy, on-the-job workers. Much of the impetus for the rising costs was traceable to new attitudes about employer responsibilities for the welfare of employees, as expressed through state and federal legislation. While each state had long since established its own workers' compensation system — laws had been on the books in some states even before World War I — state laws tended to be extremely variable regarding who and what was covered. Rarely was the primary focus of the coverage return of the worker to her or his job following injury; more often, it was in compensating the individual in dollars for proven chronic disability, an increasingly expensive solution in every sense of the word.

This focus began to change in 1970, when Congress created a new national policy covering all businesses involved in interstate commerce. Managed by the new Occupational Safety and Health Administration as a federal agency within the U.S. Department of Labor, the program was responsible for conducting research on occupational health and safety standards. Of particular relevance to physical therapists, OSHA recognized the need to review and upgrade ergonomic conditions that were potentially hazardous, such as the handling of heavy materials and poor working posture resulting from improper design of the workplace.

In the more than a quarter of a century since OSHA's creation, the developments brought about in terms of injury compensation and injury management have meant important changes for the providers of rehabilitation services, who have seen the demand for their services expand exponentially. Where many physical therapists had treated the occasional work-related musculoskeletal injury on an ad hoc basis before, they now found increasing opportunities to specialize in industrial programs that supported prevention, fitness, and on-site job safety and work-capacity analysis. Working with risk managers, ergonomic engineers, and vocational rehabilitation counselors more consistently than with physicians and other medical personnel, today's industrial physical therapists use measurement tools and diagnostic standards unique to their specialty to assess the capacity of individual workers to carry out specific tasks. They design treatments to strengthen and rehabilitate workers as appropriate, thereby enhancing worker performance and reducing the circumstances that generate workers' compensation claims. When claims are made and contested, PTs are often called upon to give expert testimony in court regarding worker function.

Throughout their nearly 75 years of formal practice, physical therapists have had a rich history both as care givers to persons with disabilities and as advocates for their integration into society. Thus, over the years, numerous disability-related state and federal laws have been passed, beginning with efforts to provide vocational education and retraining to veterans after World War I and gradually extending their reach to cover civilian adults and children.

Equal opportunity in employment was federally mandated in 1973, but it soon became apparent that lack of specific language and implementation guidelines made progress toward non-discrimination extremely slow.

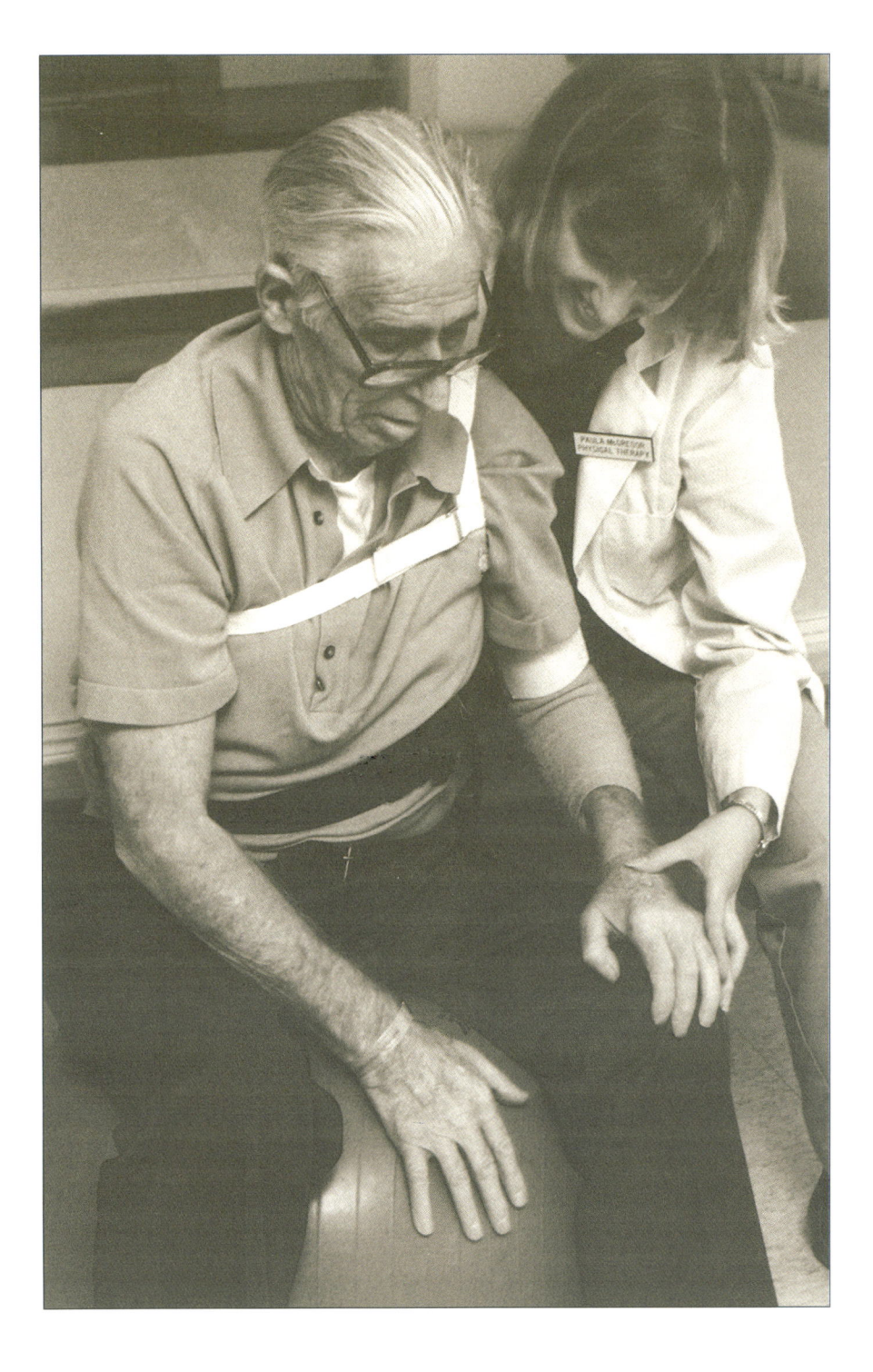

*Paula McGregor, a staff physical therapist at St. John's Mercy Medical Center, St. Louis, works to restore function in a patient recovering from stroke.*

*The 1992 Presidents' Luncheon, held during the Denver, Colorado Conference in June, brings together Mathews, Michels, Moffat, and Magistro (standing, left to right); Richardson, Bartlett and Wortley (seated, left to right).*

Subsequent efforts to make what were widely agreed to be basic human rights available culminated in 1990 in two comprehensive federal initiatives. The first was the National Institutes of Health Amendments, which created the National Center for Medical Rehabilitation Research within the National Institute of Child Health and Human Development. The other was the Americans with Disabilities Act, which recognized the rights of an estimated 40 million Americans to equal opportunities in employment and ensured physical access to a wide range of public services and accommodations. Physical therapists and APTA see the latter law opening particularly significant areas in which to do important, meaningful work. Chiefly, ADA calls upon traditional skills in evaluating function and matching patients with the physical requirements of a particular activity. Now, the matching must include developing functional job descriptions for employers, matching workers to those jobs, and helping the employer to modify other jobs to fit particular limitations. As Susan Isernhagen, a leader in industrial physical therapy, points out, ADA has the potential to become "a win/win situation" for everyone.

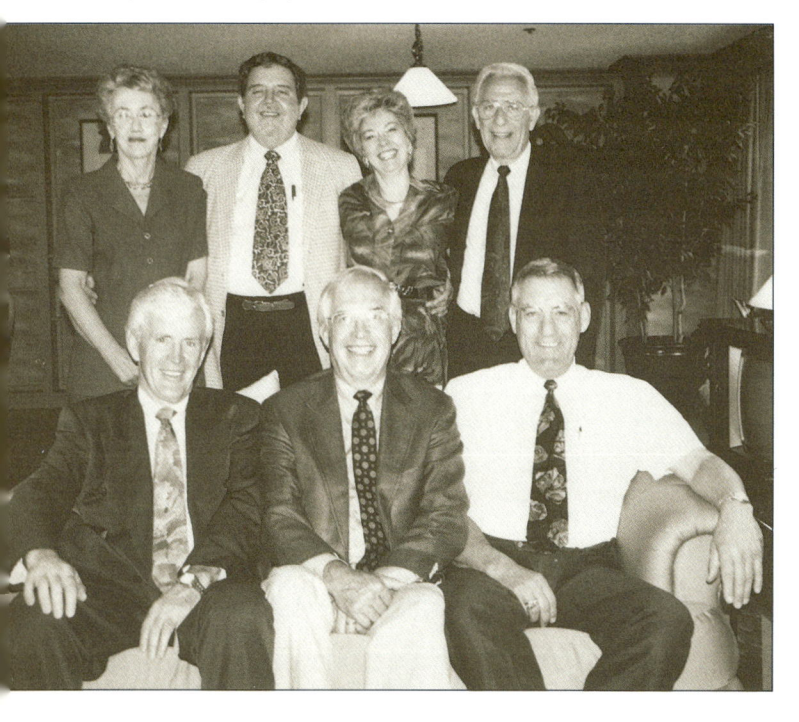

### ISSUES OF IDENTITY

During their presidencies, both Don Wortley and Bob Richardson had promoted the concept of cooperation between APTA and the American Occupational Therapy Association (AOTA). Over the years there had been considerable interaction between the two groups on the staff level in such areas as government relations, practice, and education. In the mid-eighties, as the momentum for health care reform began to gather speed, the leadership of both organizations began to discuss the possibility of formalizing certain cooperative efforts. Particularly clear was the professional interaction between PTs and OTs in clinic and school settings.

During the presidency of Jane Mathews, the executive directors and presidents of APTA and AOTA invited the leadership of the American Speech-Language and Hearing Association (ASHA), a natural partner in rehabilitation work, to join in. In 1988 these initiatives gave rise to informal meetings among the three and, in 1991, under new APTA president Marilyn Moffat, the formation of the TriAlliance of Health and Rehabilitation Professions, a coalition aimed at addressing issues of mutual concern.

In the years since formation, the TriAlliance has presented to various government agencies unified messages on public policy issues related to health, rehabilitation, and education. They also run forums at each association's annual conference to discuss a variety of topics. In 1993, for example,

240  *Healing The Generations*

the TriAlliance topic was ethics and the particular dilemmas faced when integrating good business practices with sound professional judgment and provision of high-quality care to patients. Another initiative of the TriAlliance was the building of team collaboration skills, and to this end, state/component groups within each of the three organizations were invited to submit team project proposals, with the teams chosen being supported with a series of workshops and other training resources.

One APTA staff executive who has been closely involved in the continuing activities of the TriAlliance is Frank Mallon, staff counsel and senior vice-president for Health Policy and Practice from 1981 to 1994. According to Mallon, though the three professions, serving as they do as the core of rehabilitation care, share many goals, interests, and concerns (especially in the public policy arena), each has its own identity and history. The three groups have "agreed to agree on those issues of import to all three associations and have recognized that there will be issues on which they will have to disagree."

Mallon's insights into what makes APTA the successful organization it is have served him and the profession well. In 1994 he succeeded William Coughlan as CEO. Mallon believes that one of the principal strengths of the Association today is the political and professional activism of its members, qualities that he predicts will be even more essential in the challenging years immediately ahead. This tradition of activism, says Mallon, is no chance occurrence. It arises, he believes, out of APTA's chapter structure, which has always fostered grassroots involvement on the part of members, and which has put physical therapists years ahead of most other health care professions through achieving enactment of state licensure laws.

Though his tenure in the CEO position is still relatively new, Mallon has already demonstrated that he intends to use his leadership talents to keep the Association and its individual members highly visible players in shaping the future of health care delivery.

Another issue with which APTA has grappled in recent years is that of gender. After nearly three quarters of a century in which women have dominated the profession in terms of numbers, they suffer from a disparity in professional and economic status compared with their male colleagues. This information, long suspected but made eminently clear when APTA began making regular profile surveys of active members in the early eighties, was perceived as detrimental to the entire profession.

A task force created to study the problem and make recommendations as to future actions found that, propor-

*Frank Mallon, a lawyer and former staff vice-president for health policy and practice, is the Association's current CEO. Mallon sees his task as preparing APTA's support team to meet the legislative and management challenges of the twenty-first century.*

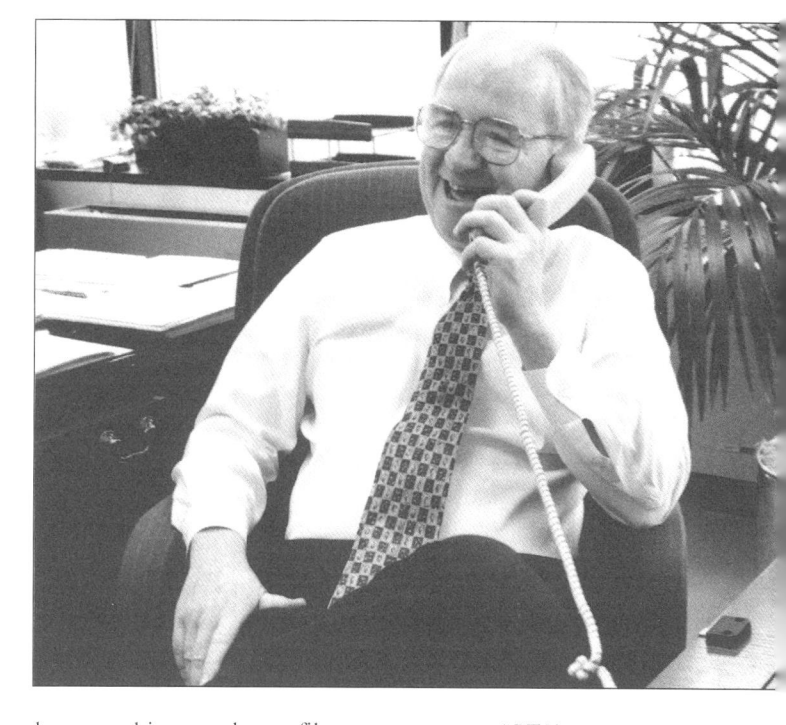

*The Diamond Jubilee Years 1980-1996*

tionately, women lagged behind men in owning their own private practices, in responsibility for administration and management in academic and institutional care settings, in holding advanced professional degrees and specialty certification, and in conducting all kinds of research. Women physical therapists were also found to participate less frequently in proportion to their numbers in sections and on professional committees, to attend fewer scientific meetings, to spend less time in continuing education programs, and ultimately to have shorter careers in physical therapy. Although the Board of Directors concluded that the reasons for the disparity were not limited to physical therapists but were societal in nature — having to do with women's traditional responsibilities as family caregivers — it also felt that outright sexual discrimination continued to be a factor. The Board further concluded that the membership would benefit as a whole if actions were taken to reduce the barriers to women's advancement wherever they lay. With this goal in mind, APTA created a new Office of Women's Issues in 1994.

### Honors and Awards

The Association has always taken pride in its members' accomplishments and the extraordinary generosity so many have shown by volunteering their time and efforts to further the profession. In recent years, several new honors and awards have been created to give due recognition.

In a special class are the Catherine Worthingham Fellows, a category of membership established in 1980 to single out persons "whose work, like the distinguished woman honored in this action, has resulted in lasting and significant advances in science, education, and the practice of the profession." The following year, the Bylaws were amended to establish a separate class of Association membership, with nominees' names submitted by individual components for final selection by the Board of Directors at its annual March meeting. Individuals so recognized are presented with a commemorative key and the right to use the initials FAPTA after their names. In 1982 Catherine Worthingham became the first recipient. Helen Hislop and Geneva Johnson joined her in 1983.

In succeeding years the number of recipients has ranged from one to six, with a current total of 41 distinguished members.

In 1981 APTA established the Dorothy Baethke-Eleanor J. Carlin Award for Excellence in Academic Teaching. Dorothy Baethke, who died in 1984, was a pioneer in physical therapy education, who taught for 25 years in the Department of Physical Therapy at the University of Pennsylvania School of Allied Medical Professions and retired as its chairman in 1972. Jane Carlin, now retired, began her long career as an educator in 1942, when she became Women's Army Corps instructor in physical therapy at Walter Reed General Hospital. In 1947 she joined Baethke and others at the University of Pennsylvania's SAMP, where she remained until her retirement in 1981. The first year's award was presented to Carlin at what turned out to be the start of another tradition: the Recognition Luncheon at Annual Conference, which was held that year in Washington, D.C.

Also inaugurated in 1981, two years after Henry Kendall's death, was the Henry O. and Florence P. Kendall Practice Award. The award which was originally developed by the Maryland Chapter to recognize excellence in clinical practice, celebrates this nationally recognized husband and wife clinician team. Through numerous publications, films, and workshops, they shared their expertise in muscle testing, posture, and physical fitness exercise regimes throughout their long careers and provided an inspiring example of dedication to the profession. The award, which is intended to go to other outstanding clinicians, was also bestowed at the Recognition Luncheon in Washington, D.C. It's first recipient was Miriam Partridge of Houston, Texas. A veteran of the WMSBC and currently in private practice, Partridge had published widely in the areas of kinesiology, therapeutic exercise, and electromyography.

The Chattanooga Research Award, like the earlier Jack Walker Award, was initiated and funded by the Chattanooga Group. First granted in 1981, it goes to the author of an outstanding physical therapy clinical research report in *Physical Therapy*.

Its first recipient was James E. Griffin, professor of physical therapy, SUNY at Buffalo, New York.

The Minority Achievement and Minority Initiative Awards were established in 1984, evolving from the earlier Award of Excellence for Minority Recruitment and Services. The former recognizes an entry-level accredited physical therapy education program for continuous and sustained achievement in recruitment, admission, retention, and graduation of minority students. The latter recognizes newly initiated programs whose designs hold the promise of sustained growth. The first awards were made in 1985 to the Universities of Puerto Rico and Connecticut, respectively. Concurrently, the first Chapter Award for Minority Enhancement, created to recognize outstanding efforts on the part of a chapter to foster minority representation and participation, was received by the Connecticut Chapter. The Minority Scholarship Award for Academic Excellence, first awarded in 1988, carries with it a scholarship of $1,000 to $2,000. The first year's recipient was Steven D. Newton of Loma Linda University. The award acknowledges and rewards academic excellence, demonstrated concerns for minority issues, and the potential for superior professional achievements.

Shortly before Signe Brunnström's death in 1988, an award for Excellence in Clinical Teaching was established to honor the Swedish-born pioneer researcher, author, clinician, and teacher. The first recipient was Linda Simonsen, senior physical therapist, Maine Medical Center, Portland, Maine, who was recognized in 1987.

Two other awards, the Margaret L. Moore Award for Outstanding New Academic Faculty Member and the Eugene Michels New Investigator Award, followed in 1989. The Moore award honors Dr. Moore who, during her many years as director of the Division of Physical Therapy at the University of North Carolina, Chapel Hill, proved a generous mentor to many young faculty members as well as a major contributor to the growth of numerous APTA faculty development programs. An early education consultant on staff, she subsequently produced a study of clinical education

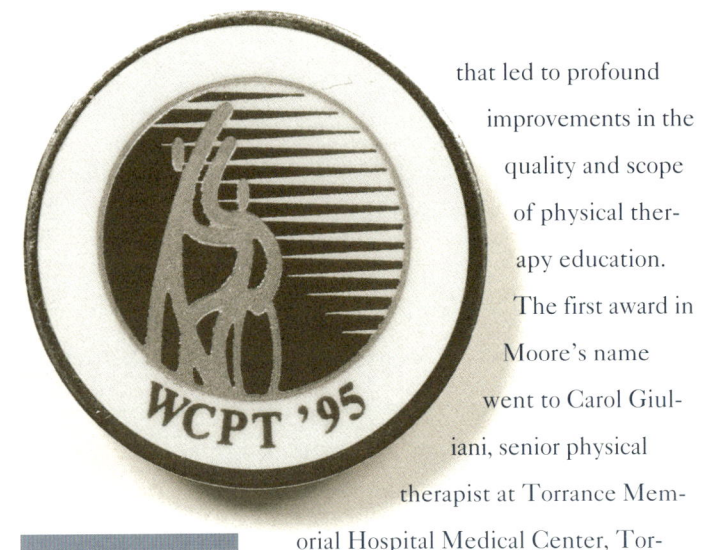

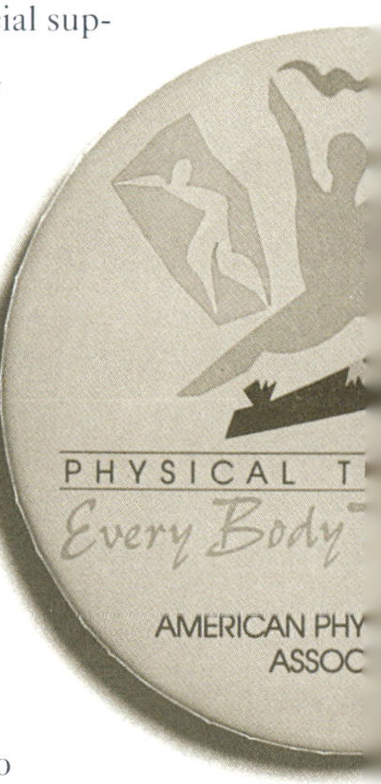

*These buttons, representing the 12th International Congress of the World Confederation for Physical Therapy (this page), the American Physical Therapy Association's National Physical Therapy Month celebrations (center), and the Uni-*
*(continued opposite)*

that led to profound improvements in the quality and scope of physical therapy education.

The first award in Moore's name went to Carol Giuliani, senior physical therapist at Torrance Memorial Hospital Medical Center, Torrance, California, in 1990.

The Michels award is named in honor of Eugene "Mike" Michels who, as APTA's associate executive vice-president for Research and Education for seven years, provided the first major impetus in the Association's plans to foster research in physical therapy. (An Annual Michels Researchers' Forum was established by the Section on Research in 1982, and the Eugene Michels Fund for Educational Research was established by the Foundation for Physical Therapy in 1984.) The New Investigator Award recognizes physical therapists engaged in independent research. In 1990, the first year the award was made, George Carvell was the recipient. On the faculty of the School of Health Related Professions, University of Pittsburgh, Carvell's research was directed to studies of the relationship between brain function and tactile behavior.

The Helen J. Hislop Award for Outstanding Contributions to Professional Literature was established to recognize a lifelong commitment to writing and publishing professional literature as demonstrated by Hislop. (Her Mary McMillan Lecture, "The Not So Impossible Dream," delivered at the 1975 annual meeting in Anaheim, California, is said to have been the most frequently cited paper ever delivered to the profession.) Jay Schleichkorn, whose writings include groundbreaking biographies of British orthopedist William John Little and of Signe Brunnström and Berta and Karel Bobath, received the first award in 1992.

### WORLD CONFEDERATION

In 1995 the World Confederation for Physical Therapy convened its 12th Congress in Washington, D.C., marking only the second time it has met in the United States since its inception in 1951. Having grown from 11 founder-member physical therapy associations to 66 today, the WCPT represents a cumulative membership of more than 200,000 physical therapists, physical therapist assistants, and students worldwide. In fulfillment of its founders' vision, the organization exists primarily to improve the quality of global physical therapy care through contacts with various world health organizations and through financial support for physical therapy education programs, particularly those in developing nations. Through its regionalized structure, the opportunities for neighbor-to-neighbor cultural and scientific exchanges between countries is also fostered.

Attendees at WCPT Congresses find the event a rich stew of experiences, both per-

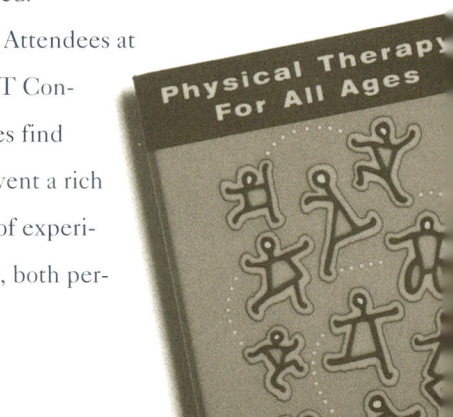

244    *Healing The Generations*

sonal and professional. Along with the opportunity to participate in a professional "hands-across-the-sea" fellowship, congress-goers also have access to an intensive program of on-site workshops, lectures, and abstract presentations. At the 1995 gathering, which drew more than 8,000 delegates from the U.S. and overseas, attendees had an opportunity to choose among exhibits, forums, lectures, and platform and poster presentations prepared by some 1,300 individuals from around the world. Fulfilling the wish that former WCPT president Eugene Michels voiced in his keynote speech to the WCPT in 1975, the World Confederation has truly found its way to becoming "a world force for good."

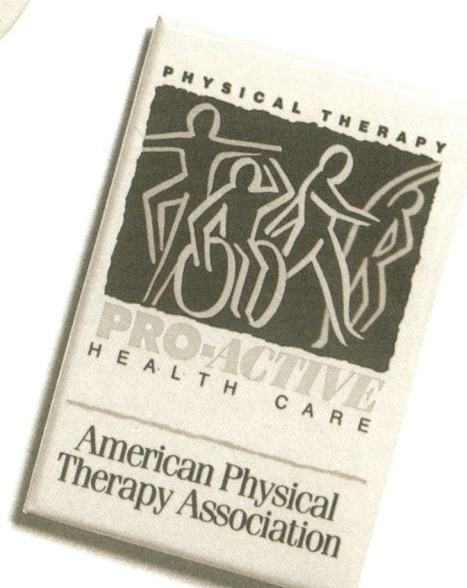

### BRAVE NEW WORLD

In 1996 the American Physical Therapy Association and the profession it represents celebrate 75 years of distinguished service to American health care. Begun by a small band of daring young reconstruction aide/technicians who saw themselves as the willing servants of the dominant medical profession, today's physical therapy profession stands on the brink of the twenty-first century with the confidence and professional capabilities to make its own autonomous way. Its possibilities are limited only by its ability to find creative ways to provide high-quality services sufficient for the demand.

While access to good health care has come to be considered a right in the United States, the growing demand from public and private agencies for cost containment is forcing changes in the manner and environment in which treatments are delivered. The rush to cost containment has significantly expanded the broad umbrella of "managed care" and its rapidly increasing appearance in both public (for example, Medicare and Medicaid) and private health insurance programs.

The changes are already evident, for example, in the trend toward outpatient surgery and early hospital discharges for patients with serious conditions, which has led to physical therapy services being delivered away from the hospital increasingly often — in private practice facilities, neighborhood clinics, or in the home — often with assistive devices that the patient can manage alone. Health care insurance systems — an alphabet soup of HMOs, PPOs, EPOs, POSs, and their variants — have put new constraints on physical therapy practice through their ability to capitate reimbursements and contract selectively with "preferred providers." This, in turn, has led to the development of "PT networks" whose aggregate size gives them access to hundreds of thousands, if not millions, of patients within their contract areas.

The scope and goals of treatments are changing, too. Where the therapeutic approach to

*versity of California at San Francisco physical therapy program (opposite page), allow the wearers to celebrate the organizations and institutions that have helped the profession overcome obstacles and thrive throughout the decades.*

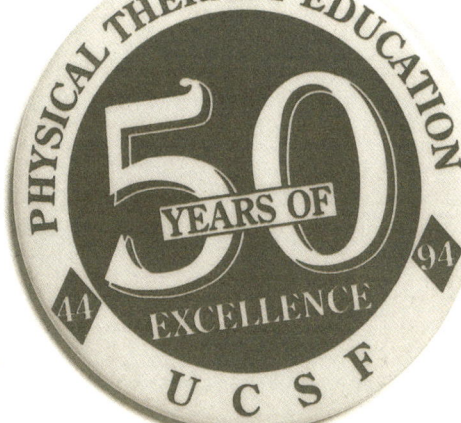

*The Diamond Jubilee Years 1980 - 1996*  245

*Marilyn Moffat, who was elected president of APTA for two terms beginning in 1991, leads the Association as it celebrates its 75th anniversary. A former editor of* Physical Therapy, *Moffat is also a Catherine Worthingham Fellow, a member of the faculty of the NYU physical therapy program, and a private practitioner.*

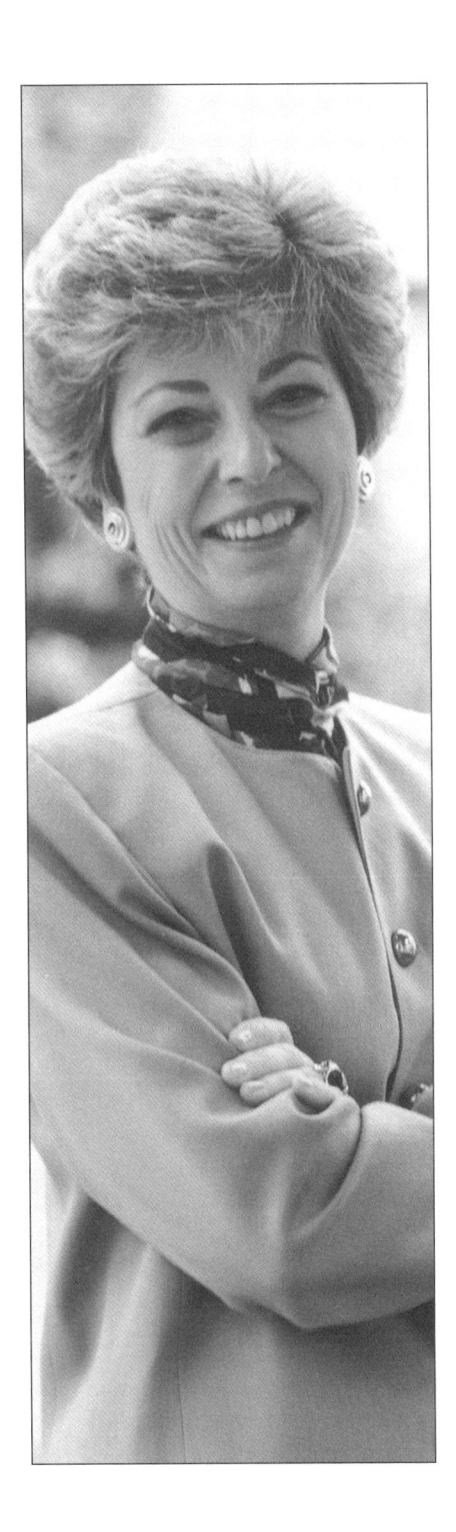

treating existing diseases and injuries was once the primary focus of the physical therapist's education and practice, health maintenance and disease prevention from the moment of birth will soon outrank this in importance as mounting research data demonstrate that many chronic diseases are either avoidable or curable through appropriate treatment. And physical therapists, who have traditionally been the quintessential "hands-on" members of the health care team, are certainly finding themselves having to balance the time spent providing hands-on care with that spent on evaluation, program design, patient education, and case management, with appropriate delegation of responsibility to assistant-level personnel and support staff.

Is the profession ready for such changes? Marilyn Moffat, who completes her second term as APTA president in 1997, has made preparing the Association for changes in the health care environment one of the central tenets of her service. High on the list of her accomplishments in this area is the strong support that she and the Board of Directors have given to public relations and advertising initiatives aimed at making physical therapy the public's choice for the prevention of injury, impairments, functional limitations, and disability and for the maintenance and promotion of health, fitness, and quality of life.

Other important accomplishments have been development of *A Guide to Physical Therapist Practice* and standardization of patient examination procedures, and launching of the Association's Resource Center for Research and Learning.

Another key activity of the Association — and one which reflects a major premise of Moffat's career as an academician and practitioner — is the move toward making the post-professional degree the normative educational model based on a consensus within the physical therapy education community.

Moffat has also worked to strengthen the Board's liaison program with the Association's components, visiting chapters with a frequency not seen in several decades and reporting back on concerns and interests at the grassroots level. She has also been highly active in APTA's recently expanded efforts at diversity and international outreach; under Moffat's aegis, the Office of Minority Affairs not only has stepped up its efforts to increase representation and participation of members from minority communities, but it has added International Affairs to its sphere of activity.

Moffat and Jane Walter (who served on the Board from 1985 to 1994 and as vice president during the last three of those years) have long championed the Association's efforts to modernize its communications. With the guidance and support of a task force on information management, empaneled shortly after she took office, the Association has been able to move swiftly and smoothly into the electronic information-distribution age. Not only is the national office broadly equipped with the tools of office automation, but communications with the Association's House of Delegates representatives are increasingly done electronically and on disk. In late 1994, in a significant break with tradition, the Board of Directors was able to conduct its first "paperless" meeting and to gain access to internal office communications via electronic mail through the marvels of notebook computers. And in 1995 APTA embarked on an Internet server system that gives every member access capability to a world of relevant professional data and bulletin boards.

More administrative in nature — but no less important to the future of the Association — were the purchase of APTA's second building, a decision for which Moffat personally campaigned and which was made within two months of her election, and an expansion of efforts to recruit and retain members — resulting in a growth of roughly 29 percent between 1991 when the number was just over 51,000 and 1995 when it reached 67,000.

All these efforts, says Moffat, are keys that are essential to keeping the profession vital and proactive in a changing environment. Says Moffat, "We must and will meet directly and forthrightly the challenges ahead — with our commitment of time, energy, financial resources, and whatever else it takes — to ensure that our patients and the clients we serve are never in want of the unique contributions we have to offer. We can do no less."

*These physical therapy students from Puerto Rico gather for a group shot at a student conclave at University of Alabama, Birmingham. Physical therapy is now ranked as one of the most desirable careers, and the membership of APTA, recorded at 67,000 in 1995, is steadily growing.*

# Timeline

**1881** Sargent School, Boston, founded by Dudley Allen Sargent. Elliott Brackett and Robert Lovett join faculty.

**1887** Forerunner of the National Institutes of Health born at Marine Hospital, Staten Island, New York.

**1889** MIT hosts first national conference on physical training, Boston Normal School of Gymnastics founded by Amy Homans.

**1893** The Cotting School, the first free day school for children with disabilities founded in Boston.

**1894** First polio epidemic in U.S. recorded in Rutland, Vermont.

**1905** Mary McMillan receives degree in physical education and goes on to take post-grad courses in electrotherapy, therapeutic exercise, massage and anatomy in London.

**1910** McMillan takes her first professional position in Liverpool, England, working with Sir Robert Jones.

**1913** First formal government survey of injuries from industrial accidents.

**1913** Pennsylvania becomes first state to license physical therapists.

**1914** R.W. Lovett, known for his novel approach to polio treatment, creates the "Vermont Plan" to treat epidemic in state. Wilhelmine Wright, his assistant trains cadre of assistants in her system of "manual muscle testing." This work becomes basis of treating patients with polio and postural deformities.

**1914** Marjorie Bouvé, Margurite Sanderson, and others found Boston School of Physical Education (future Bouvé-Boston).

**1916** McMilllan returns to U.S. to work at children's Hospital Portland, Maine. Severe polio epidemic in New York and elsewhere.

**1917** United States declares war on Germany. Division of Special Hospitals and Physical Reconstruction authorized within the Army Medical Department. Marguerite Sanderson hired as director of Reconstruction Aide program.

**1917** J.B. Mennell publishes seminal text on scientific massage, Physical Treatment by Movement, Manipulation and Massage.

**1918** First Reconstruction Aides mobilized and trained. McMillan becomes second "re-aide." Walter Reed General Hospital's program is soon joined by those at Reed College and 13 other schools. Armistice declared in November.

**1919** Sanderson retires and McMillan takes over. "Re-aides" are demobilized. Charles Lowman founds Los Angeles Orthopedic Hospital and pioneers "hydrogymnastics."

**1920** McMillan resigns to return to private practice in Boston and to complete *Massage and Therapeutic Exercise* published 1921.

**1920** Organizational meeting for American Women's, Physiotherapeutic Association held at Keen's Chop House, New York. Mary McMillan elected first President by ballot. Bimonthly *P.T. Review* makes its debut in March.

**1922** First Annual Conference held in Boston. AWPA changes name to American Physiotherapy Association.

**1923** McMillan retires and Inga Lohne elected President.

**1924** F.D. Roosevelt stricken with polio, establishes Warm Springs Foundation in Georgia.

**1926** *P.T. Review* renamed *Physiotherapy Review* and becomes monthly soon after.

**1927** NYU inaugurates first 4 year bachelor of science program to physical therapists.

**1927** Debate over what to call physical therapists arises with physicians and surgeons.

**1928** Standards for accreditation are developed with guidance of John Stanley Catilter, MD. Most accredited institutions are hospital-based and award post-baccalaureate certificates.

**1929** The Great Depression begins with the crash of the stock market.

**1933** Basil O'Connor organizes first "Birthday Ball" to raise money for polio programs.

**1933** APA asks AMA to assist with accreditation.

**1934** APA hires first paid staff member.

**1935** Social Security Act passed as part of "New Deal" package of social legislation. APA adopts first "Code of Ethics and Discipline" and American Congress of Physical Medicine and creates the American Registry for the purpose of conferring "registered" title to physical therapists who pass test.

**1937** National Foundation of infantile paralysis established.

**1938** "March of Dimes" coin collection inaugurated, and NFIP began injecting funds for various local programs related to polio.

**1938** APA gets first permanent address when office is rented in Chicago.

**1940** Educational programs shifted from hospital to university setting.

**1940** Sister Kenny arrives from Australia and is invited to Minneapolis General Hospital. NFIP asks APA to send observer team, including Florence and Henry Kendall.

**1940** Catherine Worthingham becomes wartime president of APA.

**1941** McMillan taken prisoner by Japanese at Manila's Santa Tomàs prison camp.

**1941** First special-interest "Sections" meet at Annual conference in Palo Alto, California. Schools Section survives to become permanent fixture. Coincident with Conference, first continuing education programs held at Stanford.

**1941** Emma Vogel sets up war emergency training course at WRGH.

**1942** Allied Council, consisting of 39 organizations interested in welfare of injured and disabled, organizes. APA takes leadership role.

**1942** Public Law 828 recognizes women PTs as wartime members of the Army Medical, Department with "relative" rank of 2nd Lieutenant.

**1942** Paul Campbell becomes first male physical therapist to be elected to APA national office.

**1942** NFIP begins funding APA scholarship fund.

**1943** Special Women's Medical Service Corps program for African-Americans set up at Fort Huachuca, Arizona.

**1944** House of Delegates created as legislative body within APA. APA moves into its first national office at 1790 Broadway, New York, with Mildred Elson its first salaried Executive Director. Barbara White becomes first staff Education Secretary with underwriting by NFIP.

**1944** Bolton Bill (PL 78-350) insures permanent commissioned status to women professionals serving in Army Medical Corps.

**1944** Catherine Worthingham leaves Stanford to become NFIP's Director of Professional Education.

**1946** Ida May Hazenhyer writes first formal history of the American Physical Therapy Association, which appears in four issues of the *Review*.

**1946** Council on Physical Medicine selects the term "physiatrist" to designate physicians within its specialty. APA seizes the opportunity to change its name to the American Physical Therapy Association.

**1946** Schools Section begins to meet regularly.

**1946** Hill-Burton Act passed in Congress sets off a burst of hospital construction and expansion.

**1946** Kabat-Knott collaboration begins, leading to development of their theory of proprioceptive neuromuscular facilitation (PNF).

**1947** Institute of Rehabilitation Medicine opens as an adjunct to NYU with Howard Rusk as senior director and George Deaver as medical director of physical therapy.

**1948** National Institute of Health expands to become a multidisciplinary research agency.

**1949** *Physical Therapy Review* goes from bimonthly to monthly publication.

**1949** Florence and Henry Kendall publish *Muscles, Testing and Function*.

**1949** Army Air Corps becomes separate Air Force with its own independent physical therapy program.

**1950** School of Allied Medical Professions (SAMP) becomes first full-fledged school of allied health in the U.S.

**1950** Korean War begins.

**1950** Lucy Blair joins APTA as senior consultant to the Department of Professional Services.

**1951** World Congress on Physical Therapy holds its first formal planning session in Copenhagen. Mildred Elson

is elected organization's first president.
**1952** Jane Carlin becomes editor of *Physical Therapy Review*.
**1953** Allied Health Professional Training Act passed.
**1953** Section on Self-Employed (Private Practice) formed.
**1954** APTA develops seven-hour-long professional competency examination with help of Professional Examination Service and makes it available to state licensing boards.
**1955** PL 84-294 passes, giving men physical therapists equal status with women PTs in the military.
**1956** Knott and Voss collaborate on PNF text.
**1956** Salk Vaccine is introduced in massive vaccination program.
**1956** Public Health (Community Home Health) Section is formed.
**1956** Elson resigns and is succeeded by Mary Haskell.
**1957** The Physical Therapy Fund is established to further research.
**1958** The Bobaths first tour of the U.S.
**1958** National membership dues are raised to $25.
**1959** McMillan dies at 79.
**1959** "The Return" is produced and distributed.
**1959** Lucy Blair succeeds Anetta Cornell Wood as Executive Director.
**1960** Case Western Reserve University launches 2-year graduate program in physical therapy which will be phased out 11 years later.
**1961** Voss resigns as editor of the *Review* and Helen Hislop takes over. In observance of the Association's 4th anniversary, the *Review* publishes special issue including Gertrude Beard's engaging history entitled "Foundations For Growth."
**1962** *Review* changes name to the *Journal of Physical Therapy*.
**1962** National Foundation for Infantile Paralysis ends financial support of APTA and Catherine Worthingham leaves NFIP to commence an exhaustive "Study of Physical Therapy Education" with an Office of Vocational Rehabilitation grant.
**1963** McMillan Scholarship Fund is established.

**1963** Unionism issue surfaces, starting with New York Chapter.
**1964** Committee on Research formed.
**1964** First Mary McMillan Lecture delivered by Mildred Elson.
**1965** Section an Research organized.
**1965** Medicare legislation enacted.
**1966** First physical therapists go to Vietnam.
**1967** Foundations of PTA program laid.
**1967** First Lucy Blair Service Award winners named.
**1969** Blair resigns as Executive Director.
**1970** Temporary affiliate membership offered to physical therapy (later therapist) assistants and made permanent three years later.
**1970** Sections for State Licensure and Regulation (later Health Policy, Legislation, and Regulation) and for Administration formed.
**1970** Royce Noland becomes Executive Director of APTA. National office moves to Washington, D.C.
**1970** Signe Brunnström's techniques are described in *Movement Therapy in Hemiplegia*.
**1971** American Registry dissolved by AMA.
**1972** Joint Commission on Accreditation of Hospitals attempts to interpose physiatrists between PTs and primary care physicians.
**1973** Sports Physical Therapy Section formed.
**1973** NYU inaugurates first PhD program in physical therapy.
**1974** Pediatrics, Clinical Electrophysiology, and Orthopaedic Sections formed.
**1974** Howard University, Washington, D.C., establishes the first physical therapy department at a historically black college or university and graduates eight students.
**1975** Cardiopulmonary Section formed.
**1975** At the Annual Conference in Anaheim, CA, Helen Hislop delivers McMillan lecture entitled, "The Not So Impossible Dream."
**1976** First combined Sections Meeting held in Washington D.C.
**1976** American Registry disbanded.
**1976** House of Delegates revises "Essentials of an Acceptable School of Physical Therapy."
**1977** Council on Post-Secondary Accreditation (COPA) grants recognition to APTA as a second independent accrediting agency.
**1977** Obstetrics and Gynecology (later Women's Health) Section formed; Electrophysiology, Section formed.
**1978** Geriatrics Section formed.
**1978** "Plan to Foster Clinical Research" adopted. Mechanism on "Certification of Advanced Clinical Competency" established.
**1978** Marilyn Lister begins 10-year stint as Journal editor.
**1979** Foundation for Physical Therapy set up as successor to PT Fund.
**1980** Catherine Worthingham Fellows (FAPTA) established as a new category of membership, with Catherine Worthingham as its first recipient.
**1980** House of Delegates sets 1991 as target year for raising minimum entry level of education to postbaccalaureate degree. Bylaws amended to limit size of House to 400 delegates (revised upward in 1992 to 432).
**1980** Veterans Affairs Section established.
**1981** APTA establishes formal Archives for its own history.
**1981** First Foundation for Physical Therapy research grants awarded.
**1982** Hand Rehabilitation Physical Therapy Section established.
**1983** Oncology Section established.
**1983** APTA national office moves to new building in Alexandria, Virginia.
**1983** APTA becomes sole accrediting agency for physical therapy education programs.
**1985** First examinations for Specialist Certification held. Linda Crane, Scot Erwin, and Meryl Cohen receive Advanced Certification Cardiopulmonary Physical Therapy.
**1986** *P.T. Bulletin* is launched.
**1986** First Specialist Certification in Clinical Electrophysiology and Pediatrics are awarded.
**1987** First Specialist Certifications in Neurology and Sports Physical Therapy are awarded.
**1987** Prime Timers group is created.

**1987** William D. Coughlin named Chief Executive Officer of APTA.
**1988** Steven Rose takes over as *Journal* editor.
**1988** Setting of "Goals and Objectives" becomes part of APTA's annual self-review process.
**1988** APTA Office of Minority affairs created.
**1989** First Foundation undergraduate scholarships awarded.
**1988** TriAlliance of Health and Rehabilitation Professions established
**1989** First Specialist Certifications in Orthopedics awarded.
**1989** Upon Rose's death, Jules Rothstein succeeds to Journal editorship.
**1989** Bylaws are amended to establish Affiliate Assembly for PTAs.
**1990** Two major federal initiatives affect physical therapy profession: the Americans with Disabilities Act is passed and the National Center for Medical Rehabilitation Research is created.
**1991** Student Assembly formed.
**1992** First Specialist Certification in Geriatrics awarded.
**1992** APTA expands offices, purchasing second building in TransPotomac complex.
**1992** APTA administration reorganized into seven distinct operations.
**1992** Resource Center for Research and Learning established by House action.
**1993** *PT Magazine* launched, combining quarterly *Clinical Management* and monthly *Progress Report*.
**1993** First "Impact" Conference on Postbaccalaureate Entry-level curricula held. Creighton University, Omaha, Nebraska, inaugurates pioneer "professional" D.P.T. program.
**1993** First Foundation consensus conference held.
**1994** APTA creates Office of Women's Issues. Francis J. Mallon, Esq, succeeds Coughlan as Chief Executive Officer.
**1995** American Board of Physical Therapy Specialties inaugurates nationwide electronic testing.
**1995** World Confederation for Physical Therapy convenes in Washington, D.C.
**1995** APTA celebrates 75th anniversary of Association and profession.

## PAST PRESIDENTS OF THE AMERICAN PHYSICAL THERAPY ASSOCIATION

| | | | |
|---|---|---|---|
| MARY MCMILLAN<br>Boston, Massachusetts | 1921–1923 | MARGUERITE IRVINE<br>Seattle, Washington | 1949–1950 |
| INGA LOHNE<br>Boston, Massachusetts | 1923–1924 | MARY CLYDE SINGLETON<br>Durham, North Carolina | 1950–1952 |
| DOROTHEA M. BECK<br>Montclair, New Jersey | 1924–1926 | HARRIET S. LEE<br>Washington, DC | 1952–1954 |
| GERTRUDE BEARD<br>Chicago, Illinois | 1926–1928 | MARY E. NESBITT<br>Boston, Massachusetts | 1954–1956 |
| HAZEL E. FURSCOTT<br>San Francisco, California | 1928–1930 | E. JANE CARLIN<br>Jenkintown, Pennsylvania | 1956–1958 |
| EDITH MONRO<br>Boston, Massachusetts | 1930–1932 | AGNES P. SNYDER<br>San Antonio, Texas | 1958–1961 |
| MARGARET S. CAMPBELL<br>Chicago, Illinois | 1932–1934 | MARY ELIZABETH KOLB<br>Leetsdale, Pennsylvania | 1961–1967 |
| SARAH U. COLBY<br>Los Angeles, California | 1934–1936 | EUGENE MICHELS<br>Philadelphia, Pennsylvania | 1967–1973 |
| CONSTANCE K. GREENE<br>Boston, Massachusetts | 1936–1938 | CHARLES M. MAGISTRO<br>Pomona Valley, California | 1973–1976 |
| HELEN L. KAISER<br>Cleveland, Ohio | 1938–1940 | ROBERT C. BARTLETT<br>Durham, North Carolina | 1976–1979 |
| CATHERINE WORTHINGHAM<br>Stanford, California | 1940–1944 | DON W. WORTLEY<br>Salt Lake City, Utah | 1979–1982 |
| JESSIE L. STEVENSON<br>New York City, New York | 1944–1946 | ROBERT W. RICHARDSON<br>Pittsburgh, Pennsylvania | 1982–1985 |
| SUSAN G. ROEN<br>Los Angeles, California | 1946–1948 | JANE S. MATHEWS<br>Gloucester, Massachusetts | 1985–1991 |
| LOIS RANSOM<br>Washington, DC | 1948–1949 | MARILYN MOFFAT<br>Locust Valley, New York | 1991– |

## EXECUTIVE DIRECTORS

EVELYN ANDERSON MAY
*1944*

MILDRED O. ELSON
*1944-1956*

MARY E. HASKELL
*1956-1958*

ANNETTA CORNELL WOOD
*1958-1959*

LUCY BLAIR
*1959-1960 (Acting)*
*1960-1969*

ROYCE P. NOLAND
*1969-1985*

EUGENE MICHELS
*1985-1987 (Acting)*

WILLIAM D. COUGHLAN
*1987-1994*

FRANCIS J. MALLON
*1994-*

## EDITORS OF THE JOURNAL

ISABEL H. NOBLE
*March 1921*

ELIZABETH HUNTINGTON
*1921-1922*

ELIZABETH WELLS
*1922-1924*

FRANCES PHILO MOREAUX
*1924-1927*

DOROTHEA BECK
*1927-1933*

IDA MAY HAZENHYER
*1933-1936*

MILDRED O. ELSON
*1936-1945*

LOISE REINECKE
*1945-1950*

ELEANOR JANE CARLIN
*1950-1956*

SARA JANE HOUTZ
*1956-1958*

DOROTHY E. VOSS
*1958-1962*

HELEN J. HISLOP
*1962-1968*

MARILYN MOFFAT
*1968-1970*

ELIZABETH J. DAVIES
*1970-1976*

BARBARA C. WHITE
*1976-1978*

MARILYN J. LISTER
*1978-1988*

ROBERT L. LAMB
*February-June 1988 (Acting)*

STEVEN J. ROSE
*1988-1989*

ROBERT L. LAMB
REBECCA L. CRAIK
*June-September 1989 (Acting)*

JULES M. ROTHSTEIN
*1989-*

## RECIPIENTS OF HONORS AND AWARDS

### RECIPIENTS OF THE
### *Mary McMillan Scholarship Award*

**1963**
Patricia A. McFarland
Ellen McMahon

**1964**
Martha A. Krug
Martha E. Mitchell
Suzann K. Reetz

**1965**
Janet L. Kimmey
Margaret A. Rosenkranz

**1966**
Diane Richardson
Bettyann Hyde Shuert
Ruth Ver Mulm

**1967**
Elizabeth A. Hall
Carol Ann Masemore
Sandra Kay Wright

**1968**
Sarah Lee Goodwin
Linda C. Labrecque
Susan Meibuhr
Sue Ellen Schroeder
Kathryn Ann Steyer

**1969**
Joseph H. Azbell
Glenn D. Singer

**1970**
Marcia Clifford
Margaret Lister
Linda Smith

**1971**
Emilie Jo Kallenbach
Deborah Ann Love
Barbara Weidenfeld

**1972**
Jayne Forgey
Susan Gilchrist

Jeanne Guenther

**1973**
Joan Belding
Gerald S. Coleman
Frank J. Hielema

**1974**
Ann Marie Johnson
Patricia G. Shearer
Diane Marie Siwek

**1975**
Adele Griebling
James A. McCarthy
Anthony T. Valente

**1976**
Doris A. Bourek
Betty Ann Mahoney
Ronald W. Scott

**1977**
Joel D. Benn
Elaine Rice
Jessie Van Swearingen

**1978**
Leigh Craig Anderson
Nancy J. Ensley
Ellen Anne Mahony

**1979**
Debora M. Breindel
Barbara E. Hoth
Kathleen A. McDonald

**1980**
Pamela M. Dorner
Melinda Hong
David A. McCune
Jamie B. Thurmond

**1981**
Alan J. Edmundson
Daniel E. Erb
Nancy J. Liggett
Julie Piontek
Bradley Yeung

**1982**
Marci F. Becker
Carol J. Harris

Nancy Kulikowski
Debra L. Schlenoff
Elizabeth G. Schofield

**1983**
Bradley J. Beard
Linda Sue Hanson
Natalie Sue Olson
Margaret A. Sullivan
Regis H. Turocy

**1984**
Holly A. Black
Cathy M. Butler
Karen J. Ferris
Edelle V. Field
Esther M. Haskvitz
Bonita L. Jones
Birtha J. Moses
Gay M. Naganuma
Catherine C. Roy
Pamelia S. Williams

**1985**
Michual W. Coe
Sharon A. Fultz

Elva L. Gehrke
Ronnie D. Hald
Lynne D. Hirschman
Margaret E. McNamara
Donald A. Neumann
Elisabeth G. Rice
Henry G. Rodgers
Nancy L. Stoerker

**1986**
Mari Alison Bartee
Julie Virginia Burnett
Kay Cerny
James K. Eng
Sandra Louise Jensen
David E. Johnson
Cynthia Ann Olson
Nancy D. Tarum
Annette Dianne Vollan

**1987**
John O. Barr
Beverly Sue Farmer
Manuella J. Giannini

Melinda Sue Jackson
Kathleen J. Manella
Lois F. McKillen
Susan M. Sheely

**1988**
Mark Alan Anderson
Jeffrey R. Bresnahan
Tracey Ann Byrne
Laura D. Hill
James P. McCracken
Sheri L. Poffenbarger
William S. Quillen
Bryon A. Smith
Tammy L. Sosolik
Susan F. Summergrad

**1989**
Laurie Dawn Booher
Ronald Wayne Courson
Darci Cristoffels
Mary Josephine Curran
Louise Frangale Deal
Jody Shapiro Gandy

Joan Harris
Robert Michael Kellogg
Aimee Beth Klein
Loretta Knutson Lough
Lorraine M. McMahon
Kathleen O'Dwyer
Robert Jeffrey Parker
Ingrid Frances Sparrow
Michele S. Townshend
Susan L. Whitney

**1990**
Charlene Aamodt
Jose Miguel Aldea
Lynette K. Baroutsis
Carol Bowles
Katherine M. Concilus
Pamela W. Duncan
Jamie D. Gallegos
Mary Jo Geyer
Clare Barrett Gowen
Margaret M. Hickey
Cristina D. Keller

250    *Healing the Generations*

**RECIPIENTS OF HONORS AND AWARDS**

David L. Levine
Steven Loupee
Dawne Manista
Linner Mishler
Barbara J. Norton
Barbara Sanders
Jeanne E. Sturgeon
Tamra K. Taylor

**1991**
Bryon T. Ballantyne
William D. Bandy
Kathryn M. Carlucci
Karen A. Correia
Gary L. Drilling
Walter J. Eppich
Melissa M. Gilkison
Joseph L. Gostin
Caroline M. Knebel
Teresa Rector
Leslie N. Russek
Colleen Q. Scibetta
Guy G. Simoneau
Paul A. Ullucci, Jr.
Philip J. Zarri

**1992**
Anne H. Campbell
Sandra Lee Cassady
Jeannette Cornforth
Justine Ann DeLuccio
Marian Rose Graff
Carol L. Ickes
Nancy England Kingsbury
Margaret Martinovich
Pamela M. Jinkens Rimes
Linda S. Sanabria Roberts
Nancy Ann Robertson
Lisa Lynne Slattery
Marcia B. Smith
Lisa Marie Wagner

**1993**
Joseph Cigna
Virginia Mamie Cowan
Gail S. Effken
Lisa Marie Gawen
Stacy Lynn Hite
Karen S. Kubb
Laura J. LaPorta
Kurt B. Lundquist
Terry L. McGee
Deborah A. Nawoczenski
Terri Ann Puharic
Dorian Kay Rose
Jose Luis Santos
Vicki Anne Stemmons
Lillian Taliaferro
Stacy Lee Waits
Christopher Kevin Wong

**1994**
Susan Lynn Batenhoust
Rachel Lee DeVito
Bryan C. Heiderscheit
Sandra Lynn Hogeland
Elizabeth Mostrom
Stephen J. Ryan
Mark E. Swartz

**1995**
Christine Rich Archer
Ellen L. Buckley
Julie McClure Chandler
Julia Chevan
Debra Sue Daver
Andrew D. Frank
Linda Sue Larson
Kanuja Patel
Jill Ann Sandstedt
William J. Schwarz
Pamela P. Thomasson

**RECIPIENTS OF THE**
*Mary McMillan Lecture Award*

**1964**
Mildred O. Elson
**1965**
Catherine Worthingham
**1966**
Ruby Decker
**1967**
Emma E. Vogel
**1968**
Helen Kaiser
**1969**
Margaret Rood
**1971**
Lucy Blair
**1972**
Margaret Knott
**1973**
Lucille Daniels
**1975**
Helen J. Hislop
**1976**
Eleanor Jane Carlin
**1977**
Mary Clyde Singleton
**1978**
Margaret L. Moore
**1979**
Helen Blood
**1980**
Florence P. Kendall
**1981**
Susanne Hirt
**1982**
Dorothy E. Voss
**1983**
Nancy T. Watts
**1984**
Eugene Michels
**1985**
Geneva R. Johnson
**1986**
Dorothy Pinkston
**1987**
Charles M. Magistro
**1989**
Ruth Wood

**1990**
L. Don Lehmkuhl
**1991**
Robert C. Bartlett
**1992**
Marylou R. Barnes
**1993**
Gary L. Soderberg

**RECIPIENTS OF THE**
*Marian Williams Award for Research in Physical Therapy*

**1965**
Signe Brunnström
**1967**
Mary Pat Murray
**1969**
Catherine Worthingham
**1973**
Dean P. Currier
**1978**
Gary L. Smidt
**1980**
Steven L. Wolf
**1986**
Shirley A. Sahrmann
**1988**
Gary L. Soderberg
**1989**
Fay Horak
**1991**
Suzann K. Campbell
**1992**
Susan R. Harris
**1993**
Alan M. Jette
**1994**
Joan M. Walker

**RECIPIENTS OF THE**
*Golden Pen Award*

**1965**
Jacquelin Perry
Ronald W. Lamont-Havers
**1966**
Clara Arrington
**1967**
Dorothy Briggs
(POSTHUMOUSLY)
**1969**
Helen J. Hislop
**1972**
Barbara Kent
**1973**
Marvin Tanigawa
**1974**
Mary Clyde Singleton
**1976**
Beverly Bishop

**1977**
Elizabeth Davies Carruth
Eugene Michels
**1978**
Suzann K. Campbell
**1979**
Barbara C. White
**1981**
Otto D. Payton
Dean P. Currier
**1982**
Bella J. May
Louis R. Amundsen
**1983**
Steven L. Wolf
**1984**
Gary L. Smidt
Gary L. Soderberg
**1985**
Barbara H. Connolly
**1986**
Joyce L. MacKinnon
**1987**
Ruth B. Purtilo
**1988**
Marilyn J. Lister
**1989**
Katherine F. Shepard
Jules M. Rothstein
**1990**
Robert L. Lamb
Steven J. Rose
(POSTHUMOUSLY)
**1991**
John L. Echternach
**1992**
Anthony Delitto
**1993**
Stephen M. Haley
**1994**
David Edward Krebs
**1995**
Lynn Snyder-Mackler

**RECIPIENTS OF THE**
*Lucy Blair Service Award*

**1969**
Lucy Blair
**1971**
Elizabeth C. Addoms
Clara Arrington
Gertrude Beard
Edna M. Blumenthal
Joseph M. Breuer
Shirley M. Cogland
Mary Lou Fritz
Constance Greene
Frank T. Hazelton
Dorothy G. Hoag
Jessica A. Hopkins
Muriel Kelly

Florence P. Kendall
Margaret Knott
Mary MacDonald
Margaret L. Moore
Dorothy E. Voss
Barbara C. White
Elizabeth C. Wood
Catherine Worthingham
**1972**
Eleanor Jane Carlin
Emmy Kylin
George K. Makechnie
Roxie Klema Morris
Agnes P. Snyder
**1974**
Eugene Michels
Rae M. Litaker
Dorothy E. Baethke
Frances C. Ekstam
Dorothy Frederickson
**1975**
Helen Blood
Wilbur R. Gregory
Beatrice F. Schulz
Kathryn J. Shaffer
Martha C. Wroe
**1976**
Ruby Decker
Ruth Wood
Fred M. Rutan
**1977**
Norma Fisher
Charles M. Magistro
Kathryn E. Phillips
Jeanne M. Schenck
Mary Clyde Singleton
Evelyn Walter
**1978**
James Clinkingbeard
Robert J. Hickok
Frederick A. Monaco
Inez Peacock
Dorothy Pinkston
**1979**
Ernest A. Burch, Jr.
Marjorie N. Stamm
**1980**
Marilyn J. Anderson
Robert C. Bartlett
Eleanor Flanagan Branch
Betty C. Canan
Anthony J. DeRosa
Dorothy Hewitt
Helen K. Hickey
Thelma M. Holmes
Richard V. McDougall
Helen V. Skowlund
**1981**
Jean C. Bailey
Susan Collopy
Joyce M. Flaig
Robert L. Gossett
Robert Harden
Margaret Kohli
James B. McKillip
Doris E. Porter

Thelma Pedersen
Mary Elizabeth Rexroad
Shirley Sahrmann
Virginia Wilson
**1982**
Leon Anderson
Mary E. Bennett
Roberta F. Cottman
Lucille Daniels
Sally Farrand
Paul L. Ferrara
D. LaVonne Jaeger
Nancy C. Keating
Bella J. May
Claire F. McCarthy
Mable M. Parker
Frankie L. Patton
Marilyn Moffat Salant
**1983**
Richard E. Darnell
Sally C. Edelsberg
Samuel B. Feitelberg
Jeanne L. Fischer
Geneva R. Johnson
Barbara E. Kent
Colleen M. Kigin
L. Don Lehmkuhl
Charlene M. Nelson
John W. Robinson
Steven J. Rose
Sarah Semans
Catherine Perry Wilkinson
**1984**
Justin Alexander
James A. Armour
Stanley L. Arno
O. Kennett Ball
Mary Eleanor Brown
Kay A. Clinkingbeard
Elaine M. Eckel
Jay M. Goodfarb
Clarence W. Hultgren
Marjory Wilson Johnson
Isobel L. Knoepfli
Eugene R. Lambert
Phyllis Srybnik Lehman
Jay S. Schleichkorn
Frances M. Tappan
David R. Weiler
**1985**
Robert E. Ayers
Clara P. Bright
Vilma I. Evans
Charles H. Hall
Joan M. Mills
James M. Morrow
Jean L. Roland
Peter A. Towne
**1986**
Robert L. Babbs, Jr.
Hyman L. Dervitz
Simon J. Dykstra
Carolyn B. Heriza
Barry R. Howes
Robert A. Teckemeyer
Helen Holzum Whealen

**1987**
Barbara J. Bradford
John L. Echternach
Dale H. Fitch
Helen J. Hislop
Elizabeth L. Lamberton
Betty R. Landen
Gary L. Soderberg
Ann L. Walker
**1988**
Marylou R. Barnes
Lucy J. Buckley
Susanne Hirt
Carolyn Hultgren
Otto Payton
Mable B. Sharp
Ellen F. Spake
Jeanette Winfree
**1989**
Frank L. Allender
Aurelie P. Babbitt
Andrew A. Guccione
Ruth U. Mitchell
Robert W. Richardson
Rodney W. Schlegel
Rosemary M. Scully
**1990**
Otto A. Cordero
Rebecca L. Craik
Patricia Rae Evans
Royce P. Noland
Beverly J. Schmoll
Mildred L. Wood
Lynda Woodruff
Patricia Yarbrough
**1991**
Mary S. Bowser
Carolyn A. Crutchfield
Carol M. Davis
M. Claudette Finley
Robert L. Lamb
Marilyn J. Lister
Patricia C. Montgomery
John B. Wadsworth
**1992**
Bonnie M. Blossom
Linda D. Crane
Laurita M. Hack
Harry G. Knecht
Glory Y. Sanders
Ann F. VanSant
Cynthia C. Zadai
**1993**
Carolyn L. Bloom
Jack D. Close, Sr.
Donna Joy El-Din
Marilyn R. Gossman
Jacqueline Montgomery
Joan Carol Nethery
Katherine F. Shepard
Jane K. Sweeney
**1994**
John O. Barr
Corinne T. Ellingham
Bette Horstman
Scot Irwin
Donald Jackson

Mary Ann Wharton
Don W. Wortley
**1995**
Susan S. Deusinger
Larry P. Fronheiser
Neva F. Greenwald
Dorothy Nelson
Eric D. Reuss
Jane M. Walter

**RECIPIENTS OF THE**
*Dorothy Briggs Memorial Scientific Inquiry Award*

**1970**
Mary Elizabeth Lucas
**1971**
Eugene Michels
**1972**
Martha Anne Clendenin
Shelby J. Clayson
**1973**
Nancy Urbscheit
**1974**
John B. Wadsworth
**1976**
Ronald Bugaj
**1977**
Robert M. Kantner
**1978**
Douglas D. Ely
**1979**
Jeffrey G. Rothman
Margaret Ely Pringle
**1980**
Nancy I. Kemp
Carol A. Scholz
**1981**
Carol B. Loria
Karen Kendrick Claunch
**1982**
Ellen L. Curry
**1983**
Catherine A. Hinton
**1984**
Charity Ann Johansson
D. Joyce White
**1985**
Mark W. Cornwall
Robin M. Vili
**1986**
Patricia C. Montgomery
Megan Binder Quain
Teresa M. Steffen
**1987**
Stephen M. Haley
Anthony C. Oliveri
John O. Barr
**1988**
Ann Woodward Krause
Deborah E. Lechner
Thomas M. Mohr

## RECIPIENTS OF HONORS AND AWARDS

**1989**
Stanley N. Garn
Carolyn Heriza
**1990**
M. Kathleen Kelly
**1991**
Josette A. Bettany
**1992**
Carol I. Leiper
Janet Collins Siegel
Elaine J. Tripp
**1993**
Patricia Griegel-Morris
Krissann Mueller-Klaus
Keith Taylor
Irene R. McEwen
**1995**
Heidi J. Indergand
Diane U. Jette

### RECIPIENTS OF THE
*Minority Recruitment and Services Award*

**1974**
Georgia State University
**1976**
University of Florida
**1977**
University of Florida
**1979**
University of South Carolina
**1981**
Georgia State University
**1982**
University of Connecticut
**1983**
Essex County College

### RECIPIENTS OF THE
*Jack Walker Award*

**1978**
Mary L. Baker
**1979**
Terry Hoskins Michel
**1980**
Louis R. Amundsen
**1981**
Terry R. Malone
**1982**
Susan E. Alvarez
**1983**
Sandy Moore

**1984**
Lucinda L. Baker
**1985**
Phyllis C. Wright
**1986**
Louise C. Grim
**1987**
Joyce L. MacKinnon
**1988**
David R. Sinacore
**1989**
Dolores B. Bertoti
**1990**
Julianne Wright Howell
**1991**
Michael T. Cibulka
**1992**
James A. Birke
**1994**
Judy Carmick
**1995**
Kathleen Gill-Body

### RECIPIENTS OF THE
*Dorothy E. Baethke– Eleanor J. Carlin Award for Excellence in Academic Teaching*

**1981**
Eleanor Jane Carlin
**1982**
Jo Ann Clelland
**1983**
Marianne E. McDonald
**1984**
Carolyn Ann Crutchfield
**1985**
Mary Clyde Singleton
**1986**
Shirley A. Stockmeyer
**1987**
David H. Nielsen
**1988**
Katherine F. Shepard
**1989**
Nancy T. Watts
**1990**
Darlene M. Hertling
**1991**
Pamela A. Catlin
**1992**
Mary P. Watkins
**1994**
George J. Davies

**1995**
Neal E. Pratt

### RECIPIENTS OF THE
*Chattanooga Research Award*

**1981**
James E. Griffin
**1982**
Carol I. Leiper
**1983**
Carmella Gonnella
**1984**
Dean P. Currier
**1985**
Maureen K. Holden
**1986**
Dale R. Fish
**1987**
Carl G. Kukulka
**1988**
Mary Kate McDonnell
**1989**
Luther C. Kloth
**1990**
Michael A. Smutok
**1991**
Claire Peel
**1992**
Bella J. May
**1993**
Robert J. Palisano
**1994**
Louise A. Mollinger
**1995**
Karen W. Hayes

### RECIPIENTS OF THE
*Henry O. and Florence P. Kendall Practice Award*

**1981**
Miriam J. Partridge
**1982**
Marlin N. Shields
**1983**
Martha C. Wroe
**1984**
Sarah Semans
**1985**
Charles M. Magistro
**1986**
Lyle Emery
**1987**
Jeanne L. Fischer

**1988**
Gerald N. Lampe
**1989**
Peter Towne
**1990**
Robert Green
**1991**
Rodney W. Schlegel
**1992**
H. Duane Saunders
**1993**
Susan J. Isernhagen
**1995**
Carmen Abril

### *Catherine Worthingham Fellows of the APTA*

**1982**
Catherine Worthingham
**1983**
Helen J. Hislop
Geneva R. Johnson
**1984**
L. Don Lehmkuhl
Mary Pat Murray
**1985**
Steven J. Rose
**1986**
Florence P. Kendall
Eugene Michels
Dorothy Pinkston
Shirley Sahrmann
Nancy T. Watts
**1987**
Suzann K. Campbell
Gary L. Smidt
Steven L. Wolf
**1988**
Gary L. Soderberg
**1989**
Susan R. Harris
Ruth B. Purtilo
Katherine F. Shepard
**1990**
Mary Eleanor Brown
Charles M. Magistro
Marilyn Moffat
Arthur J. Nelson
Laura K. Smith
Ruth Wood
**1991**
Richard E. Darnell
Carmella Gonnella
Marilyn R. Gossman
**1992**
Helen Blood
Ernest A. Burch, Jr.

John L. Echternach
Bella J. May
Rosemary M. Scully
**1993**
Robert C. Bartlett
Otto D. Payton
Martha C. Wroe
**1994**
Marylou R. Barnes
Jules M. Rothstein
**1995**
Rebecca L. Craik
Mary M. Edmonds
Beverly Jean Schmoll
Jane M. Walter

### RECIPIENTS OF THE
*Minority Achievement Award*

**1985**
University of Puerto Rico, San Juan
**1987**
Georgia State University
**1989**
University of Connecticut
**1992**
Langston University
**1994**
Florida International University
**1995**
Marquette University

### RECIPIENTS OF THE
*Minority Initiatives Award*

**1985**
University of Connecticut
**1986**
State University of New York at Stony Brook
**1987**
Florida A&M University
**1988**
Florida International University
**1989**
University of Pittsburgh
**1990**
New York University
**1991**
Marquette University
**1995**
Temple University

### RECIPIENTS OF THE
*Signe Brunnström Award for Excellence in Clinical Teaching*

**1987**
Linda A. Simonsen
**1988**
Kathleen J. Manella
**1989**
Madeleine A. Baker
**1990**
Carolyn Berner Kelly
**1991**
Mary C. Sinnott
**1992**
Anne-Marie Sirois
**1993**
Joanne Whipple
**1995**
Beverly J. Devine

### RECIPIENTS OF THE
*Margaret L. Moore Award for Outstanding New Academic Faculty Member*

**1990**
Carol A. Giuliani
**1991**
Michael T. Gross
Lawrence G. Pan
**1992**
Irene R. McEwen
**1993**
James E. Gordon
**1995**
Deborah S. Nichols

### RECIPIENTS OF THE
*Eugene Michels New Investigator Award*

**1990**
George E. Carvell
**1991**
Donald A. Neumann
**1992**
Carolee J. Winstein
**1993**
Stuart Binder-Macleod
**1994**
Lynn Snyder-Mackler
**1995**
Michael J. Mueller

### RECIPIENTS OF THE
*Minority Scholarship Award for Academic Excellence*

**1988**
Steven D. Newton
**1989**
Elizabeth Bluebird
**1990**
Altrece A. Arnold
Rose Del Valle
Sarah John
Laura A. McKown
**1991**
Melinda Johnson
Juanita McDavid
Kelly Ryujin
Sonya Sconiers
**1992**
Samuel T. Anaya
Becky Ann Gamino
Kimi Hasegawa
Linda Sanabria-Roberts
Darlene Y. Robinson
Joy Denise Worrell
**1993**
Maria P. Rettig
Christopher Kevin Wong
Coleen L. Dodson
Carolina A. Candelaria
Cornelio M. Pasquil
**1994**
Celeste W. Brown
James E. Trimble
Oscar Esqueda, Jr.
Anita M. Calvillo-Dietz
Denise Gobert
**1995**
Susana Areciga
Luis Hincapie
Erika Lee
Richard Nez
Stephanie West

### RECIPIENTS OF THE
*Helen J. Hislop Award for Outstanding Contributions to Professional Literature*

**1992**
Jay S. Schleichkorn
**1993**
Steven L. Wolf
**1994**
Joan M. Walker

**1995**
Neil I. Spielholz

### *Honorary Members*

**1936**
Charles LeRoy Lowman
**1947**
Melbourne G. Westmoreland
**1956**
Mildred O. Elson
**1964**
Constance Greene
**1965**
Frances A. Hellebrandt
**1966**
Walter P. Blount
Ernst Fischer
**1967**
John L. Caughey
Emma E. Vogel
**1968**
Alfred Riva Shands, Jr.
**1969**
Sarah S. Rogers
Lucy Blair
**1971**
Florence Linduff Knowles
Lister Hill
**1972**
Clara Arrington
Helen Kaiser
Jacquelin Perry
Catherine Worthingham
**1975**
Robert G. Dicus
William Darwin Paul
**1977**
Agnes P. Snyder
**1979**
Berta Bobath
Karel Bobath
**1981**
Beverly F. Bishop
James Cyriax
Robin McKenzie
**1985**
Albert B. Sabin
Jonas E. Salk
**1991**
Per-Olaf Astrand
Mark Mueller
**1992**
Patrick J. Ford
Geoffrey D. Maitland
Janet G. Travell

# Index

(**BOLD** listings indicate photograph)

### A
Abbott, Edville, 37, 44
*Activities of Daily Living*, 202
Addoms, Elizabeth, 132, 142, 203
Adkins, Hazel, 107
Allender, Frank, 209
Adler, Sue, 166-167
Allied Council. *See* National Council on Rehabilitation
Allied Health, 194-195
Allied Health Professions Training Act, 194
Alpine light treatment, 90, **90**
American Board of Physical Therapy Specialties, 200, 220
American Congress of Physical Medicine, 210
American Congress of Physical Therapy, 86
American Electro-Therapeutic Association, 25, 29, 47
American Expeditionary Force (AEF) hospitals, 44, 47, 58, 68
American Hospital Association, 212
American Medical Association (AMA), 76, 80, 81, 82, 212-213; Council on Physical Therapy, 82, 83, 85, 86, 93, 117
American Occupational Therapy Association (AOTA), 240
American Physical Therapy Association: Annual Conference, 76, 79, 120, 178, 179, 189, 190, 191, **209**, 215; Board of Directors, 207, 208, 213; chapters, 79, 80, 92; Combined Sections Meeting, 198, 209; Constitution and Bylaws, 72, 74, 75, 92, 93, 101; emblem, 86, 133; Executive Committee, 71, 93; executive director position, 130; executive secretary position, 101; governance structure and reorganization, 121, 198, 216-221, 230; House of Delegates, 121, 188, 191, 192, 197, 199, 200, 210, 211, 215; incorporation, 86; insignia, 190, 190, **193**; membership, 72-75, 92, 98, 103, 105, 139; national office, 120, 130, 154, 220, **224**; CEO position, 230; origins, 70, 77; professional title; 86; 71, 133. *See also* Association Awards; Association Divisions, Sections, and Committees
American Physiotherapy Association (APA). *See* American Physical Therapy Association
American Registry of Physical Therapists, 140-141
American Registry of Physical Therapy Technicians (ARPTT), 102
American Society of Allied Health Professionals, 195
American Women's Physical Therapeutic Association (AWPTA). *See* American Physical Therapy Association
American Registry of Physical Therapists, 140-141, 210
American Society of Allied Helath Professionals, 212
Anderson, Leon, *222*
Andry, Nicolas, 10, 11
Army Medical Specialist Corps (AMSC), 137, **138**, **146-147**, 148, 149
Arrington, Clara "Sonny," 152, 153, 170
Association awards, 242; Award for Minority Enhancement, 243; Award of Excellence for Minority Recruitment and Services, 214; Award for Excellence in Clinical Training, 174; Catherine A. Worthingham Fellow, 203; Chattanooga Research Award, 243; Doctoral Research Awards, 226; Dorothy Briggs Memorial Scientific Inquiry Award, 214; Eugene Michels New Investigator Award, 244; Golden Pen Award, 214; Gold Key Award, 127; Helen J. Hislop Award, 244; Henry O. and Florence P. Kendall Practice Award, 243; Jack Walker Award, 214; Lucy Blair Service Award, 208, 214, 229, 235; McMillan Scholarships, 177; Major Mary Elizabeth Lucas Award, 214; Margaret L. Moore Award for Outstanding New Faculty Members, 243; Marian Williams Award for Research in Physical Therapy, 213; Mary McMillan Lecture Award, **204**, 213; Minority Achievement Award, 243; Minority Initiative Award, 243
Association Divisions, Sections, and Committees: Administration Section, 198; Cardiopulmonary Section, 198; Clinical Electrophysiology Section, 198; Committee on Education and Publicity, 83, 85; Committee on Research, 188-190; Community Home Health Section, 153; Constitutional Revisions Committee, 101; Curriculum Revisions Committee, 138; Department of Minority Affairs, 230; Division of Professional Services, 192; Education Section, 122,137, 231; Geriatrics Section, 198; Health Policy and Practice Division, 236; International Affairs Department, 230; Judicial Committee, 207; Neurology Section, 198; Obstetrics and Gynecology Section, 198; Office of Vocational Rehabilitation (OVR), 146; Office of Women's Issues, 242; Orthopaedic Section, 198; Pediatrics Section, 198; Private Practice Section, 153; Research Section, 189; Sports Physical Therapy Section, 198; Standing Committee on Licensing, 93; Standing Committee on Public Laws, 141; State Licensure and Regulation Section, 198
Asklund, Shirley, 197
Ayers, Robert, 198
Ayres, Anna Jean, 168-169

### B
Baethke, Dorothy, 137, 242
Baker, Mary, 214
Barden-LaFollette Act, 146
Bartlett, Robert C. "Bob," 191, 209, **212**, 212, 225, 232, **240**
Baruch, Bernard, 130, 131
Baruch, Simon, 31, 32, **32.**
Base Hospital #8, 61, **61**
Basmajian, J.V., 187, 188
Battle Creek Medical and Surgical Sanitarium, 27, 33, 85
Battle Creek Normal School of Physical Education, 19, 47, 61
Baxter, Metta, 116, 118
Beard, Gertrude, 87, **87**, 88, 125, 183
Beck, Dorothea, 74, 80, 81, **81**, 86, 88
Bell, Josephine, 52, 75
Bennett, William, 16, 43
Benson, Herbert, 188
Black, Joseph, 233
Blair, Lucy, 98, 99, 133, 144, 155, 158-160, **161**,178-180, **178**, 206, 207
Blood, Helen, 196, 197, 222
Blumenthal, Edna, 119, 146, 164, 169
Bobath, Berta "Berti," 168, 169-171
Bobath, Karel, 169-171
Bolton Bill (Public Law 78-350), 111
Boston Children's Hospital (BCH), 19, 35, 73, **73**, **89**, 127, 128, 143, 163
Boston Normal School of Gymnastics, 19, 50, 81
Boston School of Physical Education, 19, 47, 50, 80, 85
Boutros, Henry, 220
Bouvé-Boston, 19, 100, 107
Bouvé, Marjorie, 19, 50
Brackett, Elliott, 19, 44, 46, 52, 62, 71, 76, 134
Bradford, Barbara, 197
Bradford, Edward H., 37, 38
Bradley, Helen, 61, 68
Brake, John, 198
Briggs, Dorothy, 188
Bright, Clara, 198
British Orthopaedic Association, 16
Brooke General Hospital. *See* Fort Sam Houston Station Hospital
Brown, Jefferson, **101**
Brown, Mary Eleanor, 132, 147-148, 173, 202, 243
Brunnström, Signe, 35, 110, 111, 132, 146, 147, 168, 171-174, **175**, 203, 214, 243
Burch, Ernie, 232
Burney, Leroy. *See* U.S. Army Surgeon General

### C
Campbell, Margaret S.,
Campbell, Suzann, 225
Canadian Physiotherapy Association, 160, 167
Carlin, Eleanor Jane, 107, 137, 139, 144, 154, **164**, 242
Cardiopulmonary Certified Specialty (CCS), 201
Carpenter, Cheryl, 219
Case Western Reserve University, 200, 204
Castleman, Mary Lee, 109, 113
Caton, Richard, 25, 26
Central nervous system (CNS) disorders, 162, 168
Cerebral palsy (CP), 11, 100, 101, 163-168
*Chapters Bulletin*, 209
Chartered Society of Physiotherapists (Society of Trained Masseuses), 6, 13, 21, 41-42, 76, 92, 167
Children's Rehabilitation Center. Athens, **122**
Cirullo, Judy, 220
Civil Service Commission, 44
Civil War, 36, 37
*Clinical Management in Physical Therapy*, 236
Coalition for Health Advocacy and Recruiting Minorities (CHARM), 213
Cohen, Meryl, 200, **220**
Colby, Sarah U., 99, **99**, **101**
Columbia University, 19; School of Physical Therapy, 142; Teachers College, 47, 52, 81
Coolidge, President Calvin, 78
Connolly, Jerome, 230
Corbusier, Harold, 71, 72, 183
Corrective therapists (CTs), 140
Cossoy, Barbara, 191
Cotting School, 38, **38**
Coughlan, William D., **223**, 228
Coulter, John Stanley, 89, 90, 102, 105, 106, 183
Council of Physical Therapy School Directors, 138, 185
Council on Medical Education and Hospitals, 210, 212
Couster, Wout, **223**
Covalt, Donald, 203
Craik, Rebecca, 225, 235
Crane, Linda, 200, **220**
Crothers, Bronson, 163-165
Crowell, Minerva, 55, 80
Currier, Dean, 198
Crutchfield, Carolyn, 200
Cushing, Harvey, 74

### D
D. T. Watson School of Physiatrics, 86, 159, 160, 180, 181
Daffron, Margot, 217
Daniels, Lucille, 96, 142, 222
Davies, Lt. Col. Elizabeth, 208
Day, William Lee, **227**
Deaver, George, 132, 147, 172, 202, 203
Decker, Ruby, 61, 204
deGregorio, Fred, 225
DeHaven, George, 198
Department of Health, Education and Welfare, 184
Depression, Great, 94, 98, 99
DeRosa, Anthony, 150, 191
Dervitz, Hy, 191
Diathermy, 29, 30, 48, **48**, 67
Dixon, Routh, **108**
Doctors of Osteopathy (D.O.s), 15
Donner, Mia H., 50, **50**, 65, 66
Dorando, Charles, 193, 196
Dowtin, Brenda, 217
Drinker, Philip, 98, 156
DuBois-Reymond, Emil, 23, 25
Duchenne, Guillaume, 23, **23**, 24
Dunleavy, Jim, 220
Dynomometers; Salter one-handed, 14; Graeme Hamond's, 14

### E
Earhart, Alice, **108**
Easter Seal Society, The. *See* National Easter Seal Society
Edwards, Ens. Betty, 112, **112**
Education, physical therapy: curricula, 75, 77; educational standards, 78, 79, 83; Post-baccalaureate certificate programs,

*Index* 253

137; Post-baccalaureate education, 231, 232, 234; scholarship drives, 129; tuition, 129; War Emergency Training Courses, 40, 45, 47, 50, 53, 54, 58, 65, 73, 83, **104**, 106, 107, 108;
Eischen, Clem, 192, **192**
Eisenhower, President Dwight D., 147
Elders, Joycelyn. *See* U.S. Army Surgeon General
Electrotherapy, 21, 22, 23, 24, 25, 67, 91. *See also* Diathermy
Elson, Mildred O., 97, 99, 125, 130, 135, 136, 141, 142-143, **142**, 144, 148, 153, **161**, 177, 182, 222, 213
Emery, Michael, 225
Emory University, Rehabilitation Research and Training Center, 187-188, 214
Enwemeka, Chukuka, 225
Evans, Vilma, 150, **151**, 152, 158
Exercise therapy, 7, 10, 11, 13, 14, 18, 90-91; hydrogymnastics, 32; resistive exercise, **41**

**F** Feitelberg, Sam, 111, 191, 192, 232
Fisher, Bella Abramowitz, 116, **116**, **117**
Fitzsimons General Hospital, 72, **72**
Flickinger, Mary, 109, 110
Foreign-trained program, 180
Fort Huachuca Station Hospital, 107
Fort Sam Houston Station Hospital (Brooke General Hospital), **48**, 51, 61, 63, **63**, 68
Fort Sheridan, 70, **71**, 81
Forward, Edna, 187
Foundation for Physical Therapy (Physical Therapy Fund), 144, 209, 214, 215, 225, 226, 227, 228
Franklin, Benjamin, 22, **22**
Frenkel, H. S., 13, 14
Freud, Sigmund, 163
Friz, Lt. Col. Barbara Robertson, 150
Furscott, Hazel E., 72, 77, 79, 87, 93, **93**

**G** Gaither, Ann, **108**
Garrison, Tricia, 219
Georgia Warm Springs Foundation, 95, **95**, 97, 98
Gillespie, Eleanor, 89
Goldthwait, Joel, 44, 46-47, 50, 52, 60, 67, 74, 80, 183
Gonella, Carmella, 160, 187, 189, 204
Gorgas, William. *See* U.S. Army Surgeon General
Gossman, Marilyn, 225, 232
*Government Relations Bulletin*, 209
Graham, Douglas, 15, 17
Granger, Frank B., 47, 50, 51, 60, 62, 68, 71, 72, 76, 78, 80
Graves, Dorothy, 159
Green, Fern, **108**
Green, Leila Holly, **108**, 170
Greenbank Home for Crippled Children, 43
Greene, Constance K., 61, 100, **100**
Griffin, G.V.M., **161**
Griffin, James, 243
Grunewald, Lucile, 84, **101**
Gwyer, Janet, 227

**H** Haley, Stephen, 225
Harden, Bob, 197
Harmon, Ann, **108**
Harmon, Georgianna, 160
Harvard Medical School, 47; Course 441, 73, 85, 87; Course 442, 76, 80, 85, 134
Hall, Mary Alderman, **108**
Haskell, Mary E., 144, 153, **153**, 155, 158-159
Hazenhyer, Ida May, 89, 93, 101, 102, 103, 128, 132
Health care financing, 222
Heliotherapy (artificial and natural), 26, 27, **27**, 90, 91
Hemenway, Mary, 19
Hickock, Robert, 215
Hill-Burton Act. *See* Hospital Survey and Construction Act
Hillebrandt, Frances, 144

Hines, Harry M., 144
Hippocrates, 7, 8, 22
Hirschberg, Rubens, 13, 14
Hislop, Helen, 138, 180-182, 181, 185, 188, 193, 199, 204, 211, 215, 242
Hitchcock, Lena, 56, 57
Hofkosh, Jack, 150, 203
Holmes, Thelma, 196
Homans, Amy, 19, 70
Homeopathy, 25
Horak, Fay, 225
Hospital Survey and Construction Act, 145
Hubbard, Carl, 97
Hubbard, Leroy, 95, 96
Hubbard tank, 97, **97**
Hultgren, Carolyn, 230
Huntington, Elizabeth, 55, 75, 77
Hydrotherapy, **9**, 10, **10**, 30, 31, 32, 33, **33**, **51**, 65, 91; contrast bath, 66; paraffin bath, 66-67
Hygenic Institute and School of Physical Culture. *See* Sargent School

**I** Incorporated Society of Trained Masseuses. *See* Chartered Society of Physiotherapists
*In Good Hands*, 21
Institute of Physical Medicine and Rehabilitation, 203
Industrial Physical Therapy, 43, 238
Ionta, Margaret, 129
Ionta, Marjorie, 129, 168
Iron lung, 98, 156, **156**
Irvine, Marguerite, 54, 55, 144
Irwin, Scot, 198, 200, 220

**J** Jackson, Wilmotine, 152
Jackson-Wyatt, Osa, 198
Jacobs, Miriam, 159, **161**
James Whitcomb Riley Hospital, 164, 174
Johnson, Geneva, 148, 195, 234, 242
Joint Commission on Accreditation of Hospitals (JCAH), 142, 211
Jones, Maj. Elizabeth, 149
Jones, Sir Robert, 16, 43, 44, 51
*Journal of the American Physical Therapy Association*. *See* *Physical Therapy, the Journal of the American Physical Therapy Association*

**K** Kabat, Herman, 165
Kabat-Kaiser Institute for Neuromuscular Rehabilitation, 166
Kaiser Foundation, 162, 167
Kaiser, Helen L., **106**, 172, 121, 122, **122**
Kaiser, Henry, 165
Kaiser, Henry, Jr., 165
Kaiser Rehabilitation Center. *See* Kaiser Foundation
Kalish, Ruth, 187
Kellogg, John Harvey, 19, 26, 27, **28**
Kellogg light cabinet, 27
Kelly, Muriel, 208
Kendall, Florence Peterson, 35, 98, 100, 125, 126, 155-156, 232, 242
Kendall, Henry, 35, 95, 100, 125, 126, 155-156, 242
Kenny, Elizabeth "Sister," 123-125, **125**, 123-128, 155, 157, 165
Kessler, Henry, 171-172
Kessler Institute of Rehabilitation, 171-172
Klenzak brace, 97
Klenzak, John, 96, 97
Knapp, Miland, 127
Knott, Margaret "Maggie," **162**, 166-168, 176
Kolb, Mary Elizabeth, "Mary Lib," 142, 180, **180**, 191, 197, 206
Krasnye, J. F., 78, 79
Krusen, Frank, 171, 127
Kuehlthau, Brunetta, 117
Kuckhoff, F. A., 207

**L** Lamb, Robert, 234
Lambert, Margaret, 220
Lamont-Havers, Ronald, 214
Lawrence, Maj. Mary, 120
Lawton, Edith Buchwald, 142, 203
Lee, Col. Harriet S., 149, 150
Legion of Merit, 113, 116
Legg, Arthur T., 73
Lehmkuhl, Don, 189
Letterman General Hospital, 45, 72, 77, 82, 93
Licensing and credentialing, 93, 102
Ling, Pehr Henrik, 12
Ling System. *See* Swedish Movement Treatment
Lippitt, Louisa, 52, 55
Lister, Marilyn, 234
Little, Elizabeth, 174, **228**
Little, William John, 11, 163
Little's Disease. *See* Cerebral Palsy
Long, Lillian, 142
Lohne, Inga, 52, 53, **53**, 59, 60, 77
Los Angeles Children's Hospital, 85
Los Angeles Orthopedic Hospital, 94
Lovett, Robert W., 19, 35, 37, 73, 94, 95, 96
Lowman, Charles, 94, 95
Lucas-Championnière, Just Marie Marcelin, 16, 17, 44, 60

**M** Magistro, Charles, 140, 209, **211**, 212, 215, 225, **240**
Mahoney, Helena, 96, 97
Mallon, Francis J. "Frank," 220, 223, 224, 241, **241**
Marks, A. A., 36
*Massage and Therapeutic Exercise*, 70, 74-75, **75**
Massage treatment, 7, 8, **8**, 10, 11, 16, 17, 27; "Rubbers," 9, 11, 17; spinal manipulations, 15, 16
Mathews, Jane S., 228, **231**, **240**
May, Andrew Jackson, 105
McAllister, Carroll, 82
McDonald, Harriet, 55, 59
McGarrett, Adelaide, 164, 222
McGregor, Paula, 239
McMillan, Mary Livingston "Mollie", 6, **6**, 7, 40, **40**, 42, **42**, 43, 51, 52, 71, 72, 74, 122, 134, 164, 176-177, **176**, 183, **197**; in China, 103, **103**; as president, 76, 77, 79; at Reed College, 54, **54**, 55, 59, 64, **64**; retirement, 80; in the Surgeon General's Office, 60, 67; at Walter Reed General Hospital, 70; in World War II, 116, 135
Mary McMillan Lecture, 181, 199, 203
Medicare and Medicaid programs, 192-193, 194, 209
Medico-Mechanical Institute, 13
Medlin, Oskar, 34
Mennell, James B., 16, 44, 60, 183
Mensendieck System of Functional Exercises, 147
Merrill, Janet, 35, 65, 72, 73, **73**, 77, 80, 87, **89**, 94, 127, 183
Mesmer, Franz Anton, 23
Michels, Eugene "Mike," 179, 189, 197, **197**, 208, 209, 228, **240**
Mitchell, Wier, 15, 17, 24. *See also* Wier Mitchell Rest Cure
Moffat, Marilyn, 203, 208, 217, 222, 231, **240**, 240, **246**, **246**, 247
Moffroid, Mary, 226, 234
Monro, Edith, 94, **94**, 101
Montefiore Home for Chronic Invalids, 31
Montgomery, Major James B., 68, 78
Moore, Margaret, 138, 139, 144, 204, 243
Moreaux, Frances Philo, 81
*Muscle Testing*, 96

**N** Nagelschmidt, Karl Franz, 29, 30
National Council on Rehabilitation, 121
National Easter Seal Society, 101, 139, **139** 164, 166
National Foundation for Infantile Paralysis (NFIP), 98, 99, 124-129, 139-140, 158, 159, 178, 181, 185-186
National Institutes of Health (NIH), 39, 145, 184
National Society for Crippled Children and Adults. *See* National Easter Seal Society

Nesbitt, Mary E., **154**
Neuro-Developmental Treatment (NDT), 170-171
Neuro-Developmental Treatment Association (NDTA), 171
New Haven School of Physiotherapy, 78, 85
New York University 202; Institute of Rehabilitation Medicine, 132, 143; Department of Physical Education, Health and Recreation, 202, 212; Institute of Physical Medicine and Rehabilitation, 143, 231; Testing and Advisement Center, 140
Noble, Isabel, 59, 73, 74, 75
Noland, Royce P., **206**, 206, 207, 209, 215, 217, 220, 228
Northwestern University Medical School, 85, 89, 137

**O** O'Connor, Basil, 95, 98, 151, 158
Occupational therapy, 46, 48, 49, 68, 70, **88**, 112
Office of Vocational Rehabilitation (OVR), 146
Orthoses, 32, **47**, **69**, 132
Osler, Sir William, 163
Osteosynthesis, 11
Ozburn, Sue, 205, 206

**P** Paget, Rosalind, 19, 21
Palmer, Benjamin Frank, 36
Palmer, Daniel David, 15
Palmer School of Chiropractic, 16
Paré, Amboise, 9, 37
Partridge, Miriam, 243
Peacock, Inez, 220
Perry, Jacquelin, 204, 214
Perry, Col. Miriam, 148
Phelps, Winthrop, 163-165, 169
Philadelphia Orthopedic Hospital and Infirmary for Nervous Diseases, 17, 85
*Physical Reconstruction and Orthopedics*, 78
Physical therapist (therapy) assistants (PTAs), 196, 197; Education Group (PTAEG) 197
*PT Bulletin*, 235
Physical therapy treatment: facilities, 90; 102; origins, 7; in ancient Greece, 7, 8, 26, 30; in ancient Rome, 30
*Physical Therapy Review (Physiotherapy Review)*: inaugural issue, 73, **74** ,88, 132, 150, 152, 154, 180, 183, 234, 235, **236**; Constitution and Bylaws, 74
*Physical Treatment by Movement, Manipulation and Massage*, 16
*Physical Therapy,The Journal of the American Physical Therapy Association*, 180, 181, 182, 186, 188, 203, 209, 213, 214
Pinkston, Dorothy, 192, 219
Plan to Foster Clinical Research in Physical Therapy, 189-190
Plastridge, Alice Lou, 35, 96, **96**, 97, 98, 121, 125, 126, 157
Poliomyelitis, 34, 35, 89, 94, 95-102, 123-128, 155-163, 183
Pope, Henry, 96, 97
Pope, Margaret, 96, 97
Portland Childrens Hospital, 44, 51
Practice without referal, 236, **238**
Priessnitz, Vincent, 30, 31
Prime Timers, 219, 220
*Progress Report*, 209
Proprioceptive Neuromuscular Facilitation (PNF), 167
Prostheses, 32, 33, 34, 35, **36**, 39, **39**, 63
Pugh, John, 10
Public Law 78-350. *See* Bolton Bill
Public Law 79-725. *See* Hospital Survey and Construction Act
Public Law 80-36, 137
Public Law 84-294, 149

**R** Rader, Beulah, 72, 77
Ransom, Lois, 115, 139, **139**
Reconstruction aides, 40, **45**, 45-57, **57**, 58-60, **60**, 61-69; duties, 50, 59, 60; head aides, 49; insignia, 49; living conditions, 59, 49; military status, 48; post-war employment, 68, 69, 71; qualifications, 47, 48; remuneration, 49; status of men, 82; uniforms, 42, **42**, 49, 50, 58; working conditions, 58; World War Reconstruction Aides Assembly, 70; in World War II, 113
Reed College, 40, 47, 53, 54, 59; brochure, 55; curriculum, 54

"Reedites," 54, **54**, 55, 78;
Reinecke, Louise, 130, 133
Rest Cure. *See* Wier Mitchell Rest Cure
Resource Center for Research and Learning, 228
"Return, The" 146
*Review*. *See Physical Therapy Review*
Richardson, Robert W., 220, **222**, 240, **240**
Robbins, Viola "Robbie," 193
Robertson, Lt. Barbara, 118
Roen, Susan, 95, **101**, 136, 168
Roentgen, Wilhelm, 27, 28, 29
Romberger, Phoebe, 226-227
Rood, Margaret "Roody," 174-176, 222
Roosevelt, President Franklin Delano, 95, 96, 98, 104
Rose, Steven, 190, 234
Rothstein, Jules, 156, 203, **227**, 228, 235
Rusk, Howard, 131, 132, 203

**S** Sacksteder, Maj. Mary Ellen, 158
St. Louis University, School of Nursing and Health Services, 194
Salk, Jonas, 160, **161**
Sanderson, Marguerite, 19, 51, 52, **52**, 55, 60, 74, 77, 183
Santo Tomás University, 116, 135
Sargent School, 13, 18, 19
Sargent, Dudley Allen, 13, 17, 19
Schleichkorn, Jay, 150, 165, 170, 244
Scholz, John, 226, 227
Scully, Rosemary, 222
Seater, Steve, 225
Seether, Tom, 227
Semans, Sarah, 170-171, 222
Sensory Integration (SI) therapy, 169
Shattner, Dorothy, 234
Shannon, James M., 224
Sheppard, Morris, 105
Singleton, Mary Clyde, **148**
Smith, Arretta, 151
Snyder, Lt. Col. Agnes P., 110, 150, **165**, 180
Stanford University, 137, 187, 207, 214, 232
State Board of Medical Examiners, 141
State University of New York Downstate Medical Center, 212
Sternberg General Hospital, 52-53, 116
Stevenson, Jessie L., 100, 113, **113**, 121, 129, 136, 141
Still, Andrew Taylor, 14, 15
Stromeyer, Georg F. L., 11
Surgeon General. *See* U.S. Army Surgeon General
Swedish Movement Treatment, 12, 16, 43
Swezey, Marion, 72, 77

**T** Tappan, Fran, 107, 116, 150, 174, 222
Taylor, George, 13, 15
Teekemeyer, Robert, 111, 150
Terry, Eselle, 82
Theilmann, Maj. Ethel, 149
*Therapeutic Exercise*, 96
Thomas, Hugh Owen, 43
Thomas splint, 43
Thompson, Capt. Beatrice, 184
Tillman, Ruby, 158
Tilt board, 182, **182**
Torp, Capt. Mary, 149
*Toward Independence*, 120
TENS (transcutaneous electrical nerve stimulation), 187-188
TriAlliance of Health and Rehabilitation Professions, 240, 241
Truman, President Harry, 137

**U** Ultrasound, 187
Unionism, 190-192; Local 1199 of the Drug, Hospital and Health Care Employees Union, 190, 192
University of Florida, 194

University of Iowa, 181, 227
University of Pennsylvania, School of Allied Medical Professions, 137, 181, 189, 194
United Cerebral Palsy Association (UCPA), 165
U.S. Army Division of Special Hospitals and Physical Reconstruction, 44 , 46, 60; Physical Therapy Section, 47
U.S. Army Medical Corps, 42, 44, 48, 51, 58, 59, 105, 113
U.S. Bureau of Health Manpower, 194
U.S. Public Health Service, 39, 68, 73, 99, 100, 144-145, 183, 184, 207
U.S. Army Surgeon General: office of, 6, 39, 46, 47, 51-53, 60, 61, 68, 70, 77, 104, 105, 131; Leroy Burney, 183; Joycelyn Elders, 151; William Gorgas, 44, 45, 51

**V** Veterans Administration (VA), 131, 132, 146
Veterans' Bureau, 60, 69, 104
Vietnam War, 204
Vogel, Col. Emma "Emmy Lou," 60, 69, 78, **78**, 104, **104**, 105, 107, 110, 113, 115, 120, 137, **148**
Voluntary aide detachment (VAD), 44
Voris, Anna, 55, 56
Voss, Dorothy, 163, 167-168, 180, **180**

**W** Walker, Jack (Jack Walker Award), 214
Walter, Jane, 219, 232
Walter Reed General Hospital, 41, **41**, **45**, 51-52, 53, 55, 60, 68, 69, **69**, 70, **70**, 78, 85, 98, **104**, 105
Walton, Jeri, 220
Wellesley College, Department of Hygiene and Physical Education, 19, 51, 81
Wells, Elizabeth, 73, 75, 80
Whitcomb, Lt. Col. Beatrice, 150
White, Barbara, 116, 130, 136, 139, 197, 202
Wickliffe, Col. Nell, 148, 150
Wier Mitchell Rest Cure, 17, 21
Williams, Marian, 144, 213
Williams, Thelma Petty, 151
Winters, Margaret Campbell, 98, **98**, **101**
Wolf, Steven, 187, 188
Women's Medical Specialist Corps (WMSC). *See* Army Medical Specialist Corps
Wood, Annetta Cornell, 178
Woodruff, Lynda 214
World Confederation for Physical Therapy, 142, 143, **143**, 244
World War I, 6, 40-69; Armistice, 58, 59, 61, 68, 71; hospitals, 14; physical therapy equipment, 45, 65; physical therapy treatment protocol, 48; reconstruction aide training, 7; treatment of orthopedic problems, 46
World War II, 104-121; discriminatory treatment, 105; duties, 108, 109, 114, 119; eqiupment, 117-119; facilities, 104; housing, 108; military status 105, 108, 110; physical therapy insignia, 49, 113; remuneration, 108; staffing shortage 106, 113, 114; status of men, 111; uniform, 111, **111**,112, 113
Worthingham, Catherine, 96, **101**, 108, **108**, 120, 129, 140, 141, 185-186, 193, 196, 201, 204, 242
Worthingham Report, 185, 186
Wortley, Don W., 217-218, 222, 240, **240**
Wright, Jessie, 86, 170
Wright, Wilhelmine, 35, 65, 96

**X** X-rays (Roentgen waves), 28, 29

**Y** Yang Ming Medical College, 203
Yurick, Linnea, **226**

**Z** Zander Institutes, 13
Zander, Gustav, 12, 13, 14
Zander machines, 12, 13, 14
Zernow, Leila, 113
Zimmerman, James, 191

## *Acknowledgments*

Writing about an organization that has only gradually come to recognize the value of its long and colorful history poses many challenges for the researcher. While other aspects of American medical history are exceedingly well-documented from their beginnings, the story of physical therapy's development has remained somewhat in the shadows. APTA member Ida May Hazenhyer made the first serious attempt to set the record down in 1976 coincident with the U.S. Bicentennial. Now, as the Association prepares to celebrate its own 75th Anniversary, a second, more wide-ranging history has been prepared. Containing many new facts relating to APTA, its individual chapters, and its members, this latest effort must be considered part of a work in progress. If the history is successful, it will inspire other historians to continue the search for additional historic documents, personal memoirs, letters, photographs, and other memorabilia by which the past can be known and the future more firmly charted.

*Healing the Generations* could not have been written without the contributions of a host of wise counselors whose enthusiasm, recollections, and insights have been generously shared.

Among the many friends of APTA I would like to thank are: Jean Barclay and Stuart Skyte of England's Chartered Society of Physiotherapy, now celebrating their own centenary; Mary Farrell and Edward McMillan, Jr., whose personal recollections as well as memorabilia of founder Mary McMillan have made this great lady come alive again in these pages; Lettie Gavin, whose groundbreaking researches into the history of women serving in World War I was particularly instructive in enlarging our understanding of the lives and times of the Reconstruction Aides; Garth Stoltz, whose knowledge of John Harvey Kellogg and the Battle Creek Sanitarium are unique; Hank Kanies of the Chattanooga Group, Inc., whose interest in early physical therapy devices runs deep; and Jim Heisler and Marie DeGreef, who are but two of the scores of individuals who have helped me resurrect the life stories and professional contributions of long-gone members.

Of even more sustained assistance have been many current members of APTA and Association staff. Topping this long list are Charles Magistro, Eugene Michels, and Jay Schleichkorn, who over a period of nearly two years cheerfully answered questions by phone and fax at almost any hour of the day or night. Also extremely helpful were Vilma Evans, Robert Harden, Geneva Johnson, Virginia Metcalf, Marilyn Moffat, Inez Peacock, Dorothy Pinkston, Rosemary Scully, Jane Sweeney, and Jane Walter, who helped to review the manuscript; and Col. David Greathouse, Florence Kendall, Rick Reuss, and Frank Mallon, whose expertise in their own areas of the history were invaluable. Lastly, I must extend my most sincere appreciation to Nancy Perkin Beaumont, APTA Senior Vice President of Communications, whose guidance and words of cheer have made these months of detective work always pleasurable; and to my friends at Greenwich Publishing, Mowry Mann, Bronwyn Evans, and Christine Huberty, who have always encouraged me to do my very best.

*Wendy Murphy*